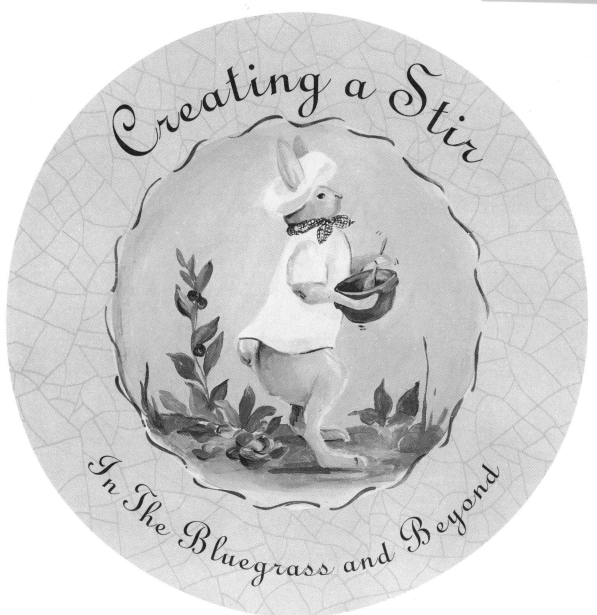

Creating a Stir

In The Bluegrass and Beyond

Published by
The Fayette County Medical Auxiliary
for the benefit of
Kentucky's children

To order additional copies of *Creating A Stir* please write or call:

Creating A Stir

FCMA Publications

2628 Wilhite Court, Suite 201

Lexington, Kentucky 40503-3304

Telephone: (859) 293-9100

Fax: (859) 277-3919

E-mail: creatingastir@mindspring.com

or visit our web page at

www.creatingastir.com

Cost per copy is $22.95, plus $4.00 shipping and handling.
Kentucky residents add $1.38 sales tax per copy.

ISBN number 0-9673442-0-4

First Printing   November 1999   10,000 copies

Second Printing   October 2000   10,000 copies

Printed in the USA by

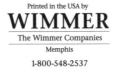

WIMMER

The Wimmer Companies

Memphis

1-800-548-2537

Table of Contents

Creating a Stir!!!!

Creating A Stir in the kitchen is easy. Creating A Stir outside of it is another matter.

To create a stir . . . is to generate excitement . . . provoke new thought . . . awaken ideas . . . passionately bring about change . . . invoke vigorous movement and transformation!

This book is about change and making a difference; changing the way we think about food and entertaining, and the way we think about our state and its people. Its about starting something new, creating excitement, and stirring things up. . . .

Within the pages of this cookbook, not only will you find recipes that incite the desire to create a "culinary stir", you will also feast on new and interesting insights into Kentuckians who have made a difference in our communities, in our great state and beyond!

Like the recipes, the list of Kentuckians is impressive and diverse! Included are the obviously famous – George Clooney, Diane Sawyer, Pee Wee Reese, Muhammed Ali and Abraham Lincoln to the more quiet and unassuming types like John Bibb, creator of Bibb lettuce, Franklin Sousley, a soldier who helped raise the flag on Iwo Jima and John Colgan, the inventor of chewing gum! You will discover tidbits and tantalizing facts touching the most revered **and** most infamous Kentucky kin who have gone out into this big ol' world of ours and made it a better place (or at least a more interesting one)!

While the recipes are tried and true, they are anything but ordinary. The staples of any good cookbook are here, like Pasta with Basil Pesto, Harvest Pumpkin Bread and Grape and Walnut Chicken Salad. But, who can resist the temptation to try something with a bit of a *twist*! Penne with Shiitake and Fresh Ginger, Dried Bing Cherry and Gorgonzola Salad, Crostini with Feta, Sun-Dried Tomatoes and Olives, Spectacular Beef Tenderloin with Port Sauce and Puff Pastry Garnish and Autumn Apple Cake with Brown Sugar Applejack Glaze more than fit the bill. Enjoy this extraordinary collection of recipes that are as inspiring and incomparable as the Kentuckians who are featured throughout.

How fitting then that the Fayette County Medical Auxiliary is sponsoring this project. The women of this organization have been Creating A Stir throughout the Bluegrass for more than 50 years. The FCMA's mission for this project is to help families and communities meet the growing needs of Kentucky's children through policy change and education. Perhaps their best known contribution is the establishment of the Ronald McDonald House of the Bluegrass, (a collaborative effort with the Fayette County Medical Society). Through tireless fundraising efforts, the house opened in 1984 and remains a haven for the families of children undergoing medical treatment at local hospitals.

Baby Health, a nonprofit organization that provides free medical care to children under 12, has also received countless hours of support from FCMA members. The Family Care Center, Children's Advocacy Center, and the Nathaniel Mission are just a few of the numerous charities that have benefited from the love, support and commitment of the women of the FCMA.

ALL PROCEEDS FROM THIS BOOK will be dedicated to worthy charities that serve the CHILDREN OF KENTUCKY.

To all those in the Bluegrass and beyond who enjoy *Creating A Stir*. . . Bon Appétit!

Melissa Rose Anthony

Melissa Rose Anthony

Melissa has a background in public relations and special event planning with Preston-Osborne Public Relations Firm, Christie's Auction House in London, England and Cross Gate Gallery. Her freelance articles have appeared in numerous publications, including The Carlyle Hotel, Louisville Magazine, The Equine Image and Symbol Magazine of the South. Melissa works from her home in Versailles, Kentucky.

About the Artist

Raised in McKinney, Texas, a suburb of Dallas, Kijsa Presley Housman planned on pursuing an art career from her childhood. Following her dream, she attended Baylor University receiving a BFA degree in painting, then onto graduate school at Vanderbilt University to study art history. Marrying, moving and settling in Lexington, Kentucky created new opportunities for her artwork. While her husband Brad Housman, from Paducah, Kentucky, completed medical school, she created murals and decorative elements for residential and commercial interiors, theatrical sets, TV sets for PBS, works commissioned by state government, and a multitude of smaller projects that include furniture, a unique line of pottery, greeting cards and invitations. With Brad currently in his last year of OB/GYN residency, Kijsa has been busy with their best creation yet . . . the birth of their first child, Talia Claire Housman born August 12, 1999!

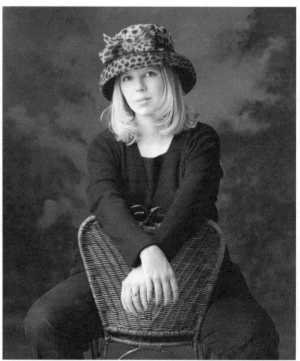

Photograph by
Walden's House of Photography

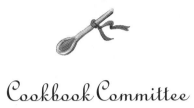

Cookbook Committee

CHAIRMAN
Jennifer Bales Waller

SECTION CHAIRMEN

Debra Ashbrook Adkins
Leslie Beebe
Karma Cassidy
Melissa Trainor Elliott
Julie Floyd
Mary Ann Gevedon

Jody Greenlee
Susan Gross
Dawn Hughes
Starr Kramer
Sydney Skinner
Melissa Toney

Ann Wheeler

COMMITTEE MEMBERS

Jane Anderson
Theresa Back
Kathy Balthrop
Barbara Bennett
Jody Bosomworth
Cheryl Broster
Kathryn Daniel
Denise Duncan
Mary Evans
Jenny Gates
Patti Geil
Alberta Gerson
Sue Gill
Alana Greenman
Hilary Halpin
Joan Hutchinson

Mischelle Isernhagen
Margee Koffler
Tracy Kostelic
Vida Laureano
Gloria Martin
Cindy McKinney
Cindy Miers
Karen Milligan
Lisa Montgomery
Kitty Moore
Martha Nicol
Sharon Nighbert
Betty Nolan
Jane Allen Offutt
Cecilia Page
Janet Peat

Shirley Read
Sharon Reed
Mary Beth Richardson
Susan Ridenour
Donna Rogers
Randy Rogers
Doris Rosenbaum
Lise Sanchez
Pat Schindler
Janet Schwartz
Karen Shank
Amy Tjoa
Genie Whayne
Judy Woods
Julie Youkilis
Connie Young

RECIPE CONTRIBUTORS AND TESTERS

Debra Ashbrook Adkins
Kristen Elizabeth Adkins
J. Thomas Adkins, M.D.
Nanci Alexander
Katie Alford
Lee Floyd Allen
Miriam Allen
Jane Anderson
Susan Anderson
Elizabeth Armstrong
Holly Arnold
Wilma Jean Ashbrook
Theresa Back
Laura Callaway Bales
Sharon Bales
Kathy Balthrop
Mary Barrett
Lisa Barton
Leslie Beebe
Carol Kennedy Behr
Nancy Bell
Jo Bellin
Barbara Bennett
Cathy Berg
Mickey Binion
Tammy Bishop
Donna Boettner
Peggy Borders
Jody Bosomworth
Barbara Bowers
C. Richard Bowers, Jr., M.D.
Jack Brady
Bernard Branch, M.D.
Cheryl Broster
Tracy Browning
Dolores Bsharah
Patty Burchett
Alan Bush
Barbara Bush
Mrs. William Bush
Brenda Cannon

Forrest Cannon
Emma Elizabeth Carter
David Cassidy, M.D.
Karma Cassidy
Terry Caudill
Ellen Chapman
Isobel Chewning
Marianne Christie
Jody Clark
Stephanie Clowers
Tiffany Cobb
Debby Coleman
Connie Collis
Chef Chris Cox
Marian Cox
Phyllis Cronin
Jordan Bales Cross
Karen Dailey
Kathryn Daniel
Linda Daugherty
Barbara Davis
Jane DeMartini
Connie Dick
Geneva Donaldson
Melanie Dowell
Denise Duncan
Phil Dunn
Harriet Dupree, Dupree Catering
Carrie Elliott
Jerry Elliott
Jill Elliott
Melissa Trainor Elliott
Meredith Elliott
Mitchel Elliott
Linda Ellis
Mary Evans
William M. Evans, M.D.
Virginia Fairchild
Julie Floyd
Mary Floyd
Abe Fosson, M.D.

Charlene Foster
Merlene Furr
Pam Gee
Patti Geil
Betty Gentry
Alberta Gerson
Larry Gevedon, M.D.
Mary Ann Gevedon
Susan Gex
Mildred Gillespie
Lida I. Givens
Peggy Graddy
Karen Graves
Jody Greenlee
Alana Greenman
Joan Greenman
Cissy Gregg
Joan Gross
Leslie Gross
Stephanie Eads Gross
Susan Gross
Dolores Guiler
J. Mike Guiler, M.D.
Sherry Guiler
Mary Hampton
Susan Hart
Pat Haven
Shirley Hayes
Mary Herms
Chef Jerry Hester
Barb Hickey
Vicki Huckeba
Dawn Hughes
Joan Hutchinson
Pat Issel
Jean Jacobs
Martha Jenkins
Grace Johnson
Magdalene Karon, M.D.
John Kennan

8

Paige Kikuchi
Margee Koffler
Tracy Kostelic
Starr Kramer
Sherry Kyker
Vida Laureano
Beverly Lewgood
Rosemarie Lewis
Betty Lloyd
Mary Ann Evans Lochridge
Carolyn Sands Looff
Katrina Louck
Susan Marterie
Gloria Martin
Judy Mathis
Pat Mayo
St. Claire McIntyre
Cindy McKinney
Wendy McNevin
Frankie Meeks
Monika Mentzer
Betty Michel
Karen Milligan
John Michael Montgomery
Lisa Montgomery
Kitty Moore
Mousetrap, The
Sandra Myers
Tootsie Nelson
Andrea Newton
Bruce R. Nicol, M.D.
Joan Nicol
Martha Nicol
Jackie Nicolson
Richard Niemi
Betty Nolan
Jane Allen Offutt
Jane Oliver
Susan Oliver
Connie Orck
Ann Orr
Julie Osetinsky

Connie Ott
Arlene Parks
Mrs. Stanley S. Parks, Sr.
Julie Payne
Janet Peat
Julia Pezzi
Carolyn Plumlee
Beth Porter
Beth Poulton
Marilyn Prevel
Jacquie Purdy
Shirley Read
Sharon Reed
Eileen Regan
Shirley Regan
Victor Regan
Lisa Richards
Mary Beth Richardson
Susan Ridenour
Julie Riegger
Donna Rogers
Mildred Rogers
Randy Rogers
Annie Ronald
Doris Rosenbaum
Amy Rukavina
Linda Rukavina
Becky Saha
Lise Sanchez
Kate Savage
Janet Schwartz
Susan Scott
Elise Scully
Sydney Skinner
Sheila Sekela
Karen Shank
Ethelene Slabaugh
Sugar Slabaugh
Lori Solvik
Something Special Catering
Lavinia Spirito
Pam Stephenson

Jane Stilz
Chef Kellie Stoddart
Chef Michael Stoddart
Lois Summers
Linda Swartz
Susan Taylor-Mitchel
Sherrill Thomas
Jane Floyd Tipton
Amy Tjoa
Melissa Helms Toney
Priscilla Caye Trainor
Lorine Trosper
Heather VanDeren
Sue Vaughan
Lyn Purdy Voige
Fernita Wallace
Claire McKay Waller
Eliza Grace Waller
Eugenia Waller
Jennifer Bales Waller
Mildred Waller
Roy M. Waller III, M.D.
Helen Walton
Lauren Ward
Jane Warner
Henry Wells, Jr., M.D.
Mrs. Henry Wells, Sr.
Susan Wells
Mary Jane Whaley
Genie Whayne
Ann Wheeler
Clarice White
Alma Wichman
Edith Wiesel
Tom Wiesel
Adele Williams
Bookie Wilson
Charlotte Wilzbach
Elizabeth Love Wolford
Michelle Woolum
Julie Youkilis
Connie Young

Special Thanks

I am especially grateful to the following individuals.
What they did to encourage and refine this project is immeasurable!

A special thanks to . . .

Carolyn Kurz and Staff, The Fayette County Medical Society Office
Charlie Stone, The Stone Advisory
Chef Chris Cox
Chef David Larson, The Pampered Chef
Chef Harriet Dupree, Dupree Catering Inc.
Chef Jerry Hester
Chefs Michael and Kellie Stoddart, The Kitchen at Chevy Chase
Debbie Adkins
Diane Sawyer, ABC-TV
Dr. Charles L. Shearer, President Transylvania University
Dr. George Zack, Conductor–The Lexington Philharmonic
Former President and Mrs. George Bush
Greg Michel, Michel Consulting
Jane Allen Offutt
John Kennan, The Mousetrap
John-Michael Montgomery
June Mumme
Kijsa Housman
Laura Freeman, Laura's Lean Beef
Labrot and Graham Distillers
Mary Beth Van Uum, Joseph Beth Booksellers
Mayor Pam Miller
Melanie Glasscock–Simpson, WLEX-TV
Melissa Rose Anthony
Phyllis George
Ralph Hacker
Robert Taylor
Roy and Lucie Meyers, á la lucie, Pacific Pearl, Roy and Nadine's Restaurants
Shelley and Bruce Richardson, Historic Elmwood Inn
Sonny, Claire and Eliza Waller
Spindletop Productions
Suki Wright
Susan Harkins, Friends of the Farmer's Market
Sydney Skinner
The John J. Greeley Family
Tim and Beverly Walden, Walden's House of Photography

Thanks so much!
Jennifer Bales Waller, Cookbook Chairman

Appetizers & Beverages

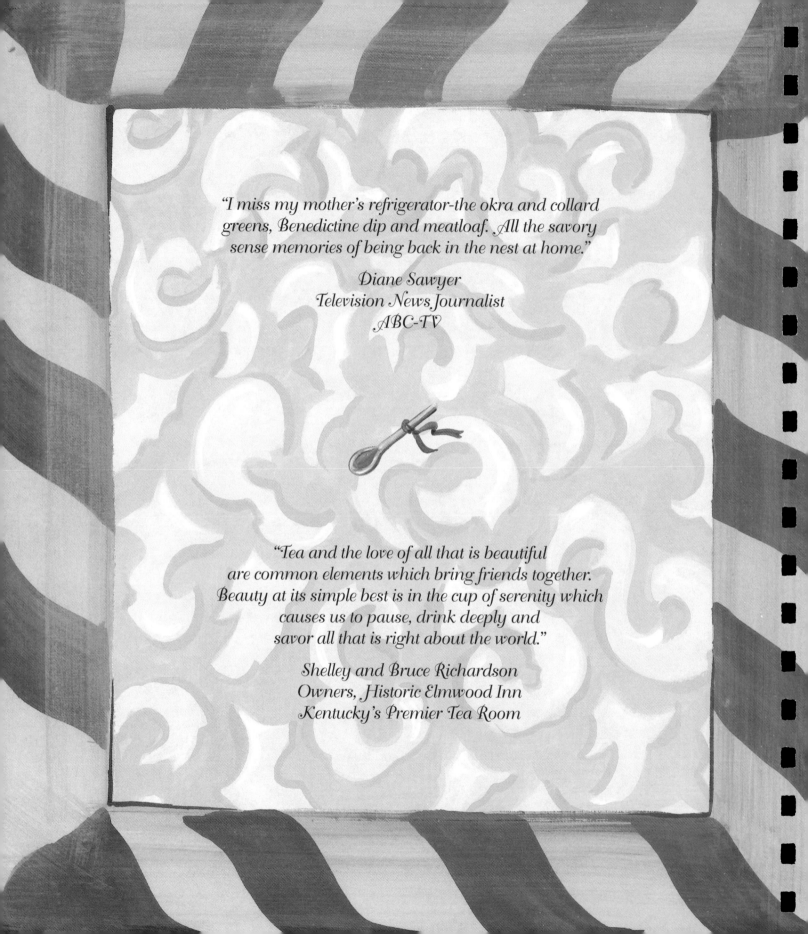

"I miss my mother's refrigerator-the okra and collard greens, Benedictine dip and meatloaf. All the savory sense memories of being back in the nest at home."

Diane Sawyer
Television News Journalist
ABC-TV

"Tea and the love of all that is beautiful
are common elements which bring friends together.
Beauty at its simple best is in the cup of serenity which
causes us to pause, drink deeply and
savor all that is right about the world."

Shelley and Bruce Richardson
Owners, Historic Elmwood Inn
Kentucky's Premier Tea Room

Crostini with Feta, Olives, and Sun-Dried Tomatoes

Crostini is a popular Italian appetizer that literally means "little toasts."
These simple toasts are topped with various combinations of cheese and other
extraordinary bits of color and flavor. This one is outstanding!

4 ounces cream cheese, softened	4 ounces sun-dried tomatoes packed in oil, chopped
1 cup feta cheese	½ teaspoon garlic salt
2 tablespoons milk	1 baguette, cut into ½-inch slices
¼ cup pitted ripe olives, finely chopped	½ cup butter, melted
	Fresh basil leaves for garnish

- Combine cream cheese, feta, and milk, beating just until smooth.

- Combine olives, sun-dried tomatoes, and garlic salt in a separate bowl; set aside.

- Place baguette slices on a baking sheet. Bake at 425° for 5 minutes. Remove from oven, turn, and brush generously with melted butter. Return to oven and bake an additional 5 minutes or until golden and crispy.

- Spread a dollop of cream cheese on buttered side of each bread slice; top evenly with olive mixture. Garnish each slice with a fresh basil leaf.

Makes 24

Blue Cheese-Pecan Wafers

12 ounces blue cheese, crumbled	1 cup plus 2 tablespoons finely chopped pecans
¾ cup butter, softened	¼ teaspoon cayenne pepper
2 cups all-purpose flour	

- Beat blue cheese and butter at medium speed with an electric mixer until fluffy; add flour, pecans, and red pepper, beating well.

- Shape dough into 2 (10-inch) rolls; chill 2 to 3 hours or until firm.

- Cut dough into ¼-inch slices and place on ungreased baking sheets.

- Bake at 350° for 15 minutes.

Makes 6 dozen wafers

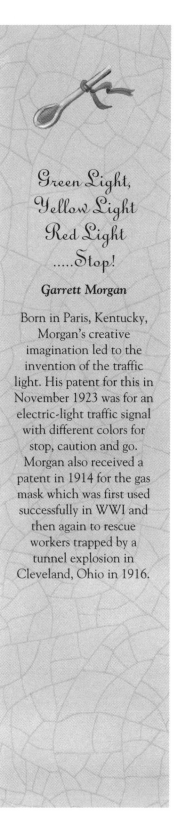

Green Light, Yellow Light Red Light .....Stop!

Garrett Morgan

Born in Paris, Kentucky, Morgan's creative imagination led to the invention of the traffic light. His patent for this in November 1923 was for an electric-light traffic signal with different colors for stop, caution and go. Morgan also received a patent in 1914 for the gas mask which was first used successfully in WWI and then again to rescue workers trapped by a tunnel explosion in Cleveland, Ohio in 1916.

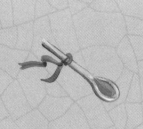

Boy Scouts Honor

Daniel Carter Beard

Better known as "Uncle Dan", Beard grew up in Covington, Kentucky. In 1905, Beard organized the Sons of Daniel Boone, the forerunner of the Boy Scouts of America and in 1909, the Boy Pioneers of America. In 1910, the Boy Scouts of America was founded and he headed the organization for 31 years. He created the Scout hat, shirt, neckerchief and several merit badges. He was an associate editor of *Boy's Life Magazine*. In 1922, he received the only gold eagle badge ever awarded by the Boy Scouts and the first for outstanding citizenship by the state of Kentucky. Alaska's Mount Beard was named for him.

Nantucket Scallop Puffs

An appetizer that will have guests raving!

3 tablespoons unsalted butter	Freshly ground pepper to taste
1 pound bay scallops, quartered	12 dozen 1-inch bread rounds cut from
2½ teaspoons finely minced lemon zest	white toasting bread (we used
3 garlic cloves, minced	Pepperidge Farm Toasting Bread)
3 tablespoons chopped fresh dill	Sweet Hungarian paprika
2 cups (8 ounces) shredded Swiss or	Lemon slices and fresh dill sprigs
Gruyère cheese	for garnish
2 cups mayonnaise	

- Melt butter in a skillet over medium-high heat; add scallops, lemon zest, and garlic. Cook, stirring constantly, 2 to 3 minutes or until scallops are just barely done.

- Add dill and cook 30 seconds. Remove from heat and let cool to room temperature.

- Add cheese, mayonnaise, and pepper to scallop mixture, stirring well. Cover and chill up to 5 days, if desired.

- Place bread rounds on baking sheets ½ inch apart; top each round with a heaping teaspoon of scallop mixture. Sprinkle lightly with paprika. Broil 5 inches from heat 2 to 3 minutes or until puffed and golden.

- Transfer scallop puffs to serving platters and garnish with lemon slices and fresh dill sprigs. Serve warm.

Makes 12 dozen puffs

Swiss and Chive Spread

Unbelievably easy for such a fabulous result!

3 cups (12 ounces) finely shredded Swiss cheese	¼ cup chopped chives
	½ teaspoon salt
¾ cup mayonnaise	¼ teaspoon ground white pepper

- Combine Swiss cheese and mayonnaise in a bowl; add chives, salt, and pepper, stirring well. Cover and chill until ready to serve.

- Serve spread with rich buttery crackers.

Spinach Quiche Appetizer Squares

1 cup all-purpose flour	½ medium onion, minced
1 teaspoon baking powder	4 cups (16 ounces) finely shredded
1 teaspoon salt	sharp cheddar cheese
2 large eggs, lightly beaten	1 (10-ounce) package frozen chopped
6 tablespoons butter, melted	spinach, thawed and well drained
1 cup milk	

- Combine flour, baking powder, and salt in a large bowl; add eggs, butter, and milk, stirring well. Stir in onion, cheese, and spinach.

- Pour spinach mixture into a lightly greased 9 x 13 x 2-inch pan.

- Bake at 350° for 40 to 45 minutes or until golden. Let stand at room temperature 3 to 5 minutes before cutting into squares.

Makes 24 to 36 squares

Sausage and Cheese Tartlets

Watch them disappear!

1 pound mild sausage	1 teaspoon cayenne pepper
1¼ cups (5 ounces) shredded Monterey Jack cheese	1 cup Ranch dressing
	4 ounces pitted ripe olives, chopped
1¼ cups (5 ounces) shredded sharp cheddar cheese	3 packages phyllo tart shells

- Brown sausage in a skillet over medium heat, stirring until it crumbles and is no longer pink; drain and return to pan.

- Add Monterey Jack and cheddar cheese, cayenne pepper, Ranch dressing, and olives and cook over low heat, stirring until cheese is melted. Spoon mixture into phyllo shells and place on baking sheets.

- Bake at 350° for 8 to 10 minutes. Serve warm.

Makes 36 tartlets

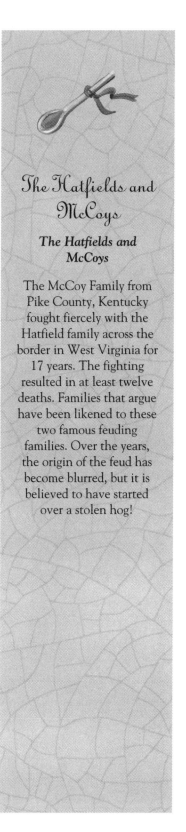

The Hatfields and McCoys

The Hatfields and McCoys

The McCoy Family from Pike County, Kentucky fought fiercely with the Hatfield family across the border in West Virginia for 17 years. The fighting resulted in at least twelve deaths. Families that argue have been likened to these two famous feuding families. Over the years, the origin of the feud has become blurred, but it is believed to have started over a stolen hog!

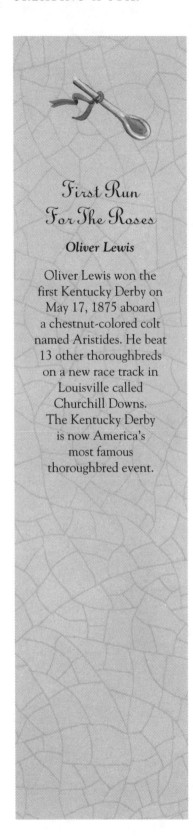

Hot Baked Pizza Dip

The ultimate "game day" dip! Hearty and satisfying . . . everyone loves it!

1	(8-ounce) package cream cheese, softened	5	ounces pepperoni, finely chopped
1	(14-ounce) jar pizza sauce	2	cups (8 ounces) shredded mozzarella or pizza blend cheese
½	cup chopped green onions		Tortilla chips or toasted bread rounds
½	cup chopped green bell pepper		
½	cup green or ripe olives, chopped		

- Preheat oven to 350°.

- Spread cream cheese in the bottom of a 10-inch pie plate or quiche dish; top with pizza sauce.

- Layer toppings in the following order over pizza sauce: green onions, bell pepper, olives, pepperoni, and cheese.

- Bake at 350° for 30 to 35 minutes or until bubbly and cheese is golden.

- Serve dip with tortilla chips or toasted bread rounds.

Serves 8 to 12

Goat Cheese and Roasted Red Pepper Crostini

1	baguette, cut into ½-inch slices	6	ounces roasted sweet red peppers, drained and chopped
4	tablespoons butter, melted	½	teaspoon olive oil
3	ounces goat cheese, softened	1	cup pitted ripe olives, coarsely chopped
3	ounces cream cheese, softened		Fresh oregano leaves for garnish
2	teaspoons lemon juice		
1	teaspoon dried oregano		

- Place bread slices on a baking sheet; bake at 450° for 5 minutes. Remove from oven, turn, and brush with melted butter. Return to oven and bake an additional 5 minutes or until golden and crisp.

- Combine goat cheese, cream cheese, lemon juice, and oregano; mix well.

- Toss together red peppers and oil; set aside.

- Spread buttered side of bread with a dollop of cheese mixture; top evenly with red peppers and olives. Garnish each slice with a fresh oregano leaf. Serve warm or at room temperature.

Makes 24

Antipasto Kabobs

Excellent for a summer buffet

1-2 (9-ounce) packages refrigerated cheese-filled tortellini
1 pint ripe cherry tomatoes
1 cup pimiento-stuffed or kalamata olives
1 pound prosciutto or salami slices, folded in half and then in half again

1 pound provolone or mozzarella cheese, cut into 1-inch cubes
1 (14-ounce) can artichoke hearts, drained and quartered
16 ounces Italian dressing

- Thread tortellini, tomatoes, olives, meat slices, cheese, and artichokes onto 6-inch wooden skewers; place in a 9 x 13 x 2-inch baking dish.
- Drizzle dressing over kabobs, turning to coat. Cover and chill 4 to 6 hours, turning occasionally. Drain and serve.

Makes 24 kabobs

Pesto and Sun-Dried Tomato Pâté

Very pretty, the colors make it especially nice for holiday gatherings.

1 (8-ounce) package cream cheese, softened
1 cup unsalted butter, softened
1 garlic clove, chopped
½ cup tightly packed fresh spinach
½ cup fresh basil

¼ cup fresh parsley
¼ teaspoon salt
¼ cup olive oil
½ cup freshly grated Parmesan cheese
¼ cup chopped pine nuts
Chopped sun-dried tomatoes

- Combine cream cheese and butter, stirring until smooth; set aside.
- Process garlic, spinach, basil, parsley, salt, oil, and Parmesan cheese in a blender until a thick paste forms; add pine nuts and blend.
- Line a 4-inch container with damp cheese cloth; spread one-fourth of cream cheese mixture in bottom. Top with half of pesto and another one-fourth of cream cheese mixture; sprinkle with a layer of tomatoes. Repeat layers once. Cover and chill 1 hour and 30 minutes.
- Invert pâté onto a serving plate and serve with crackers.

Serves 10 to 12

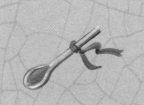

Give Me Liberty or Give Me Death!

Patrick Henry

The famous Virginian, once owned the land that is now the Kentucky Horse Park. The Kentucky Horse Park was the brainchild of noted horseman **John R. Gaines** from Lexington. The idea was championed by Representative **William G. Kenton, Jr.** The Park opened on September 7, 1978 and remains a major tourist attraction for the Lexington area. The park includes . . . A 28,000 square-foot visitor's center a 52,000 square-foot International Museum of the Horse, a model farm, the Breed's Barn which houses the thirty two represented breeds, the daily Parade of Breeds attraction, the Kentucky Equine Institute, the Hall of Champions-home to racing and show-ring greats, an equestrian vocational school, the draft and carriage horse barns that support the park's tours by horse-drawn carriage, a campground with swimming, tennis, basketball and volleyball facilities and the 3,500 seat Frederick L. Van Lennep Arena. The park also plays host to the annual Rolex Three Day Event that attracts international riders to compete on this prestigious cross-country course.

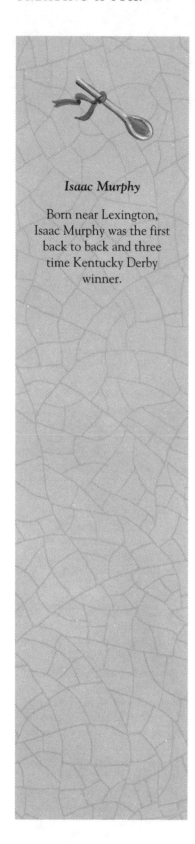

Isaac Murphy

Born near Lexington, Isaac Murphy was the first back to back and three time Kentucky Derby winner.

Feta and Walnut Spread

Quick, easy, and delicious!

1	pound feta cheese	4	ounces pitted ripe olives, chopped
¼-½	cup extra-virgin olive oil	2	garlic cloves, minced
½	cup ground walnuts		

- Process cheese in a food processor; with machine running, add ¼ cup oil in a slow, steady stream. Add ground walnuts, olives, and garlic and process until soft, adding more oil as needed.
- Chill up to 30 minutes before serving. Serve with crackers or bread rounds.

Makes 1½ cups

Crab and Swiss Stuffed Shrimp

Absolutely delicious! These are wonderful for a cocktail buffet.

1	can crabmeat		Salt and pepper to taste
1	cup mayonnaise		Hot sauce to taste
1	cup fine, dry breadcrumbs	16-20	large fresh shrimp, peeled,
1	cup (4 ounces) shredded Swiss cheese		deveined, and butterflied

- Combine crabmeat, mayonnaise, breadcrumbs, Swiss cheese, salt, pepper, and hot sauce; stuff each shrimp with 1 tablespoon mixture. Place on a baking sheet.
- Bake at 400° for 7 to 10 minutes.

Makes 16 to 20

Black Bean Hummus

Hummus with a twist!

30	ounces black beans, rinsed and drained	2	garlic cloves, minced
¾	cup tahini (sesame seed paste)	2	tablespoons olive oil
¼	cup fresh lemon juice	4	green onions, sliced
¼	cup chopped fresh parsley	½	teaspoon ground cumin
			Salt and pepper to taste

- Combine all ingredients except salt and pepper in a food processor and blend until smooth; season with salt and pepper.
- Spoon hummus into a serving bowl and serve with assorted raw vegetables or pita bread triangles.

Cincinnati Chili Dip

The unique flavor of Cincinnati-style chili highlights this dip.
Fans of the famous chili will ask for it again and again!

2 (8-ounce) packages cream cheese,
    softened
26 ounces frozen Cincinnati-style chili

1 medium onion, diced
3 cups (12 ounces) finely shredded
    mild cheddar cheese

- Spread cream cheese in the bottom of a 9 x 13 x 2-inch baking dish lightly coated with vegetable cooking spray.
- Heat chili according to package directions, blotting all liquid with paper towels. Add onion, stirring well.
- Spread chili over cream cheese. Top with shredded cheddar cheese.
- Bake at 350° for 30 minutes or until cheese is bubbly.
- Serve with corn chips.

Serves 10 to 12

Terrace Scallops

2 large eggs, lightly beaten
½ cup milk
    Salt and pepper to taste
¾ pound bay scallops, cleaned and
    dried

⅓ cup sesame seeds, toasted
½ pound bacon, each slice cut in half
    Lime wedges

- Combine eggs, milk, salt, and pepper in a bowl. Dip scallops in egg mixture and dredge in sesame seeds.
- Wrap each scallop in a strip of bacon, securing with a wooden pick. Place scallops in a 9 x 13 x 2-inch baking dish.
- Broil scallops 4 to 5 inches from heat (with electric oven door partially open) 2 minutes on each side, watching carefully to prevent burning.
- Serve scallops immediately with lime wedges.

Serves 6 to 8

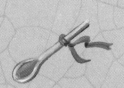

Proud To Be a Coal Miner's Daughter

Loretta Lynn

Born in Butcher Holler, Kentucky in 1935, Loretta Lynn is one of the most famous and well loved country singers/composers. Lynn's father was a coal miner and her famous song "Coal Miner's Daughter" speaks of her pride in her poor but hard-working Kentucky family. She was the first female to be named Entertainer of the Year by the Academy of Country Music and the Country Music Association. She won Top Female Artist by fans for twelve years.

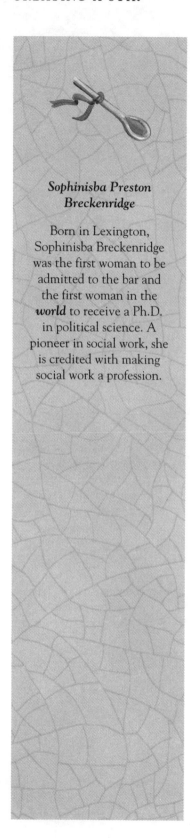

Texas Crabgrass

The combination of spinach and hot pepper cheese makes this warm dip a winner.

1	cup White Sauce	2	(10-ounce) packages frozen spinach, cooked and well drained
2	cups (8 ounces) shredded Monterey Jack cheese with peppers	1	teaspoon Worcestershire sauce
		5	drops hot sauce (optional)

- Combine white sauce, cheese, and spinach in a saucepan over medium heat, stirring until well blended. Stir in Worcestershire sauce and hot sauce.
- Serve dip warm with corn chips.

White Sauce

2	tablespoons butter	1	cup milk
2	tablespoons all-purpose flour		

- Melt butter in a medium saucepan over medium heat; add flour, stirring well. Add milk and cook, stirring constantly, until thick and bubbly.

Serves 8 to 12

Blue Cheese and Onion Focaccia

A really tasty combination!

1	tablespoon butter	¼	cup sun-dried tomatoes packed in oil, chopped
2	cups sliced onion	3	ounces blue cheese, crumbled
½	teaspoon dried sage		
1	(10-ounce) Italian bread shell (we used Boboli thin pizza crust)		

- Melt butter in a skillet over low heat; add onion and cook until tender and lightly browned. Stir in sage.
- Arrange onion on bread shell and sprinkle with sun-dried tomatoes and cheese.
- Bake at 350° for 15 minutes or until cheese is melted.

Serves 10 to 12

Baked Fiesta Dip

Chiles put the heat on in this hearty dip!

2 cups (8 ounces) shredded Monterey Jack cheese
2 cups (8 ounces) shredded cheddar cheese
½ cup plus 2 tablespoons mayonnaise
¾ cup whole kernel corn, drained
8 ounces canned chopped green chiles

1 tablespoon finely chopped chipotle chile pepper
½ teaspoon garlic salt
¾ cup seeded chopped ripe tomato
⅓ cup sliced green onions
2 tablespoons chopped fresh cilantro

- Combine Monterey Jack and cheddar cheese, mayonnaise, corn, green and chipotle chile peppers, and garlic salt; spread in a 10-inch fluted quiche dish or 1-quart baking dish. Cover and chill 24 hours.

- Combine tomato, green onions, and cilantro; set aside.

- Bake cheese mixture at 350° for 25 to 30 minutes or until thoroughly heated.

- Spoon tomato mixture into center of dip and serve with tortilla chips.

Serves 10 to 12

Cream Cheese-Chutney Pâté

Simple ingredients and easy preparation don't short change this appetizer, on taste . . . it is excellent!

2 (8-ounce) packages cream cheese, softened
1 cup (4 ounces) shredded cheddar cheese
2 tablespoons sherry
1 teaspoon salt

2 teaspoons curry powder (optional)
1¼ cups chutney
¼ cup finely chopped pecans
1 pound bacon, cooked crisp and finely crumbled
½ cup chopped fresh chives

- Combine cream cheese, cheddar cheese, sherry, salt, and curry; mix well and mold into a rectangle on a serving tray or place in a plastic wrap-lined 4-cup mold. Chill at least 1 hour.

- If using a mold, invert onto a serving tray. Spoon chutney over top. Sprinkle with pecans, bacon, and chives.

- Serve pâté with crackers.

Serves 10 to 12

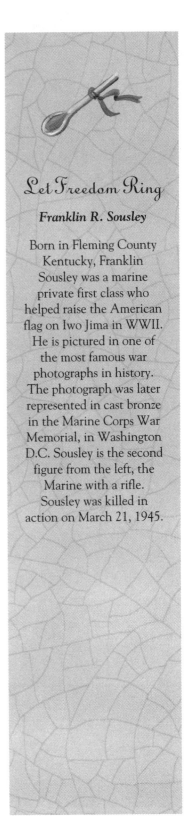

Let Freedom Ring

Franklin R. Sousley

Born in Fleming County Kentucky, Franklin Sousley was a marine private first class who helped raise the American flag on Iwo Jima in WWII. He is pictured in one of the most famous war photographs in history. The photograph was later represented in cast bronze in the Marine Corps War Memorial, in Washington D.C. Sousley is the second figure from the left, the Marine with a rifle. Sousley was killed in action on March 21, 1945.

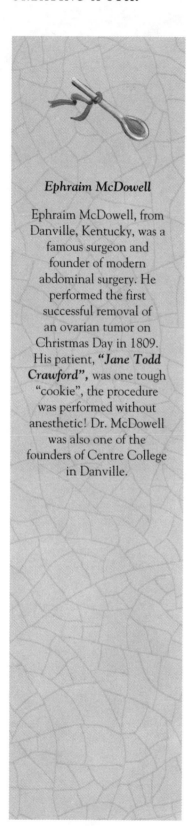

Three Cheese-Pecan Terrine

2 cups (8 ounces) finely shredded cheddar cheese, softened	4 ounces cream cheese, softened
1 cup (4 ounces) finely shredded Swiss cheese, softened	⅓ cup sour cream
	¼ teaspoon onion powder
	⅔ cup pecans, chopped

- Combine cheddar and Swiss cheese, cream cheese, sour cream, and onion powder and beat at medium speed with an electric mixer until slightly fluffy.

- Sprinkle half of pecans in a plastic wrap-lined 4-cup mold or 3 x 7 x 2-inch loaf pan; spread half of cheese mixture over nuts. Top with remaining nuts and cheese mixture, pressing to level. Cover and chill overnight or up to 48 hours.

- Unmold terrine on a serving plate and let stand at room temperature 10 minutes. Serve with crackers or fresh fruit.

Serves 12

Roasted Beef and Blue Cheese Pinwheels

Attractive and easy-especially good for casual gatherings

1 cup whipped butter, softened	8 large flour tortillas
1 (8-ounce) package cream cheese, softened	13 ounces roasted sweet red peppers, drained and cut into ¼-inch strips
1 teaspoon seasoned salt	1½ ounces fresh basil leaves
¼ cup blue cheese, crumbled	½ pound roast beef, thinly shaved

- Beat butter, cream cheese, salt, and blue cheese at medium speed with an electric mixer until creamy; spread 2 to 3 tablespoons mixture in the center of each tortilla.

- Place sliced peppers in rows 1 inch apart over cheese mixture to within ½ inch of edge. Place basil between rows of peppers (do not overlap).

- Place roast beef over peppers and basil, covering tortilla to within ½ inch of edge. Roll up tightly, jelly roll fashion; cover with plastic wrap and chill.

- Unwrap rolls; cut off and discard ½ inch from each end. Cut rolls into ¾-inch slices. Place pinwheels, cut side down, on a serving platter.

Makes 6 dozen pinwheels

Awesome South of the Border Dip

*Make this impressive dip when company is coming
and you're short on time. It always wins lots of compliments!*

1 (8-ounce) container sour cream
1 (8-ounce) package cream cheese, softened
1 can jalapeño bean dip
¼ cup picante sauce

2 teaspoons dried parsley
2 cups (8 ounces) shredded cheddar cheese, divided
2 cups (8 ounces) shredded Monterey Jack cheese, divided

- Beat sour cream and cream cheese at medium speed with an electric mixer until smooth. Add bean dip, picante sauce, parsley, 1¼ cups cheddar, and 1¼ cups Monterey Jack cheese, beating well.

- Pour mixture into a 10-inch fluted quiche dish. Sprinkle with remaining cheddar and Monterey Jack cheeses.

- Bake at 325° for 35 to 45 minutes. Let stand at room temperature 10 minutes before serving.

- Serve dip with tortilla chips.

Serves 12

Dean Fearing

Dean Fearing, from Ashland, Kentucky wrote the cookbook ***Mansion on Turtle Creek*** and is regarded as the Chef responsible for starting many of the Southwestern food trends in America.

Sausage-Spinach Balls

2 (10-ounce) packages frozen chopped spinach, cooked and well drained
2 cups herb-seasoned stuffing mix
6 ounces grated Parmesan cheese
2 tablespoons minced onion
6 large eggs, lightly beaten

½ cup butter, melted
2 garlic cloves, minced
1½ teaspoons salt
½ teaspoon pepper
6 ounces bulk sausage, cooked and drained

- Preheat oven to 350°.

- Combine all ingredients, stirring well. Form mixture into walnut-size balls and place on ungreased baking sheets.

- Bake at 350° for 20 minutes or until golden. Serve immediately.

Makes 4 to 5 dozen balls

Uncooked sausage balls can be frozen on a baking sheet; store in zip-top plastic bags. Thaw and cook as directed.

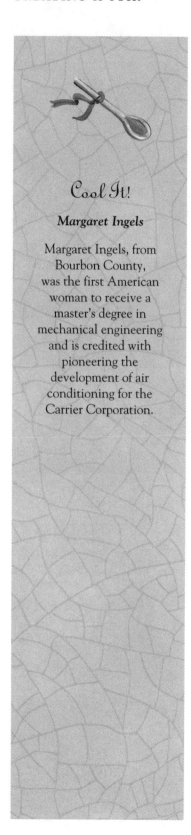

Baby Maryland Crab Cakes

These bite-size cakes are big on flavor! Serve with your favorite spicy cocktail or rémoulade sauce.

1	pound lump or claw crabmeat, drained		Cracked pepper to taste
2	large eggs, lightly beaten		Dash of Worcestershire sauce
¼	cup chopped onion		Dijon mustard
½	cup cracker crumbs		Chopped green bell pepper (optional)
3	tablespoons mayonnaise		Butter or margarine
1	tablespoon prepared mustard		

- Combine first 9 ingredients and, if desired, green bell pepper in a large bowl, stirring well; shape mixture into small 2-inch cakes and flatten slightly.

- Melt butter in a skillet over medium heat; add patties in batches and fry until brown. Serve hot with spicy seafood sauce.

Serves 6

Baked Santa Fe Dip

Men love this!

1	(8-ounce) package cream cheese, softened	1	(2.25-ounce) can sliced ripe olives, drained
1	can chili without beans (we used Old El Paso)	1	bunch green onions, chopped
2	cups (8 ounces) shredded Monterey Jack cheese with peppers	1	(4.5-ounce) can chopped green chiles, drained
		2	cups (8 ounces) shredded cheddar cheese

- Layer cream cheese, chili, Monterey Jack cheese, olives, green onions, green chiles, and cheddar cheese in a fluted quiche pan.

- Bake at 350° for 20 minutes or until bubbly.

- Serve dip warm with tortilla chips.

Serves 6 to 8

Hot Swiss Crab Dip with Crispy Pita Triangles

6 tablespoons butter
1 cup chopped green onions, divided
2 tablespoons all-purpose flour
1 cup clam juice
1 cup half-and-half
1 (8-ounce) package cream cheese, softened

1½ cups tightly packed shredded Swiss cheese
1 tablespoon prepared horseradish
2 teaspoons Worcestershire sauce
1 teaspoon cayenne pepper
½ cup chopped fresh parsley
1 pound fresh lump crabmeat, drained Crispy Pita Triangles

- Melt butter in a large heavy saucepan over medium-high heat; add ¾ cup green onions and sauté 2 minutes. Add flour, whisking 1 minute.

- Gradually whisk in clam juice and half-and-half and bring mixture to a boil; boil, stirring constantly, until thickened.

- Reduce heat and add cream cheese, Swiss cheese, horseradish, Worcestershire sauce, and cayenne pepper, stirring until melted. Stir in remaining ¼ cup green onions, parsley, and crabmeat and cook until thoroughly heated.

- Serve dip warm with Crispy Pita Triangles.

Crispy Pita Triangles

¼ cup chopped fresh parsley
3 tablespoons olive oil
2 tablespoons chopped green onions

1 (12-ounce) package pita bread, cut into wedges

- Combine parsley, oil, and green onions in a small bowl; brush over pita wedges and place on a baking sheet.

- Bake wedges at 350° for 20 minutes or until crispy.

Serves 12

Toasted Pecans

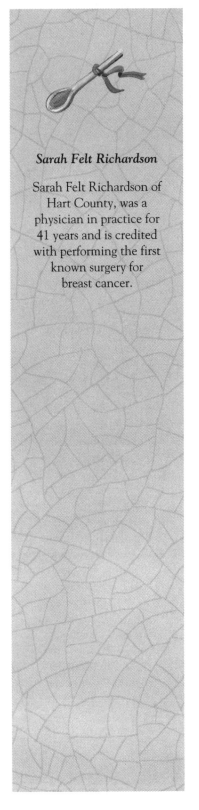

Sarah Felt Richardson

Sarah Felt Richardson of Hart County, was a physician in practice for 41 years and is credited with performing the first known surgery for breast cancer.

Too yummy! These make a great gift when packaged in decorative bags or tins.

2 pounds large pecan halves (good quality)

1½ cups butter, melted
Salt to taste

- Place pecans in a shallow roasting pan. Bake at 200° for 1 hour or until pecans take on a shiny coat.

- Pour melted butter over pecans and salt generously, stirring well. Bake 2 to 3 more hours, stirring well every hour.

- Drain pecans on paper towels. Let cool slightly and salt generously again.

Makes 2 pounds.

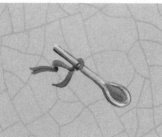

America's Favorite Frontiersman

Daniel Boone

The quintessential American frontiersman. Boone was originally led to Kentucky after agreeing to lead a hunting and trapping expedition. In 1777, while on a salt-making excursion at Blue Licks, Boone and 30 others were captured by the Shawnee Indians. Boone ingratiated himself with Chief Black Fish and along with sixteen others, was adopted into the tribe, Boone becoming the "son" of Black Fish himself. He was free to hunt alone which enabled him to hoard enough supplies for his escape. He escaped in 1778 and traveled 160 miles in four days to Boonesboro, saving it from Indian attack. Boone County and Boone, Kentucky are named for this great American pioneer.

Spicy Shrimp Spread

1	pound medium-size fresh shrimp, steamed, peeled, and deveined	1	teaspoon grated onion
2	(3-ounce) packages cream cheese, softened	1	teaspoon prepared horseradish
⅓	cup ketchup	½	teaspoon cayenne pepper
		½	teaspoon Worcestershire sauce
			Hot sauce to taste

- Coarsely chop shrimp.
- Beat cream cheese, ketchup, onion, horseradish, red pepper, Worcestershire sauce, and hot sauce at medium speed with an electric mixer until smooth; stir in chopped shrimp. Cover and chill at least 2 hours.
- Serve dip with assorted crackers.

Makes 1¼ cups

Southern Cheese Straws

"Straws" are a staple on any Southern cocktail buffet table. Serve these crispy, cheesy tidbits with your favorite drinks. Careful, they're addictive!

½	cup margarine (do not use butter)	1½	cups all-purpose flour
2	cups (8 ounces) shredded cheddar cheese	½	teaspoon salt
		⅛	teaspoon cayenne pepper (optional)

- Beat margarine and cheese at medium speed with an electric mixer until creamy; add flour, salt, and, if desired, red pepper, beating well.
- Spoon dough into a cookie press fitted with a sawtooth disc; press out in long strips on greased cookie sheets. Cut strips into 2- to 3-inch pieces.
- Bake at 325° for 20 to 30 minutes or until golden.

Makes 4 dozen

Crispy Cheese Rounds

1 pound sharp cheddar cheese, softened overnight	1 teaspoon salt
1 cup butter or margarine	1 tablespoon sugar
3 cups all-purpose flour	1 teaspoon cayenne pepper

- Shred cheese. Beat butter and cheese at medium speed with an electric mixer until creamy; add flour, salt, sugar, and cayenne pepper, beating well.

- Roll dough to ¼- to ⅛-inch thickness on a lightly floured surface. Cut with a small round cookie cutter and place on baking sheets.

- Bake at 325° for 20 to 25 minutes.

Makes 6 dozen rounds

Fruit Salsa with Cinnamon-Sugar Tortillas

This is a must try!

2 medium Granny Smith apples, chopped	2 tablespoons brown sugar
1 kiwifruit, sliced and chopped	Juice of 1 orange
1 cup sliced fresh strawberries	1 package flour tortillas
2 tablespoons apple jelly	Ground cinnamon
	Granulated sugar

- Combine apple, kiwi, strawberries, jelly, and brown sugar; squeeze juice of 1 sweet orange over salsa and stir gently.

- Brush tortillas with water and sprinkle with cinnamon and granulated sugar.

- Bake tortillas at 350° for 5 minutes.

- Cut tortillas into pieces and serve with fruit salsa.

Serves 8 to 10

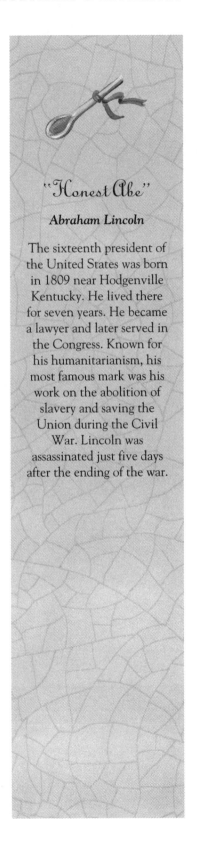

"Honest Abe"

Abraham Lincoln

The sixteenth president of the United States was born in 1809 near Hodgenville Kentucky. He lived there for seven years. He became a lawyer and later served in the Congress. Known for his humanitarianism, his most famous mark was his work on the abolition of slavery and saving the Union during the Civil War. Lincoln was assassinated just five days after the ending of the war.

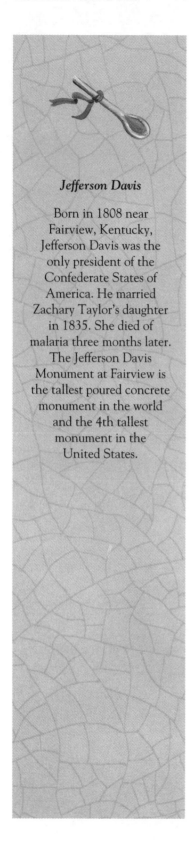

Jefferson Davis

Born in 1808 near Fairview, Kentucky, Jefferson Davis was the only president of the Confederate States of America. He married Zachary Taylor's daughter in 1835. She died of malaria three months later. The Jefferson Davis Monument at Fairview is the tallest poured concrete monument in the world and the 4th tallest monument in the United States.

Hot Mushroom Empanadas

3	tablespoons butter	2	tablespoons all-purpose flour
8	ounces minced fresh mushrooms	¼	cup sour cream
1	large onion, minced		Pastry Dough Rounds
1	teaspoon salt	1	large egg, lightly beaten
¼	teaspoon dried thyme		

- Melt butter in a skillet over medium heat; add mushrooms and onion and sauté 5 minutes or until tender. Add salt, thyme, and flour, stirring until blended. Stir in sour cream.

- Place 1 teaspoon filling on half of each Pastry Dough Round; brush edges with beaten egg. Fold pastry over and press edges with a fork to seal.

- Prick the top of each 3 times and brush again with egg. Place on baking sheets.

- Bake at 450° for 12 to 15 minutes or until golden.

Pastry Dough Rounds

1	cup butter, softened	2	tablespoons heavy cream
1	(8-ounce) package cream cheese, softened	1	teaspoon salt
		2½	cups all-purpose flour

- Beat butter and cream cheese at medium speed with an electric mixer until creamy; add cream, beating well. Stir in salt and enough flour to make a soft dough.

- Divide dough into 2 portions; chill several hours or overnight.

- Roll 1 portion dough to ¼-inch thickness on a lightly floured surface. Cut into 12 circles with a 2¾-inch round biscuit cutter. Repeat procedure with remaining portion.

Makes 24 empanadas

Artichoke Bake au Fromage

Wonderful-not your traditional artichoke bake!

1	cup mayonnaise	1	cup grated Parmesan cheese
1	(8-ounce) package cream cheese, softened	1	(14-ounce) can artichoke hearts, drained and chopped

- Combine mayonnaise, cream cheese, and Parmesan cheese, stirring well; stir in artichoke hearts. Spoon mixture into a small 1-quart round glass baking dish.

- Bake at 350° for 30 to 35 minutes or until golden and bubbly.

- Serve dip warm with corn chips.

Serves 8

Mini Curried Pizza Wedges

Another good one for casual gatherings, these spicy wedges disappear quickly!

1	cup (4 ounces) shredded sharp cheddar cheese	1	teaspoon curry powder
1	cup chopped olives	1	teaspoon salt
1	cup chopped green onions	1	teaspoon pepper
		6	English muffins, halved

- Combine cheddar cheese, olives, green onions, curry powder, salt, and pepper in a bowl; spread evenly on English muffin halves. Quarter halves and place on a baking sheet
- Bake at 400° for 20 minutes.

Makes 24

Eggplant Terrine

Takes a little extra time to prepare but is well worth the incredibly delicious results! You could actually make a meal of it.

2	medium eggplants, peeled and thinly sliced	1	(24-ounce) can roasted sweet red peppers, torn into pieces
	Salt and pepper to taste	1	(11-ounce) package goat cheese, crumbled
	Olive oil		Freshly grated Parmesan cheese
	Minced garlic	1	baguette, sliced and toasted
1	(7-ounce) jar black olive tapenade		

- Layer eggplant slices on a large baking sheet, salting generously. Let stand at room temperature 30 minutes.
- Rinse eggplant with cold water and layer on paper towels.
- Sauté eggplant in hot oil, seasoning with salt, pepper, and garlic on both sides. Drain on paper towels.
- Place a layer of eggplant in a 2-quart baking dish; spoon a thin layer of tapenade over top. Place a layer of roasted red pepper pieces over tapenade.
- Sprinkle a layer of goat cheese over red pepper. Repeat layers with remaining ingredients, ending with eggplant. Press down on top.
- Sprinkle terrine with Parmesan cheese.
- Bake at 400° for 25 to 30 minutes. Serve with toasted baguette slices.

Makes 15 to 20

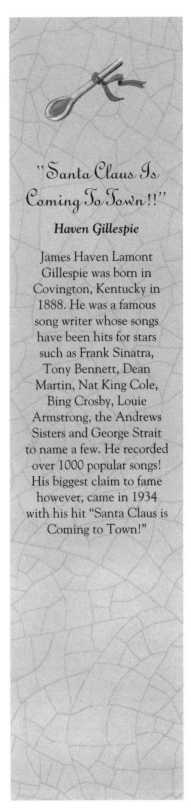

"Santa Claus Is Coming To Town!!"
Haven Gillespie

James Haven Lamont Gillespie was born in Covington, Kentucky in 1888. He was a famous song writer whose songs have been hits for stars such as Frank Sinatra, Tony Bennett, Dean Martin, Nat King Cole, Bing Crosby, Louie Armstrong, the Andrews Sisters and George Strait to name a few. He recorded over 1000 popular songs! His biggest claim to fame however, came in 1934 with his hit "Santa Claus is Coming to Town!"

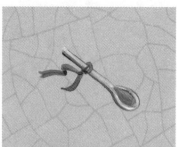

Spicy Southwest Spinach Dip

A real crowd pleaser! . . . Ordinary spinach dip teams up with the lively flavors of the Southwest for a quick and easy appetizer that won't last long!

1	(10-ounce) package frozen chopped spinach, thawed and drained well	1	bunch green onions, chopped
8	ounces cream cheese, softened	1	teaspoon cumin
½	cup salsa	2	cups Monterey Jack and cheddar blend cheese

- Combine all ingredients except cheese and cook in a saucepan until heated through, stirring constantly.
- Pour into a 10-inch quiche plate and top with cheese.
- Bake at 350° for 20 minutes until cheese is bubbly.
- Serve with sturdy tortilla chips.

Serves 12

Broccoli-Cheddar Appetizer Spread

Quick and easy to prepare, everyone loves this dip . . . including the hostess!

1	(16-ounce) container sour cream	1	(10-ounce) package frozen chopped broccoli, cooked and drained
3	cups (12 ounces) shredded cheddar cheese	1	round dark pumpernickel loaf (optional)
1	package Knorr vegetable soup mix		Corn chips

- Combine sour cream, cheddar cheese, and soup mix in a bowl; stir in broccoli.
- Scoop out center of bread, if desired. Spoon dip into hollowed bread.
- Serve dip with corn chips.

Serves 8 to 10

Romano-Ricotta Stuffed Triangles

Easy preparation for a "stuffed" appetizer. They'll dazzle your guests!

1	(17¼-ounce) package frozen puff pastry sheets, thawed	2	tablespoons minced fresh parsley
¾	cup ricotta cheese	1	teaspoon crushed oregano
1	cup grated Romano cheese	½	teaspoon black pepper
½	cup chopped roasted sweet red pepper	¼	cup milk
		¼	cup grated Romano cheese

- Unfold pastry sheets and cut each into 9 (3-inch) squares.
- Combine ricotta cheese, Romano cheese, red pepper, parsley, oregano, and black pepper in a bowl, stirring well.
- Brush edges of pastry squares with milk to moisten; spoon 2 teaspoons filling on half of each square. Fold pastry over filling, forming a triangle, and press edges with a fork to seal. Prick top of each triangle with a fork.
- Brush tops of triangles with milk. Sprinkle with Romano cheese and place on baking sheets.
- Bake at 400° for 20 to 25 minutes or until golden.

Makes 18

Cheese-Mushroom Canapés

This recipe always wins lots of compliments.
"Regulars" at the party are always looking for it!

1	cup (4 ounces) shredded cheddar cheese	1	cup mayonnaise
1	cup (4 ounces) shredded Monterey Jack cheese	1	(7-ounce) can pitted ripe olives, chopped
1	cup minced green onions	1	cup chopped fresh mushrooms
		40	cocktail rye bread slices

- Combine cheddar and Monterey Jack cheese, green onions, mayonnaise, olives, and mushrooms in a bowl, stirring well; spread evenly on bread slices and place on a baking sheet.
- Bake at 350° for 10 minutes.

Makes 40 canapés

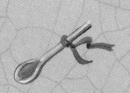

Floats Like a Butterfly and Stings Like a Bee!

Muhammad Ali

Born Cassius Clay in Louisville Kentucky in 1942. Ali won the world heavyweight title four straight years, the first coming in 1964. He won six Golden Gloves tournaments in Kentucky, two national Golden Gloves and an Olympic Gold medal in 1960. The total number of amateur fights is unknown. He got his start at the age of twelve, when seeking help from a policeman at a nearby gym after his new bike had been stolen. The policeman encouraged and obviously persuaded Ali to join his boxing class. They never found his bike; but, Ali became one of the most celebrated prize fighters in sport's history.

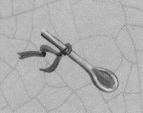

Kentucky produced four Vice-Presidents. They included both the oldest and the youngest.

Richard M. Johnson

A Scott County native was born in 1781. Campaigning as Martin Van Burren's running mate, Johnson was elected vice-president from 1837-1841.

Youngest Vice-President

John Cabell Breckinridge

Running on the ticket with James Buchanan, Breckenridge was elected vice-president in 1856. At the time of his inauguration in March of 1857, he became the youngest vice-president in the nation's history. A charismatic leader, he was known for his charming and personal manner and for his exceptional oratory skills.

Gorgonzola-Walnut Spread

You'll love the classic European pairing of blue cheese and walnuts in this incredibly easy and delicious spread!

¼ cup very finely chopped or grated walnuts	5 ounces Gorgonzola or other favorite blue cheese
16 ounces cream cheese, softened at room temperature	1 tablespoon Cognac
	1 bunch fresh chives, finely chopped
	Salt and pepper to taste

- Combine cream cheese and Gorgonzola mixing very well.
- Add Cognac, salt and pepper, mix well until very smooth.
- Add walnuts and chives and mix until well blended.
- Spoon into serving bowl.

Serves 8 to 10

Pico de Gallo

This is the real thing . . . fresh and wonderfully spicy!

1 medium to large sweet onion, minced	⅓ cup minced fresh cilantro
	Juice of 1 lime
3 large ripe tomatoes, minced	1 tablespoon sugar
2-4 jalapeño peppers, seeded and minced	¼ teaspoon ground cumin
1 teaspoon minced garlic	

- Combine all ingredients, stirring well; cover and chill several hours. Serve with tortilla chips.

Hot Parmesan Puffs

4	ounces cream cheese, softened	⅛	teaspoon cayenne pepper
¾	teaspoon grated onion		Dash of hot sauce
¼	cup homemade mayonnaise	2	tablespoons grated Parmesan cheese
1	tablespoon chopped fresh chives	1	baguette, cut into 1½-inch rounds

- Combine cream cheese, onion, mayonnaise, chives, cayenne pepper, hot sauce, and Parmesan cheese in a bowl, stirring well; spread evenly on bread slices.

- Freeze unbaked puffs, if desired.

- Thaw and place on baking sheets. Bake at 350° for 15 minutes or until golden and puffed.

Makes 18 to 24 puffs

Artichoke Bites

A yummy new way to serve artichokes.

2	(6-ounce) jars marinated artichoke hearts	⅛	teaspoon pepper
1	small onion, diced	¼	teaspoon dried oregano
1	garlic clove, minced	⅛	teaspoon hot sauce (optional)
4	large eggs, lightly beaten	2	cups (8 ounces) shredded cheddar cheese
¼	cup fine, dry breadcrumbs	2	tablespoons minced fresh parsley
¼	teaspoon salt		

- Drain marinade from artichoke hearts, reserving liquid from 1 jar. Chop artichoke hearts and set aside.

- Sauté onion and garlic in hot reserved marinade in a skillet over medium heat 5 minutes.

- Combine eggs, breadcrumbs, salt, pepper, oregano, and, if desired, hot sauce in a large bowl, stirring well with a fork. Fold in cheese and parsley. Stir in artichoke hearts and onion mixture. Pour into a 9 x 13 x 2-inch pan.

- Bake at 325° for 30 minutes.

- Let cool slightly and cut into 1-inch squares. Serve hot or cold.

Makes 6 dozen

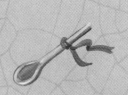

Adlai E. Stevenson

Born in Christian County, Kentucky in 1835. He was elected vice-president during Grover Cleveland's second administration in 1892.

Oldest Vice-President

Alben W. Barkley

Alben Barkley from Paducah, Kentucky, took the oath of vice-president on January 20, 1949, and became the oldest man to do so. He served as vice-president under Harry S. Truman. He was regarded as one of the most popular Democrats and was the recipient of numerous awards. He even vied with General Dwight D. Eisenhower for Look magazine's most "fascinating" American. April 30, 1956 "I would rather be a servant in the house of the Lord than to sit in the seats of the mighty" (Alben W. Barkley during the key note address at a mock convention organized by students of Washington and Lee University.) Following the conclusion of the speech, Barkley suffered a fatal heart attack.

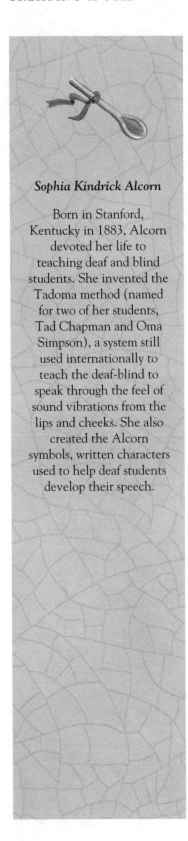

Sophia Kindrick Alcorn

Born in Stanford, Kentucky in 1883, Alcorn devoted her life to teaching deaf and blind students. She invented the Tadoma method (named for two of her students, Tad Chapman and Oma Simpson), a system still used internationally to teach the deaf-blind to speak through the feel of sound vibrations from the lips and cheeks. She also created the Alcorn symbols, written characters used to help deaf students develop their speech.

Roasted Pepper and Artichoke Puffs

A fabulous combination of color and flavor meld together in this savory appetizer.

2	tablespoons butter	1	tablespoon lemon juice
1	bunch green onions, minced		Freshly ground black pepper to
2	garlic cloves, minced		taste
1	(13¾-ounce) can artichoke	½	cup mayonnaise
	bottoms, diced	3	red bell peppers, cut into
3	ounces thinly sliced prosciutto,		2- x 1½-inch pieces
	minced	3	yellow bell peppers, cut into
3	tablespoons chopped fresh basil		2- x 1½-inch pieces
½	cup grated Parmesan cheese	¼	cup olive oil
½	cup (2 ounces) shredded Gruyère or	2	tablespoons balsamic vinegar
	Jarlsberg cheese		Salt to taste

- Melt butter in a skillet over medium heat; add green onions and garlic and sauté 2 to 3 minutes.

- Combine green onion mixture, artichoke bottoms, prosciutto, basil, Parmesan and Gruyère or Jarlsberg cheese, tossing well. Sprinkle with lemon juice and pepper. Stir in mayonnaise and chill 1 hour.

- Preheat oven to 400°.

- Place bell pepper pieces in a large shallow baking dish; drizzle with oil and vinegar and season with salt and pepper.

- Bake at 400° for 15 minutes.

- Spoon 2 teaspoons artichoke mixture on each bell pepper piece. Broil 4 inches from heat (with electric oven door partially open) until cheese is bubbly.

Makes 36 to 48

Zesty Pecans

The combination of Worcestershire sauce and hot sauce really gives these pecans a kick!

1	pound pecans	3	tablespoons Worcestershire sauce
	Salt to taste		Dash of hot sauce or cayenne
1	tablespoon butter, melted		pepper

- Combine pecans, salt, and butter, stirring well. Place in a 10 x 15-inch jelly-roll pan.

- Bake at 300°, stirring often, 15 to 20 minutes. Remove from oven and sprinkle with Worcestershire sauce and hot sauce, stirring well. Return to oven and bake an additional 5 to 10 minutes.

Makes 1 pound

Olivada Ann

Olivada refers to the black olive paste in this recipe.
This mixture makes a delicious crostini!

1	can pitted ripe olives, drained	⅓	cup olive oil
2	tablespoons capers, drained	1	baguette, sliced
2	teaspoons minced garlic		Roasted sweet red pepper slices
¼	cup fresh or 2 tablespoons dried cilantro		Shredded Gorgonzola cheese

- Process olives, capers, garlic, cilantro, and oil in a food processor until pureed.
- Place bread slices on a baking sheet. Broil 4 inches from heat (with electric oven door partially open) until browned. Turn and brown other side.
- Spread olive paste evenly on bread slices. Top each with a red pepper slice and sprinkle with cheese.
- Return to oven and broil until cheese is lightly browned.

Makes 18 to 24

Crabmeat Remick

Rich and elegant! A grand beginning to any meal.

1	pound lump crabmeat, drained	½	teaspoon hot sauce
6	bacon slices, cooked crisp	½	cup chili sauce
1	teaspoon dry mustard	1	teaspoon tarragon vinegar
½	teaspoon paprika	1½	cups mayonnaise
½	teaspoon celery salt		

- Place crabmeat evenly in 6 ramekins of crab shells. Bake at 350° until thoroughly heated.
- Top each ramekin with a bacon slice.
- Combine dry mustard, paprika, celery salt, and hot sauce in a bowl; add chili sauce and vinegar, stirring well. Whisk in mayonnaise. Spoon evenly over bacon.
- Broil 4 inches from heat (with electric oven door partially open) until glazed.

Serves 6

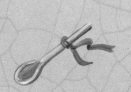

Oh Say Can You See?!!!

Thomas Hunt Morgan

Born in Lexington, Kentucky in 1866. Morgan influenced more than any other, the direction of biological science in this country. Internationally, he ranks as the most important contributor to the knowledge of genetics following Gregor Mendel. In 1910 he established the chromosomal theory of inheritance (the discovery that genes are on the chromosomes of all organisms.) This led to the advanced understanding of the physical basis of heredity. He became the first American non-physician to win the Nobel prize in physiology or medicine. His awards and honors, and his national and international recognition is incalculable. Morgan was the great-grandson of **Francis Scott Key**, the composer of the "Star-Spangled Banner".

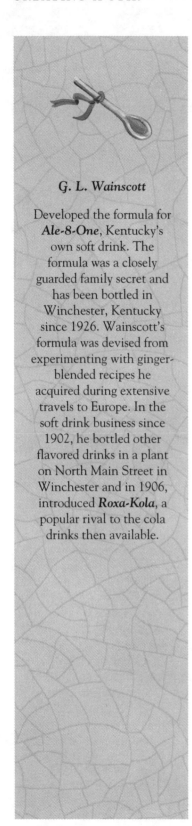

G. L. Wainscott

Developed the formula for **Ale-8-One**, Kentucky's own soft drink. The formula was a closely guarded family secret and has been bottled in Winchester, Kentucky since 1926. Wainscott's formula was devised from experimenting with ginger-blended recipes he acquired during extensive travels to Europe. In the soft drink business since 1902, he bottled other flavored drinks in a plant on North Main Street in Winchester and in 1906, introduced **Roxa-Kola**, a popular rival to the cola drinks then available.

Herbed Feta Appetizer Torte

Slice this "cheesecake" appetizer thin . . . it's rich!

1¼ cups ground walnuts
¾ cup finely crushed zwieback
¼ cup butter, melted
1½ cups herb-seasoned feta (basil, tomato)
15 ounces ricotta cheese
3 large eggs

½ cup finely chopped olives
1 cup finely chopped mushrooms
⅓ cup milk
½ teaspoon pepper
½ teaspoon salt
Sliced ripe olives, fresh basil or oregano leaves for garnish

- Combine walnuts, zwieback, and butter; mix well and press into the bottom of a 9-inch springform pan.

- Beat cheeses at medium speed with an electric mixer until well blended; add eggs, beating at low speed until blended.

- Fold olives and next 4 ingredients into cheeses. Pour into prepared pan. Place pan on a 10 x 15-inch jelly-roll pan.

- Bake at 325° for 45 to 50 minutes or until center appears set. Remove from oven and let cool 15 minutes.

- Run knife around sides of pan. Let cool 30 minutes. Remove sides of pan; cover and chill at least 4 hours or overnight.

- Cut torte into thin slices and garnish with a fresh oregano or basil leaf and olive slices.

Serves 16 to 20

Indian Chicken Curry Balls

Very unusual and very tasty

4 ounces cream cheese, softened
2 tablespoons mayonnaise
1 cup chopped cooked chicken
1 cup chopped roasted almonds

½ teaspoon salt
2 teaspoons curry powder
1 tablespoon chopped chutney
½ cup flaked coconut

- Combine cream cheese and mayonnaise in a bowl, stirring well. Add chicken, almonds, salt, curry powder, and chutney, stirring well.

- Form chicken mixture into balls; roll in coconut. Cover and chill at least 24 hours.

Makes 30 balls

Iced Mint Tea

Very refreshing! The perfect way to temper the heat!

1   cup sugar
6   cups boiling water, divided
    Juice of 2 lemons
10 fresh mint sprigs

10 regular-size tea bags
2   cups cold water
    Lemon slices and fresh mint sprigs
    for garnish

- Combine sugar, 2 cups boiling water, and lemon juice in a bowl; cover and let steep 30 minutes.
- Combine 10 mint sprigs, tea bags, and remaining 4 cups boiling water in a separate bowl; cover and let steep 30 minutes. Drain, discarding solids.
- Combine sugar mixture, mint mixture, and 2 cups cold water in a pitcher; pour into glasses over ice and garnish, if desired.

Serves 6 to 8

Holiday Cheer

A festive punch without the alcohol

2   quarts cranberry juice
¾   cup lemon juice
1   quart orange juice
2   quarts ginger ale, chilled

½   cup sugar
    Oranges and lemons, thinly sliced
    for garnish

- Combine cranberry juice, lemon juice, orange juice, ginger ale, and sugar, stirring well. Stir in fruit slices.

Serves 12 to 18

Spicy Bloody Marys

2   quarts vegetable juice
3   cups vodka
1   tablespoon salt
½   tablespoon pepper

2½   ounces Worcestershire sauce
     Juice of 5 lemons
     Celery stalks with leaves for
     garnish

- Combine juice, vodka, salt, pepper, Worcestershire sauce, and lemon juice in a pitcher, stirring well.
- Serve in tall glasses over ice; garnish with celery stalk.

Serves 6 to 8

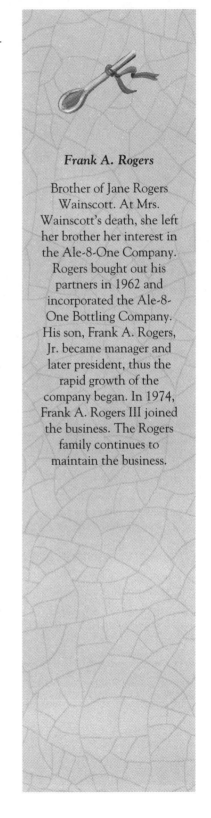

Frank A. Rogers

Brother of Jane Rogers Wainscott. At Mrs. Wainscott's death, she left her brother her interest in the Ale-8-One Company. Rogers bought out his partners in 1962 and incorporated the Ale-8-One Bottling Company. His son, Frank A. Rogers, Jr. became manager and later president, thus the rapid growth of the company began. In 1974, Frank A. Rogers III joined the business. The Rogers family continues to maintain the business.

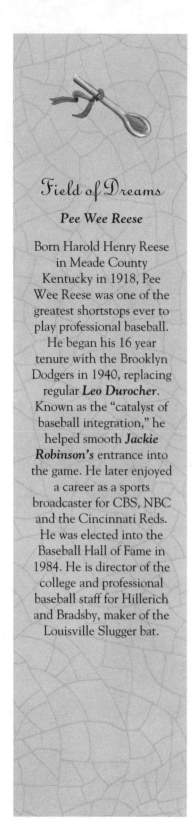

Angel Tea

1	bottle dry white wine, chilled	1	tablespoon angostura bitters
1	bottle club soda, chilled		Sliced lemon or lime for garnish

- Combine wine, club soda, and bitters in a pitcher, stirring well.
- Serve over ice and garnish with a slice of fresh lemon or lime.

Serves 6 to 8

Mimi Hillenmeyer's Eggnog

*"The following recipe has been passed down 4 generations.
I cannot remember a Christmas day without this fabulous eggnog.
It is the grand tradition in our family one that everyone looks forward to."*
The John J. Greeley Family

6	egg yolks, beaten until light	6	egg whites, whip until stiff
1	cup sugar, add to yolks and beat	1	quart whipping cream
1½	cups bourbon, add and beat		

- Whip until stiff and fold into mixture. Serve with grated nutmeg.

Serves 8

Georgetown Eggnog

6	large eggs, separated	1	pint bourbon whiskey
1	cup sugar	1	quart heavy whipping cream

- Beat egg yolks at medium speed with an electric mixer until light and pale; add ⅔ cup sugar, beating well. Slowly add the whiskey, beating continuously.
- Beat egg whites in a large bowl with clean beaters at medium speed until stiff but not dry; gradually add remaining sugar, beating well.
- Very slowly add whiskey mixture to egg whites, folding in gently so the eggnog will not separate.
- Beat whipping cream in a separate bowl at medium speed until stiff peaks form; gently fold into egg white mixture.
- Serve eggnog immediately in chilled julep cups.

Serves 12

Sparkling Pink Lemonade

Fresh squeezed lemonade with a zing!

1½ cups sugar
1½ cups fresh lemon juice
    Fresh fruit pieces (strawberries,
    melon balls, pineapple chunks)

1   quart club soda, chilled
5   teaspoons grenadine

- Combine sugar and lemon juice in a 2-quart pitcher, stirring well; chill at least 30 minutes.
- Thread fruit onto 6-inch wooden skewers.
- Stir club soda and grenadine into lemon mixture when ready to serve.
- Place fruit kabobs in glasses; fill with ice and pour lemonade over top.

Serves 6 to 8

Kentucky Mint Juleps

*Absolutely divine! Do not reserve these for
Derby Day-they are refreshing all summer long!*

4   cups shaved or crushed ice (do not
    use ice cubes)
    Sugar Syrup

1   pint quality bourbon whiskey
6   fresh mint sprigs for garnish
    Powdered sugar

- Pack ice into 6 julep cups to within ½ inch from top; add 1 jigger Sugar Syrup and 1 to 2 jiggers bourbon to each cup, stirring until cup frosts.
- Dip mint sprigs in powdered sugar and place 1 in each serving. Serve with a cocktail napkin (cups are quite chilly).

Sugar Syrup

1   cup sugar
1   cup water

1   bunch fresh mint

- Bring sugar and 1 cup water to a boil in a small saucepan, stirring until sugar is dissolved. Remove from heat and add mint.
- Cover and let steep 15 minutes, stirring occasionally. Drain, discarding solids.
- Place sugar syrup in a jar and chill until ready to serve.

Serves 6

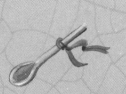

Mint Julep

The word julap or julep originally referred to a nonalcoholic medicinal syrup. However, by the mid eighteenth century, when the average American, including women and children, consumed two and a half gallons of spirits a year (much of it before breakfast!), the julep was made primarily with spirits and in our country most often with mint. Many times, the julep was taken after waking in the morning because it was thought to aid in fighting fevers that might have arisen from the night air and hot climates. Juleps were originally made with Madeira but postbellum Southerners replaced that with bourbon whiskey. Julep ingredients usually include bourbon whiskey, sugar, water, fresh mint and crushed ice, mixed and typically served in a frosted silver julep cup. They are a Kentucky tradition often associated with the Kentucky Derby.

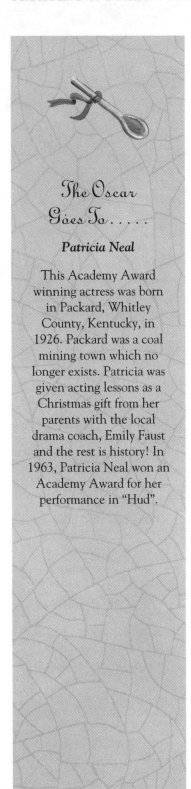

*The Oscar
Goes To.....*

Patricia Neal

This Academy Award winning actress was born in Packard, Whitley County, Kentucky, in 1926. Packard was a coal mining town which no longer exists. Patricia was given acting lessons as a Christmas gift from her parents with the local drama coach, Emily Faust and the rest is history! In 1963, Patricia Neal won an Academy Award for her performance in "Hud".

Irish Cream

Always a hit! Great for holiday get-togethers!

1 (14-ounce) can sweetened condensed milk	1 cup Irish whiskey
1½ cups whipping cream	¼ teaspoon coconut extract
¾ cup egg substitute	1½ tablespoons chocolate syrup

- Process all ingredients in a blender 30 seconds or until smooth. Pour into a jar or bottle and chill up to several weeks.
- Serve chilled mixture in glasses.

Serves 4

Zingy Fruit Punch

Use equal parts of all ingredients.

Cranberry-raspberry juice drink	Ginger ale
Grape juice	Crushed ice
Pineapple juice	

- Combine juices in a pitcher, stirring well. Chill until ready to serve.
- Stir in ginger ale and crushed ice and serve immediately.

Island Yellowbirds

A taste of the tropics!

2 cups ice cubes	¼ cup banana liqueur
½ cup light rum	¼ cup Galliano
¼ cup Triple Sec	

- Process all ingredient in a blender until frothy.

Serves 4

Kentucky Bourbon Slush

Wow . . . are these good!

2 cups boiling water
1 cup sugar
4 regular-size tea bags
1 (6-ounce) can frozen orange juice concentrate, undiluted
1 (6-ounce) can frozen limeade concentrate, undiluted

1 (6-ounce) can frozen lemonade concentrate, undiluted
2 cups bourbon whiskey
1 jar cherries, without stems
  Lemon-lime soda or ginger ale

- Combine 2 cups boiling water and sugar in a bowl, stirring until sugar is dissolved. Add tea bags; cover and let steep 10 minutes. Drain, discarding tea bags.
- Combine tea mixture, orange juice concentrate, limeade, lemonade, bourbon, and cherries in a large bowl. Freeze, stirring every 2 to 3 hours.
- Place a spoonful of slush in each glass and fill to top with lemon-lime soda or ginger ale.

Serves 8

Wassail

2 quarts apple juice
1 (6-ounce) can frozen orange juice concentrate, undiluted
1 (6-ounce) can frozen lemonade concentrate, undiluted
4 cups water

2 cups pineapple juice
3 cinnamon sticks
2 teaspoons whole cloves
1 whole allspice
2 cups red wine (optional)

- Combine apple juice, frozen orange juice and lemonade, 4 cups water, and pineapple juice in a Dutch oven.
- Place cinnamon, cloves, and allspice in the center of a piece of cheesecloth; bring ends together and tie securely. Place in Dutch oven.
- Bring mixture to a simmer and simmer until thoroughly heated.
- Stir 2 cups red wine to mixture to make a true wassail, if desired.

You can also make this recipe in a percolator; place juices and water in base and spices in top. Perk until thoroughly heated.

Serves 16 to 20

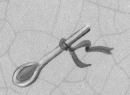

America's Native Spirit Historic Labrot and Graham

Labrot and Graham Distillery

In 1797, *Elijah Pepper* founded the perfect spot amid white oaks and dogwoods to build a distillery in the heart of the bluegrass. Located in Versailles, Kentucky amid the state's most famous horse farms, it is the only distillery where you can see the state's two most famous products maturing side by side: thoroughbred horses and Bourbon whiskey. Bourbon, America's only native spirit, has been crafted on this same site for almost 200 years. The property assumed its name in 1878 when *James Graham* and *Leopold Labrot* bought the property. The property remained in the Labrot family until purchased in 1941 by *Brown-Forman* who owned it until 1972. Brown-Forman has repurchased and restored Labrot and Graham, Kentucky's oldest operating distillery, to its past glory.

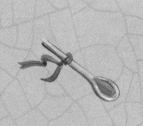

Diane Sawyer

Journalist, and television news correspondent, Diane Sawyer was born in Glasgow, Kentucky in 1945. Soon after she was born, Sawyer's family moved to Louisville, Kentucky. She began her media career in 1969 as a weathermaid for WLKY TV in Louisville then on to reporter for the same network. After working as a reporter for CBS News, she became co-anchor on CBS's "Morning with Charles Kuralt and Diane Sawyer". In 1984, she became the first woman hired as a "60 Minutes" correspondent. Her hard work and diligence paid off when she landed the co-host position on "Prime Time Live" with Sam Donaldson.

Peppermint Eggnog Punch

½ gallon peppermint ice cream (if available use ice cream that is not pink)

2 quarts eggnog
1 (2-liter) bottle lemon-lime soda
Miniature candy canes for garnish

- Place ice cream in a punch bowl; add eggnog and lemon-lime soda. Let stand 30 minutes before serving, spooning liquids over ice cream occasionally to blend.
- Hang a candy cane on the inside of each cup and serve punch in cups.

Serves 12 to 16

"Stinky's" Perfect Margarita

The authentic way!

Juice of 1 lime
1½ teaspoons powdered sugar
1½ ounces Sauza Conmemorativo Anejo Tequilla

¾ ounce Cointreau
Fresh lime wedge

- Pour all ingredients into a shaker filled with ice. Shake vigorously until well blended.
- Strain into a glass. Can be served straight up or over ice. Salt rim of the glass, if desired. Garnish with fresh lime wedge.

Serves 1

Mock Champagne Punch

2 (25.4-ounce) bottles sparkling white grape juice, chilled
2 (2-liter) bottles ginger ale, chilled
1 (32-ounce) bottle white grape juice, chilled

1 (6-ounce) can frozen lemonade concentrate, thawed and undiluted
Ice ring

- Combine sparkling grape juice, ginger ale, white grape juice, and lemonade in a large punch bowl; add ice ring and serve immediately.

Makes 6½ quarts

Caribbean Watermelon Splash

Evokes wonderful memories of brunch served ocean side in the Caribbean

2 cups freshly squeezed watermelon juice (¼ standard-size watermelon, cubed)
Juice of ½ lime

2 teaspoons superfine sugar or equivalent amount of artificial sweetener

- Cube watermelon, squeezing out juice using your hands or pressing the fruit against the inside of a bowl with a heavy spoon. Pour mixture through a wire-mesh strainer into a glass liquid measuring cup to measure 2 cups, discarding solids.

- Combine watermelon juice, lime juice, and sugar in a pitcher, stirring well. Chill until ready to serve.

- Stir mixture well and serve over crushed ice.

Serves 4

Tropical Citrus Slush

Outstanding!

3 cups sugar
2 cups water
3 (46-ounce) cans pineapple juice
2 (12-ounce) cans frozen orange juice concentrate, thawed and undiluted

1 (12-ounce) can frozen pink lemonade concentrate, thawed and undiluted
Lemon-lime soda

- Cook 3 cups sugar and 2 cups water in a saucepan over medium-low heat until sugar is dissolved. Let cool.

- Combine syrup, pineapple juice, and juice concentrates, stirring well. Pour into small freezer-safe containers and freeze until ready to serve.

- For individual servings, fill each glass with equal parts citrus mixture and lemon-lime soda.

Makes 2 gallons citrus mixture

To serve in a punch bowl, pour a portion of the citrus mixture into a mold; freeze until slushy. Push cherries into slush and freeze until firm. Combine remaining citrus mixture and 3 quarts lemon-lime soda in a punch bowl, stirring well; add ice ring and serve immediately.

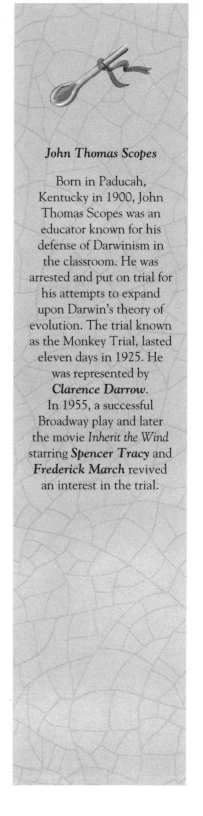

John Thomas Scopes

Born in Paducah, Kentucky in 1900, John Thomas Scopes was an educator known for his defense of Darwinism in the classroom. He was arrested and put on trial for his attempts to expand upon Darwin's theory of evolution. The trial known as the Monkey Trial, lasted eleven days in 1925. He was represented by *Clarence Darrow*.
In 1955, a successful Broadway play and later the movie *Inherit the Wind* starring *Spencer Tracy* and *Frederick March* revived an interest in the trial.

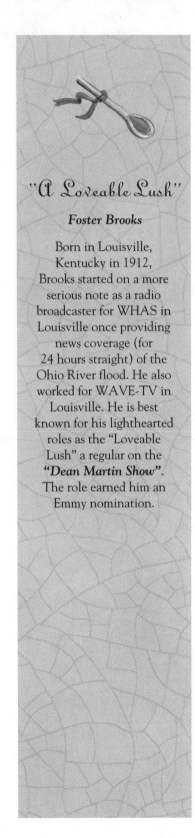

Orange Smoothie

1	cup milk	1	(6-ounce) can frozen orange juice concentrate, undiluted
1	cup water	1	teaspoon vanilla extract
½	cup sugar	12	ice cubes

- Process all ingredients in a blender until smooth.

Serves 4

White Sangría

4	cups ice cubes	1	cinnamon stick
1	(6-ounce) can frozen lemonade concentrate	½	cup superfine sugar
1	lemon, sliced and seeded	2	ounces brandy (optional)
1	orange, sliced and seeded	1	(12-ounce) bottle club soda

- Combine ice cubes and frozen lemonade in a large pitcher; mix well.

- Add lemon slices, orange slices, cinnamon stick, sugar, and, if desired, brandy; chill 1 to 2 hours, stirring occasionally.

- Remove and discard cinnamon stick. Stir in wine and chill 1 to 2 hours.

- Stir in club soda just before serving. Serve over ice.

Serves 6 to 8

Sonny's Summertime G & T

Campari adds color and sparkle to this otherwise ordinary summertime favorite.

3	ounces gin (we used Bombay Sapphire London Dry Gin)	2	teaspoons Campari
4½	ounces tonic water		Fresh lime wedges, orange slices, or lemon twists for garnish

- Pour gin into an 8 ounce highball glass that is almost filled with ice cubes.

- Add tonic and Campari. Garnish with a lime wedge, orange slice, or twist of lemon.

Serves 1

One jigger equals 1½ ounces which equals 1 shot which equals 1 bar glass. Do not alter quantities; tonic can easily overwhelm the gin!

Breakfast & Brunch

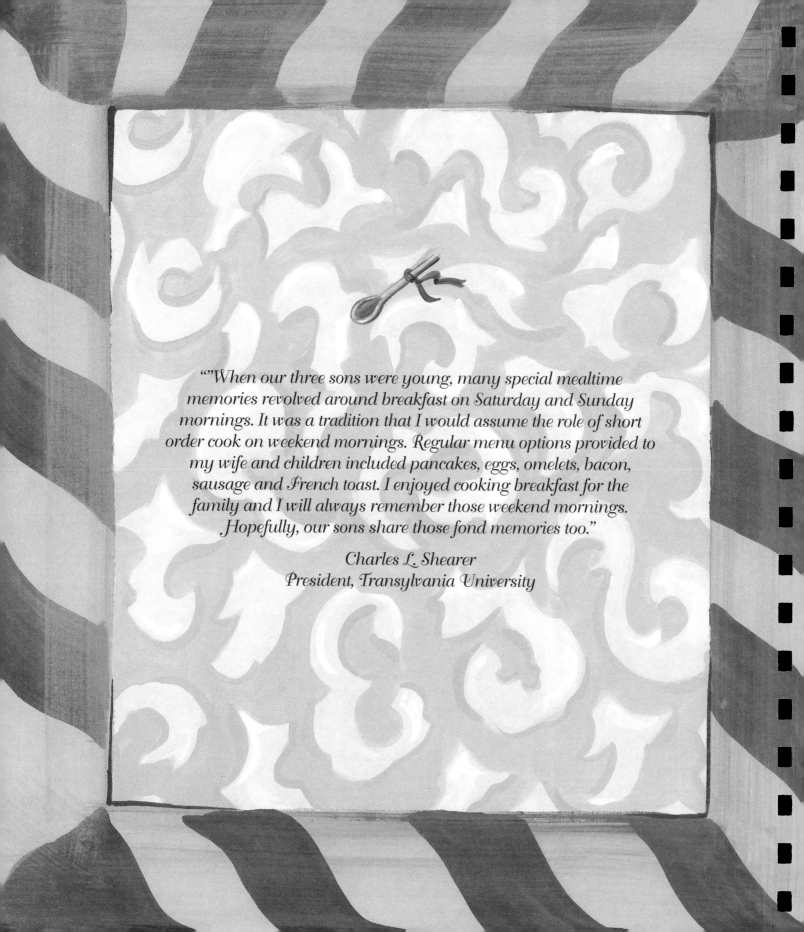

""When our three sons were young, many special mealtime memories revolved around breakfast on Saturday and Sunday mornings. It was a tradition that I would assume the role of short order cook on weekend mornings. Regular menu options provided to my wife and children included pancakes, eggs, omelets, bacon, sausage and French toast. I enjoyed cooking breakfast for the family and I will always remember those weekend mornings. Hopefully, our sons share those fond memories too."

Charles L. Shearer
President, Transylvania University

Streusel Glazed Blueberry Coffee Cake

Rise and shine with this outstanding cake! It is exceptional when served warm!

2	cups all-purpose flour	1	cup milk
1	cup sugar	1	large egg
3	teaspoons baking powder	1½	cups fresh blueberries
1	teaspoon salt		Walnut Streusel
⅓	cup butter, softened		Glaze

- Beat flour, sugar, baking powder, salt, butter, milk, and egg at low speed with an electric mixer 30 seconds; increase speed and beat 2 minutes. Pour half of batter into a 9 x 13 x 2-inch pan lightly coated with vegetable cooking spray.

- Sprinkle blueberries over batter in pan; top with remaining half of batter. Sprinkle Walnut Streusel over top.

- Bake at 350° for 40 to 45 minutes. Let cool.

- Prepare glaze and drizzle over cooled cake.

Walnut Streusel

½	cup chopped walnuts or pecans	3	tablespoons butter, softened
⅓	cup firmly packed brown sugar	½	teaspoon cinnamon
¼	cup all-purpose flour		

- Combine all ingredients, stirring well.

Glaze

1	cup powdered sugar	¼	teaspoon vanilla extract
2	tablespoons milk		

- Combine all ingredients, stirring until smooth.

Do not use frozen blueberries.

Serves 12

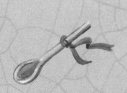

Take Me Out To The Ballgame...

Earle Bryan Combs

Professional baseball star, Earle Combs was born in Pebworth, Kentucky in 1899. In 1924 Combs became the center fielder for the New York Yankees flanked by two Yankee greats, **Babe Ruth** and **Bob Meusel**. He had a reputation for his speed and reckless base stealing. He scored the winning run in the final game of the World Series in 1927. Some of his nicknames included "Kentucky Greyhound", "Kentucky Colonel" and "Gray Fox". A very introspective, religious man, Combs was considered one of the few real gentlemen on the fun-loving, boisterous Yankee teams of the time. After suffering several game related injuries, he resigned in 1935. Combs' trained his young replacement. The "new guy" turned out to be **Joe DiMaggio,** another baseball legend. Combs was inducted into the Baseball Hall of Fame in 1970.

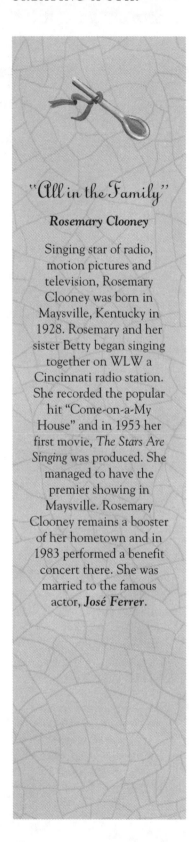

Giant Sunday Morning Pancakes

What fun! These cakes truly are giant, and they are some of the best you have ever put in your mouth.

3	large eggs		1	cup milk
½	cup sugar		1	tablespoon baking powder
6	tablespoons butter, melted		¼	teaspoon salt
1½	cups all-purpose flour			

- Whisk together eggs, sugar, and melted butter in a medium bowl. Gradually add flour alternately with milk, whisking well after each addition.
- Whisk in baking powder and salt.
- Ladle ¾ cup batter onto a hot griddle; cook 1 minute or until bubbles form on the surface and bottom is lightly browned. Turn and cook 1 minute or until done. Repeat procedure with remaining batter.
- Serve pancakes with syrup.

Makes 6 giant pancakes

It's fun to vary these by sprinkling ¼ cup blueberries, raisins, or chocolate morsels over each pancake before turning to finish cooking.

Old English Breakfast Strata

The savory combination of ham and Old English cheese offers a nice change from the traditional sausage breakfast casserole.

6	slices white bread, trimmed and buttered on each side		2	cups milk
				Salt and pepper to taste
6	slices Old English cheese		1	cup ham, chopped
6	whole eggs, slightly beaten		1	(4-ounce) can sliced mushrooms

- Grease a 13 x 9 x 2-inch casserole. Line the bottom of the casserole with broken bread pieces.
- Layer the cheese over the bread to cover the casserole.
- Add the eggs to the milk and pour over the cheese and bread.
- Place ham and mushrooms over the eggs.
- Cover and refrigerate overnight. Remove 1 hour before baking.
- Bake uncovered at 350° for 45 minutes.

Serves 6 to 8

Sausage Gravy and Angel Biscuits

Whoaaa . . . are these good! Rich and incredibly delicious!

1	pound bulk sausage	1	teaspoon salt
¼	cup plus 2 tablespoons all-purpose flour	½	teaspoon pepper
2¼	cups half-and-half		Angel Biscuits

- Brown sausage in a skillet over medium heat, stirring until it crumbles and is no longer pink. Drain, reserving ¼ cup drippings in skillet.

- Add flour to drippings, whisking until smooth. Add sausage, half-and-half, salt, and pepper; cook over medium heat, stirring occasionally, until thickened and bubbly.

- Serve sausage gravy over Angel Biscuits.

Serves 6 to 8

Angel Biscuits

1	(¼-ounce) envelope active dry yeast	1	teaspoon salt
2	tablespoons warm water	¼	cup sugar
5	cups all-purpose flour	1	cup shortening
1	teaspoon baking soda	2	cups buttermilk
3	teaspoons baking powder		

- Combine yeast and 2 tablespoons warm water, stirring to dissolve.

- Sift together flour, baking soda, baking powder, salt, and sugar in a large bowl; cut in shortening with a fork or pastry blender until mixture is crumbly. Add buttermilk, mixing well. Add yeast mixture, stirring well.

- Knead dough until smooth; transfer to a greased bowl, turning to coat. Chill.

- Roll out dough on a lightly floured surface and cut biscuits using a round cookie cutter. Place on a greased baking sheet. Let rise in a warm place (85°), free from drafts, 30 minutes.

- Bake at 400° for 15 minutes.

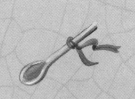

Nick Clooney

Actor and host of American Movie Classics. He is also the father of ER's George Clooney.

George Clooney

Born in Lexington, Kentucky in 1961, the famous actor is best known for his role as heart throb Dr. Doug Ross on TV's **ER** and his motion picture roles in **Batman and Robin**, and **One Fine Day** starring Michelle Pfeifer. Clooney attended Northern Kentucky University.

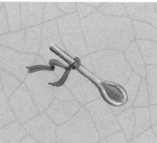

Man O' War

Man O' War

Most would argue that some of the most famous Kentuckians are horses! Man O'War was foaled at the Nursery Stud, near Lexington. He was originally purchased by August Belmont II. In 1918, he was sold at the Saratoga Sales to Louis Feustel for Samuel Riddle, owner of Faraway Farm, a small racing stable near Lexington. Riddle paid a mere 5,000 for what would be one of the most famous thoroughbreds to ever race. Man O'War set numerous world records and won 20 out of 21 races! He was also known as "Big Red" for his color. He won the hearts of all those who watched him race and captivated the American public. He was the feature not only on the sports pages of daily newspapers, but editorial pages as well. Papers turned from politics and war to celebrate his victories. Close to 1,000 people attended the burial services for Man O'War and thousands more listened to the radio broadcast of the eulogies.

Easy Orange Sticky Rolls

These rolls are beautiful and go wonderfully with ham.

3   (10- to 12-ounce) cans refrigerated flaky buttermilk biscuits
1   orange
½   cup butter, melted
1   cup sugar

• Place biscuits around and on the sides of a Bundt pan coated with vegetable cooking spray, forming a ring.

• Grate zest of orange and squeeze juice. Combine orange zest, juice, butter, and sugar, stirring well. Pour over biscuits.

• Bake at 350° for 25 to 30 minutes.

• Invert onto a serving platter (with edges). Serve immediately.

Serves 6 to 8

Stuffed French Toast

¼   cup butter, melted
1   (8-ounce) package cream cheese, softened
¼   cup orange marmalade
¼   cup chopped walnuts
12   white bread slices
3   large eggs
½   cup milk
½   teaspoon vanilla extract
¼   teaspoon ground nutmeg
    Powdered sugar

• Pour butter in the bottom of a 10 x 15 x 1-inch jelly-roll pan.

• Beat cream cheese at medium speed with an electric mixer until light and fluffy; add marmalade and walnuts, beating well.

• Spread 3 heaping teaspoons cream cheese mixture on each of 6 bread slices; top with remaining bread slices. Press lightly and cut in half diagonally.

• Lightly whisk eggs in a medium bowl; add milk, vanilla, and nutmeg, whisking well. Dip bread triangles into egg mixture, coating well. Place in buttered pan.

• Broil 4 inches from heat (with electric oven door partially open) 5 to 6 minutes on each side or until golden brown.

• Sprinkle with powdered sugar and serve immediately.

Serves 6

Orange-Raisin Scones with Orange Butter

Relax with these delicious scones and a steaming pot of tea!

1¾ cups all-purpose flour
2½ teaspoons baking powder
3 tablespoons sugar
2 teaspoons grated orange zest
⅓ cup butter, cut into pieces

½ cup raisins
1 large egg, lightly beaten
4-6 tablespoons half-and-half
1 large egg, lightly beaten
Orange Butter

- Preheat oven to 400°.

- Combine flour, baking powder, sugar, and orange zest in a medium bowl; cut in butter with a fork or pastry blender until crumbly.

- Stir in raisins, 1 egg, and enough half-and-half just until ingredients are moistened.

- Turn dough out onto a lightly floured surface; knead lightly 10 times. Roll into a 9-inch circle and cut into 12 wedges.

- Place wedges 1 inch apart on a lightly greased baking sheet; brush with beaten egg.

- Bake at 400° for 10 to 12 minutes or until golden brown. Remove from baking sheet immediately and serve with Orange Butter.

Makes 12 scones

Orange Butter

½ cup butter, softened

2 tablespoons orange marmalade

- Combine butter and marmalade, stirring well.

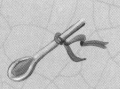

John Sherman Cooper

A U.S. senator and diplomat, John Sherman Cooper was born in Somerset, Kentucky in 1901. Cooper's political career is impressive and his accomplishments are immeasurable. In 1960, a Newsweek poll of fifty Washington correspondents named Cooper the ablest Republican in the Senate. He served under *General George Patton* in France, Luxembourg, and Germany during World War II. Kentuckians may remember him accompanying President *Dwight D. Eisenhower* from the airport on Eisenhower's only visit to Lexington in 1954. A cheering crowd of 55,000 lined the seven- mile route to the UK campus. He was appointed to the Warren Commission by President Johnson in 1963 to investigate the assassination of President Kennedy. President Ford appointed him as the first U.S. ambassador to the GDR.

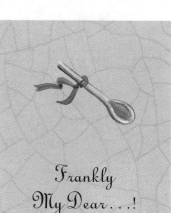

Grilled Banana Bread

A tasty twist on a traditional favorite!

1½	cups sugar	1	tablespoon warm water
⅔	cup vegetable oil	¼	teaspoon salt
2	large eggs	1	teaspoon banana flavoring
1	cup mashed ripe banana	1½	cups all-purpose flour
¼	cup buttermilk	½	cup chopped pecans
1	teaspoon vinegar	¼	cup butter
1	teaspoon baking soda	½	cup toasted flaked coconut

- Preheat oven to 325°.

- Beat sugar and oil at medium speed with an electric mixer until blended; add eggs, 1 at a time, beating well after each addition. Add banana, beating well.

- Combine buttermilk and vinegar; stir into banana mixture.

- Combine baking soda and 1 tablespoon warm water; stir into banana mixture. Add salt and banana flavoring, stirring well.

- Gradually add flour, beating until blended after each addition. Stir in nuts. Pour batter into a greased and floured 9½ x 5-inch loaf pan.

- Bake at 325° for 1 hour.

- Let cool and cut into ½-inch slices.

- Melt butter in a skillet over medium heat; add slices and sauté until lightly golden on both sides. Sprinkle with toasted coconut and serve warm.

Makes 1 loaf

Mini Cinnamon Crescents

These tiny treasures are delicious!
They have the look and taste of gourmet but without all the fuss!

1	(8-ounce) can refrigerated crescent rolls	2	teaspoons ground cinnamon
¼	cup margarine, softened	½	cup chopped nuts and/or raisins
4	teaspoons granulated sugar	1	cup powdered sugar
		2	tablespoons apple juice or milk

- Separate crescent dough into 4 rectangles, pressing perforations to seal. Spread margarine evenly over rectangles.

- Combine granulated sugar and cinnamon and sprinkle over dough. Sprinkle with nuts.

- Roll up rectangles, starting at a short end. Cut each roll into 5 slices and place, cut side down, in an ungreased 9-inch square pan.

- Bake at 375° for 18 to 22 minutes or until golden brown.

- Combine sugar and apple juice, stirring well. Drizzle over warm rolls.

Makes 20 rolls

To reheat, wrap rolls in aluminum foil and bake at 350° for 10 to 15 minutes.

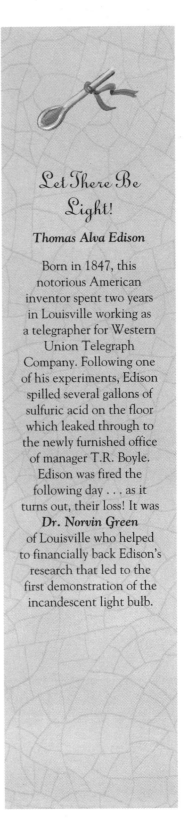

Let There Be Light!

Thomas Alva Edison

Born in 1847, this notorious American inventor spent two years in Louisville working as a telegrapher for Western Union Telegraph Company. Following one of his experiments, Edison spilled several gallons of sulfuric acid on the floor which leaked through to the newly furnished office of manager T.R. Boyle. Edison was fired the following day . . . as it turns out, their loss! It was **Dr. Norvin Green** of Louisville who helped to financially back Edison's research that led to the first demonstration of the incandescent light bulb.

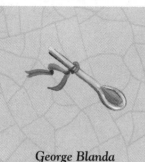

George Blanda

Professional football player and University of Kentucky alumni. Blanda played football for UK under Bernie Shively and Paul "Bear" Bryant from 1945-1948 and graduated in 1951. Blanda is recognized as one of football's greatest players playing more seasons and more games, making more consecutive appearances, scoring more lifetime points and more lifetime field goals and attempts, and scoring in more consecutive games than any other player. He was inducted into the Football Hall of Fame in 1981.

Breakfast Macaroon Cake

1	cup instant oatmeal	1	teaspoon baking soda
1½	cups boiling water	1	teaspoon ground cinnamon
1	cup firmly packed brown sugar	1	cup vegetable oil
1	cup granulated sugar	2	large eggs
1½	cups sifted all-purpose flour		

- Combine oatmeal and 1½ cups boiling water, stirring well; let stand.

- Combine brown sugar, granulated sugar, flour, baking soda, cinnamon, and oil; add eggs, stirring well. Add oatmeal to mixture, stirring well. Pour batter into a greased and floured 9 x 13 x 2-inch baking dish.

- Bake at 350° for 40 minutes.

- Sprinkle Coconut Topping over cake and broil 30 to 45 seconds or until topping is golden.

Coconut Topping

½	cup margarine	1	cup chopped nuts
1	tablespoon milk	7	ounces flaked coconut
¾	cup firmly packed brown sugar		

- Combine all ingredients, stirring well.

Serves 12 to 16

Pumpkin-Sour Cream Coffee Cake

The pumpkin makes this coffee cake outstanding!

½ cup margarine
¾ cup sugar
1 teaspoon vanilla extract
3 large eggs
2 cups all-purpose flour
1 teaspoon baking powder
1 teaspoon baking soda

1 cup sour cream
1 (16-ounce) can pumpkin
1 large egg, lightly beaten
⅓ cup sugar
1 teaspoon pumpkin pie spice
Brown Sugar Streusel

- Beat margarine, ¾ cup sugar, and vanilla at medium speed with an electric mixer until creamy; add 3 eggs, beating well.

- Combine flour, baking powder, and baking soda. Add dry ingredients alternately with sour cream to sugar mixture, beating well after each addition.

- Combine pumpkin, egg, ⅓ cup sugar, and pumpkin pie spice, stirring well; set aside. Prepare Brown Sugar Streusel.

- Spoon half of batter into a 9 x 13 x 2-inch pan lightly coated with vegetable cooking spray; sprinkle with half of Brown Sugar Streusel. Spread all of the pumpkin mixture over streusel. Spread remaining batter over pumpkin mixture and sprinkle with remaining streusel.

- Bake at 325° for 50 to 60 minutes or until golden brown.

Brown Sugar Streusel
1 cup firmly packed brown sugar
2 teaspoons ground cinnamon
⅓ cup margarine, softened
1 cup pecans, chopped

- Combine all ingredients, stirring well.

Serves 12

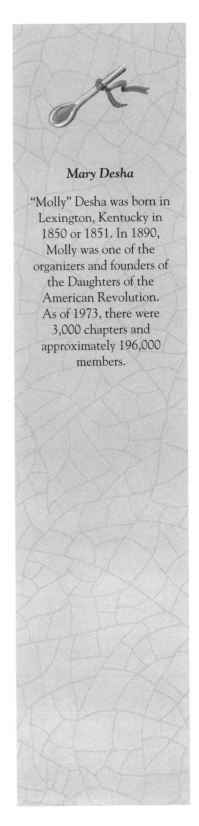

Mary Desha

"Molly" Desha was born in Lexington, Kentucky in 1850 or 1851. In 1890, Molly was one of the organizers and founders of the Daughters of the American Revolution. As of 1973, there were 3,000 chapters and approximately 196,000 members.

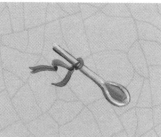

Hadley Pottery

Mary Alice Hadley

Mary Alice Hadley was born in 1911 in Terre Haute, Indiana. While living in New York with her husband, George Hadley, Mary Alice took art classes at Columbia University. In 1939 the Hadleys moved to Louisville, Kentucky and the earthenware empire was born! It all started when Mary Alice couldn't find appropriate dinnerware for use on her boat. Mary Alice decided to make her own and when friends in New York and Chicago saw her work, they were quite impressed! These same friends showed her work to others, and before long, orders started to arrive at her home. The whimsical pieces feature horses, farmers, pigs, sheep and other characters typically painted in signature colors of blue and green with a glazed finish. Hadley Pottery continues to thrive today.

Streusel Layered Sour Cream Coffee Cake

1	cup butter	2	cups sifted all-purpose flour
2	cups sugar	1	teaspoon baking powder
2	large eggs	¼	teaspoon salt
1	cup sour cream		Streusel Topping
1	teaspoon vanilla extract		

- Preheat oven to 350°.
- Beat butter and sugar at medium speed with an electric mixer until creamy; add eggs, beating well. Fold in sour cream and vanilla.
- Sift together flour, baking powder, and salt; add to butter mixture, beating well.
- Pour one-third of batter into a greased Bundt pan; sprinkle with half of Streusel Topping. Repeat layers ending with batter.
- Bake at 350° for 45 to 60 minutes.

Streusel Topping

¼	cup firmly packed brown sugar	1	cup chopped nuts
⅓	cup granulated sugar	1	teaspoon ground cinnamon

- Combine all ingredients, stirring well.

Serves 12

Overnight Breakfast Strata

*Serve this flavorful strata with fresh fruit and
coffee cake for a satisfying breakfast or brunch!*

2	pounds mild pork sausage	2	teaspoons salt
9	large eggs	3	white bread slices, cut into ¼-inch cubes
3	cups milk		
2	teaspoons dry mustard	3	cups (12 ounces) shredded cheddar cheese

- Brown sausage in a skillet over medium heat, stirring until it crumbles and is no longer pink. Drain.
- Whisk together eggs, milk, mustard, and salt; stir in sausage, bread cubes, and cheese.
- Pour mixture into a greased 9 x 13 x 2-inch baking dish. Cover and chill overnight.
- Bake at 350° for 1 hour or until golden.

Serves 8 to 12

Perfect Pumpkin Roll

1	cup powdered sugar	¾	cup all-purpose flour
1	(8-ounce) package cream cheese, softened	1	teaspoon baking powder
		2	teaspoons ground cinnamon
¼	cup butter, softened	1	teaspoon ground ginger
½	teaspoon vanilla extract	½	teaspoon ground nutmeg
3	large eggs	½	teaspoon salt
1	cup granulated sugar	1	teaspoon lemon juice
¾	cup canned pumpkin		Powdered sugar

- Beat powdered sugar, cream cheese, butter, and vanilla at medium speed with an electric mixer until creamy; set aside.

- Beat eggs in a separate bowl at high speed 5 minutes; add granulated sugar. Gradually add pumpkin, beating well.

- Add flour, baking powder, cinnamon, ginger, nutmeg, salt, and lemon juice, beating well. Pour batter into a greased and floured 10 x 15 x 1-inch jelly-roll pan.

- Bake at 350° for 15 minutes.

- Sprinkle powdered sugar on a clean dish towel; turn pumpkin roll out onto towel. Trim hard edges and sprinkle with more powdered sugar. Roll up towel and pumpkin cake together, starting at a long side; let cool.

- Gently unroll cake and spread cream cheese filling to edges. Reroll without towel. Sprinkle with powdered sugar. Chill at least 2 hours.

- Store in the refrigerator.

Serves 12

Swiss Oven Omelet

8	large eggs	2	tablespoons minced onion
1	cup milk	8	bacon slices, cooked and crumbled
2	teaspoons salt	4	cups (16 ounces) shredded Swiss cheese
½	teaspoon pepper		
2	tablespoons minced fresh parsley		

- Whisk together eggs, milk, salt, pepper, parsley, and onion; pour into a 9 x 13 x 2-inch baking dish.

- Sprinkle bacon over the top and cover with cheese.

- Bake at 350° for 40 to 45 minutes.

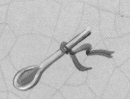

Tom Ewell

Born Yewell Tomkins in Owensboro, Kentucky in 1909, Ewell's first featured role was in 1949 as a philanderer in Adam's Rib. He went on to specialize in portraying inept woman-chasers and starred with two of Hollywood's biggest leading ladies of the 50's, *Marilyn Monroe* in *The 7 Year Itch* and *Jane Mansfield* in *The Girl Can't Help It.*

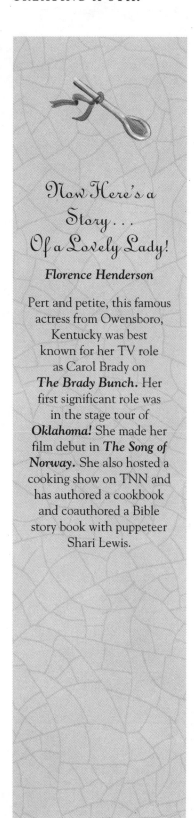

Glazed Holiday Nut Ring

A beautiful coffee cake!

½ cup warm water	5 cups all-purpose flour
1 (¼-ounce) envelope active dry yeast	2 cups finely chopped nuts
	1 cup raisins
⅓ cup granulated sugar	½ cup firmly packed brown sugar
1½ teaspoons salt	1 teaspoon salt
1 cup sour cream	1 cup powdered sugar
½ cup melted margarine	2 tablespoons milk
2 large eggs	¼ teaspoon vanilla extract

- Combine ½ cup warm water and yeast in a large bowl, stirring to dissolve. Add granulated sugar, salt, sour cream, margarine, and eggs, stirring well. Add flour, stirring well until blended. Add additional flour, if necessary, to make a soft dough.

- Turn dough out onto a lightly floured surface and knead until smooth and elastic. Place in a greased bowl, turning to grease top. Cover and let rise in a warm place (85°), free from drafts, 1 hour.

- Punch dough down and turn out onto a floured surface. Divide dough into 2 portions; roll 1 portion into a 20 x 10-inch rectangle. Brush lightly with margarine.

- Combine nuts, raisins, brown sugar, and salt; sprinkle half of mixture over dough. Roll up, starting at a long side; press edges to seal.

- Place on a lightly greased pizza pan forming a 9-inch circle. Make slits half way to center 1½ inches apart. Repeat procedure with remaining dough, margarine, and nut mixture.

- Cover rings and let rise in a warm place 1 hour.

- Bake at 350° for 20 to 25 minutes.

- Combine powdered sugar, milk, and vanilla extract to make a glaze. Pour glaze evenly over baked rings.

Serves 24 (makes 2 rings)

Lemon Soufflé Pancakes

Absolutely delicious! A wonderful way to make weekend guests feel special.

1	cup all-purpose flour	1	tablespoon grated lemon zest
1½	teaspoons baking powder	2	tablespoons fresh lemon juice
½	teaspoon salt	2	teaspoons vanilla extract
5½	tablespoons sugar	3	tablespoons melted butter
1	cup buttermilk	4	egg whites
2	egg yolks		

- Sift together flour, baking powder, salt, and sugar.
- Combine buttermilk, egg yolks, lemon zest, lemon juice, vanilla, and melted butter in a large bowl; add flour mixture, stirring just until dry ingredients are moistened.
- Beat egg whites at medium speed with a hand held mixer until medium peaks form; fold into batter.
- Drop batter by tablespoonfuls onto a medium hot griddle; cook 2½ minutes on each side or until golden.

Makes 16 pancakes

This pancake requires less batter than most, because the egg whites will expand when heated on the griddle.

Quick and Easy Italian Breakfast Casserole

This breakfast casserole doesn't need to be prepared the night before like many others. The Italian seasoning and mozzarella give this one a deliciously distinct flavor!

1	(8-ounce) can refrigerated crescent rolls	6	large eggs
1	pound mild pork sausage	¼	teaspoon dried oregano
2	cups (8 ounces) shredded mozzarella cheese	¾	cup milk

- Press crescent dough in the bottom of a greased 9 x 13 x 2-inch baking dish.
- Brown sausage in a skillet over medium heat, stirring until it crumbles and is no longer pink; drain. Spoon over dough. Sprinkle cheese over sausage.
- Whisk together eggs, oregano, and milk; pour over cheese.
- Bake at 425° for 20 minutes or until eggs are set and cheese is lightly browned. Let stand at room temperature 5 to 10 minutes before serving.

Serves 6 to 8

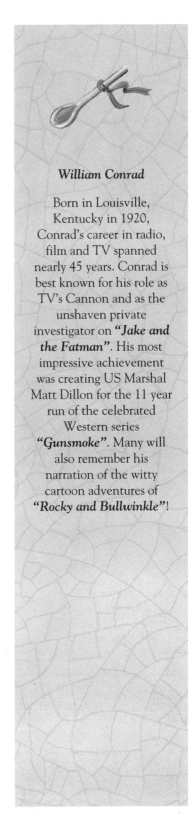

William Conrad

Born in Louisville, Kentucky in 1920, Conrad's career in radio, film and TV spanned nearly 45 years. Conrad is best known for his role as TV's Cannon and as the unshaven private investigator on *"Jake and the Fatman"*. His most impressive achievement was creating US Marshal Matt Dillon for the 11 year run of the celebrated Western series *"Gunsmoke"*. Many will also remember his narration of the witty cartoon adventures of *"Rocky and Bullwinkle"*!

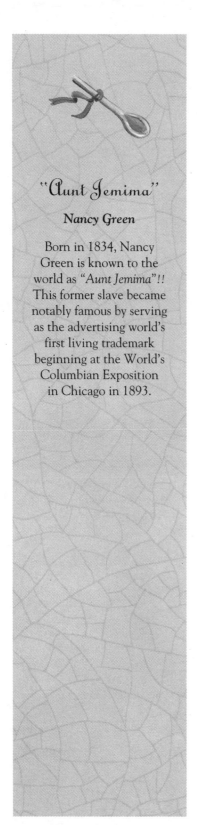

"Aunt Jemima"

Nancy Green

Born in 1834, Nancy Green is known to the world as *Aunt Jemima*!! This former slave became notably famous by serving as the advertising world's first living trademark beginning at the World's Columbian Exposition in Chicago in 1893.

Pecan Waffles with Warm Blackberry Sauce

A wonderful summertime breakfast when blackberries are in season.

2	cups all-purpose flour	2	large eggs, separated
3	teaspoons baking powder	1½	cups milk
½	teaspoon salt	6	tablespoons butter, melted
¾	cup chopped pecans		Blackberry Sauce

- Combine flour, baking powder, and salt; stir in pecans.
- Beat yolks at medium speed with an electric mixer until pale; add milk and butter, blending well.
- Add dry ingredients to butter mixture, beating just until smooth.
- Beat egg whites at medium speed in a separate bowl with clean beaters until stiff peaks form; fold into batter.
- Spoon batter on a greased waffle iron; cook 4 minutes or until done.
- Serve with warm Blackberry Sauce or plain with warm maple syrup!

Serves 6 to 8

Blackberry Sauce

4	cups fresh blackberries, washed drained, and divided	2	tablespoons honey
		2	tablespoons water
½	cup sugar	1	teaspoon lemon juice

- Crush 3 cups blackberries with a potato masher.
- Combine crushed berries, sugar, honey, and 2 tablespoons water in a saucepan. Cook over medium-high heat, stirring constantly, until bubbly.
- Cook 3 to 4 minutes or until thickened. Remove from heat and stir in lemon juice.
- Let cool slightly and stir in remaining berries, mixing well.

Blackberry Sauce can be stored in the refrigerator up to 1 week.

Basil Breakfast Strata

The unique combination of ingredients results in a superb strata-just listen to the raves!

1 cup milk
½ cup dry white wine
1 loaf day-old French bread, cut into ½-inch slices
8 ounces thinly sliced prosciutto
2 cups spinach or arugula leaves
3 tablespoons olive oil

1 pound basil torta, Swiss or smoked Gouda cheese, thinly sliced, divided
3 ripe tomatoes, sliced thin, divided
½ cup basil pesto, divided
4 large eggs
½ cup heavy whipping cream
Salt and freshly ground pepper to taste

- Combine milk and wine; dip bread slices in mixture, 1 or 2 at a time, coating well. Squeeze as much liquid from bread as possible without tearing.

- Place bread slices in a 12-inch round or oval au gratin dish; top with prosciutto. Place spinach or arugula leaves over prosciutto and drizzle with olive oil. Layer with half of cheese slices and half of the tomato slices. Top with half of the basil pesto. Repeat layers of cheese, tomatoes and pesto.

- Whisk together eggs, cream, and salt and pepper; pour over layers. Cover and chill overnight.

- Let stand at room temperature 30 minutes before baking.

- Preheat oven to 350°.

- Bake at 350° for 45 minutes to 1 hour, until puffed and golden.

Basil torta cheese can be found at any local gourmet food or cheese shop.

Serves 8 to 12

German Baked Eggs

Welcome the morning with this scrumptious egg dish!

12 large eggs, lightly beaten
4 cups (16 ounces) shredded Monterey Jack cheese
2 cups cottage cheese

¼ cup all-purpose flour
1 teaspoon baking powder
½ cup butter, melted

- Mix all ingredients in a large bowl. Pour into a 9 x 13 x 2-inch pan.

- Bake at 350° for 40 to 45 minutes or until eggs are set and top is lightly browned.

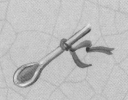

Irvin Shrewsbury Cobb

Journalist, humorist and fiction writer, Irvin Shrewsbury Cobb was born in Paducah, Kentucky in 1876. Cobb was a writer for the Saturday Evening Post and is well known for his short stories (more than fifty) depicting post-Civil War Paducah. *Sinclair Lewis* wrote, "Cobb has made Paducah, and all the other Paducahs-in Kentucky, Minnesota, California and Vermont-from which the rest of us come, live in fiction". Cobb later wrote for Cosmopolitan Magazine. Between 1900 and 1950, Cobb held the eminence (along with Alben Barkley) of being the American celebrity most widely associated with his home state of Kentucky.

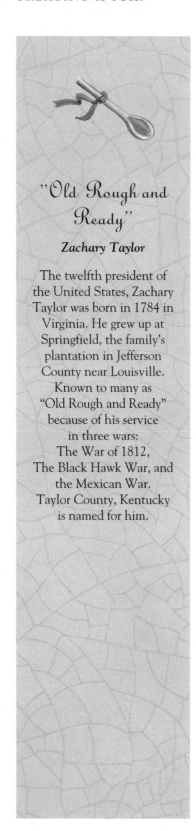

"Old Rough and Ready"

Zachary Taylor

The twelfth president of the United States, Zachary Taylor was born in 1784 in Virginia. He grew up at Springfield, the family's plantation in Jefferson County near Louisville. Known to many as "Old Rough and Ready" because of his service in three wars: The War of 1812, The Black Hawk War, and the Mexican War. Taylor County, Kentucky is named for him.

Scrambled Eggs and Mushrooms Gratinéed with Three Cheeses

1	pound fresh mushrooms, trimmed and quartered		1	cup heavy cream
				Several drops fresh lemon juice
¾	cup butter, divided		12-16	large eggs
2	tablespoons minced shallots or green onions		¼	cup grated Parmesan cheese
	Salt and pepper to taste		¼	cup (1 ounce) finely shredded cheddar cheese
2	cups milk		¼	cup (1 ounce) finely shredded Swiss cheese
6	tablespoons all-purpose flour			

- Melt 3 tablespoons butter in a saucepan over high heat; add mushrooms and sauté 5 to 6 minutes or until beginning to brown.

- Add shallots to mushrooms and cook 1 to 2 minutes. Season with salt and pepper; set aside.

- Bring milk to a simmer in a small saucepan over medium-low heat.

- Melt 5 tablespoons butter in a heavy saucepan over low heat; stir in flour with a wooden spoon and cook until frothy for 2 minutes without browning. Remove from heat and whisk in simmering milk until blended.

- Whisk in half of cream and season with salt and pepper. Bring to a boil, stirring constantly, 4 to 5 minutes. Gradually beat in additional cream to thin.

- Cook mixture until sauce thinly coats the back of a spoon. Season to taste and beat in drops of lemon juice to taste. Clean sides of pan with a spatula. Float 1 tablespoon cream on top of sauce to prevent skin from forming.

- Beat eggs and salt and pepper in a bowl just until blended.

- Melt 3 tablespoons butter in a skillet over medium heat; add eggs and cook 2 to 3 minutes. Stir rapidly until soft curds form. Immediately remove from heat (eggs should be soft) and stir in 1 to 2 tablespoons butter. Season with salt and pepper.

- Spoon a thin layer of sauce in the bottom of an oval dish; sprinkle 2 tablespoons cheese over top. Top with half of eggs.

- Fold 1 cup sauce into mushroom mixture and spoon over eggs. Sprinkle with 4 tablespoons cheese. Cover with remaining eggs and sauce. Sprinkle with remaining cheese and dot with butter.

- Let stand at room temperature up to 1 hour or chill overnight, if desired.

- Bake on a baking sheet at 350° for 25 to 35 minutes or until bubbly.

Serves 8

Baked Cheddar and Garlic Grits

These versatile grits go well with just about everything!

1   cup quick-cooking grits
½   cup butter, cut into pieces
6   ounces garlic cheese, cut into pieces
½   cup milk

1   large egg, lightly beaten
2   cups (8 ounces) finely shredded cheddar cheese

- Prepare grits according to package directions; add butter and garlic cheese, stirring until melted.

- Combine milk and egg; stir into grits. Pour mixture into buttered round or oblong 2-quart baking dish. Top with cheddar cheese.

- Bake at 350° for 1 hour. Let stand at room temperature 15 minutes before serving.

Serves 8 to 10

Ultimate Grits!

Very filling and satisfying, these delicious grits are great for serving a large crowd!

1   pound sausage (we used Jimmy Dean)
1   cup grits (not quick cooking)
2   cups water
    Dash of hot sauce
    Salt and pepper to taste

¼   cup melted butter
8   ounces diced green chiles
2   large eggs, lightly beaten
1½ cups (6 ounces) shredded sharp cheddar cheese

- Brown sausage in a skillet over medium heat; drain.

- Cook grits in 2 cups water according to package directions. Stir in sausage.

- Season with hot sauce, salt, and pepper; add butter, green chiles, eggs, and cheese, stirring well. Pour mixture into a 9 x 13 x 2-inch baking dish.

- Bake at 325° for 1 hour.

Serves 8 to 10

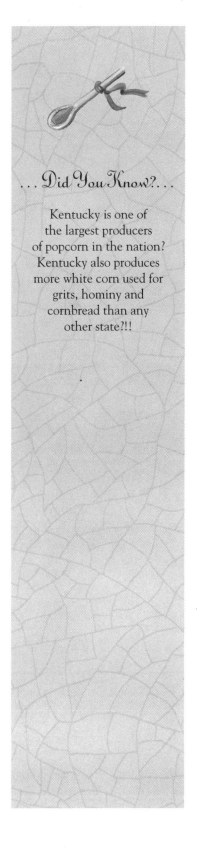

...Did You Know?...

Kentucky is one of the largest producers of popcorn in the nation? Kentucky also produces more white corn used for grits, hominy and cornbread than any other state?!!

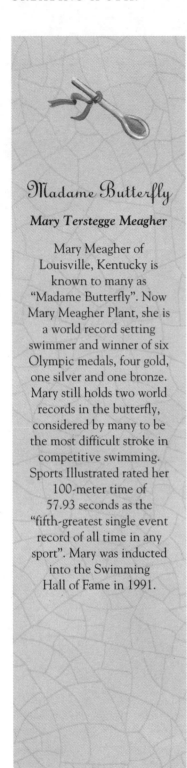

Madame Butterfly

Mary Terstegge Meagher

Mary Meagher of Louisville, Kentucky is known to many as "Madame Butterfly". Now Mary Meagher Plant, she is a world record setting swimmer and winner of six Olympic medals, four gold, one silver and one bronze. Mary still holds two world records in the butterfly, considered by many to be the most difficult stroke in competitive swimming. Sports Illustrated rated her 100-meter time of 57.93 seconds as the "fifth-greatest single event record of all time in any sport". Mary was inducted into the Swimming Hall of Fame in 1991.

Awesome Layered Grits

Fabulous! These grits are especially tasty with summer ripe tomatoes.

4	cups water	2-3	tomatoes, sliced
1	cup uncooked grits	1	cup chopped fresh basil
1	teaspoon salt	1	large Vidalia onion, shredded
1	(6-ounce) roll garlic cheese	2	cups (8 ounces) shredded Monterey Jack cheese
½	cup butter	2	cups (8 ounces) shredded cheddar cheese
2	large eggs, lightly beaten		
¼	cup milk		

- Preheat oven to 350°.

- Bring 4 cups water to a boil in a saucepan; stir in grits and salt. Cover, reduce heat, and simmer until done.

- Add garlic cheese, butter, eggs, and milk to grits, stirring well. Transfer to a 2-quart baking dish.

- Bake at 350° for 40 to 60 minutes. Let cool.

- Layer tomato slices, basil, onion, Monterey Jack and cheddar cheeses over grits.

- Bake 20 minutes or until thoroughly heated. To serve, cut into squares.

Serves 8 to 10

Individual Quiche Lorraine Tarts

1	pound bacon, cooked and crumbled	½	teaspoon pepper
2	cups (8 ounces) shredded Swiss cheese	3	large eggs, lightly beaten
½	cup chopped onion	1	cup evaporated milk
1	teaspoon salt	8	tart shells

- Preheat oven to 400°.

- Combine bacon, Swiss cheese, onion, salt, pepper, eggs, and milk, stirring well. Pour evenly into tart shells.

- Bake at 400° for 10 minutes.

- Reduce oven temperature to between 300° and 325° and bake 25 to 30 minutes. Let stand at room temperature 5 to 10 minutes before serving.

Makes 8 tarts

Three-Cheese Italian Quiche

1 unbaked 9-inch deep-dish pie crust	½ cup chopped pepperoni
2 tablespoons butter	2 tablespoons chopped green onions
1 cup fresh mushrooms, sliced	3 large eggs
¾ cup (3 ounces) shredded cheddar cheese	1 cup half-and-half
¾ cup (3 ounces) shredded Swiss cheese	1 teaspoon salt
¾ cup (3 ounces) shredded mozzarella cheese	½ teaspoon dried oregano
	½ teaspoon dried parsley

- Bake pie crust at 375° for 5 minutes.
- Melt butter in a skillet over medium heat; add mushrooms and sauté until soft and golden brown.
- Combine mushrooms, cheddar cheese, Swiss cheese, mozzarella cheese, pepperoni, and green onions; sprinkle in baked pie crust.
- Whisk together eggs, half-and-half, salt, oregano, and parsley; pour over cheese mixture.
- Bake on a baking sheet at 325° for 45 to 55 minutes. Let stand at room temperature 10 minutes before serving.

Serves 6 to 8

Rosemary-Chive-Potato Quiche

2 russet potatoes, sliced	5 large eggs
1 tablespoon chopped fresh rosemary	1½ cups half-and-half
1 tablespoon chopped fresh chives	Salt and pepper to taste
1 baked 9-inch deep-dish pie crust	

- Preheat oven to 350°.
- Sauté potato slices, rosemary, and chives in a skillet coated with vegetable cooking spray until soft. Spoon into pie crust.
- Whisk together eggs, half-and-half, and salt and pepper. Pour over potato slices.
- Bake at 350° for 20 to 30 minutes or until set.

Serves 6 to 8

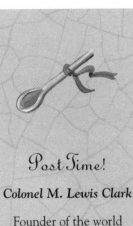

Post Time!

Colonel M. Lewis Clark

Founder of the world famous Kentucky Derby, Colonel Clark raised $32,000 in capital to build the track and in 1875 the first Derby was run. Churchill Downs was named after Clark's two uncles, **John and Henry Churchill** from whom he leased the land. **W.H. Thomas** later lent Clark the money to build the first grandstand. In 1895 **William Schulte** became president and along with his group was responsible for building a new grandstand that accommodated 1,500 seated spectators and standing room for up to 2,000. It is **Colonel Matt J. Winn** that is credited with promoting the race into what is known around the world as "the greatest two minutes in sports"!

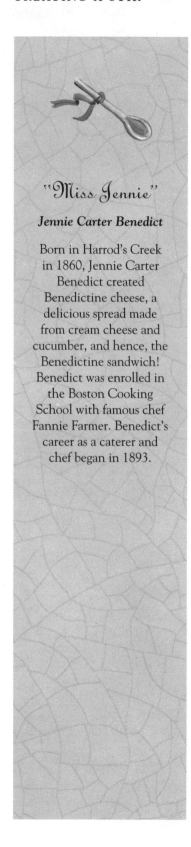

"Miss Jennie"

Jennie Carter Benedict

Born in Harrod's Creek in 1860, Jennie Carter Benedict created Benedictine cheese, a delicious spread made from cream cheese and cucumber, and hence, the Benedictine sandwich! Benedict was enrolled in the Boston Cooking School with famous chef Fannie Farmer. Benedict's career as a caterer and chef began in 1893.

Green Chile Quiche

This quiche is more like a cheese pie.
Its texture is dense, not light and fluffy like typical quiche filling.

2   unbaked 9-inch deep-dish pie crusts
1½ cups (6 ounces) shredded cheddar cheese, divided
1½ cups (6 ounces) shredded mozzarella cheese
1½ cups (6 ounces) shredded Monterey Jack cheese
1   cup (4 ounces) shredded pizza blend cheese
1   cup canned chopped green chiles
2¼ cups half-and-half
6   large eggs
2   teaspoons salt

- Bake pie crusts at 400° for 5 minutes.
- Combine ¾ cup cheddar, mozzarella, Monterey Jack, and pizza blend cheeses, stirring well. Sprinkle evenly in baked pie crusts.
- Whisk together half-and-half, eggs, and salt; pour evenly into pie crusts. Sprinkle evenly with remaining ¾ cup cheddar cheese.
- Bake on baking sheets at 375° for 50 to 60 minutes. Let stand at room temperature 15 minutes before serving.

Makes 2 (9-inch) pies

Scalloped Pineapple Casserole

Easy and delicious . . . this casserole goes well with ham.

1   cup butter, softened
1½ cups sugar
2   large eggs
40 ounces pineapple chunks, undrained
½   cup heavy cream
5   cups French bread cubes

- Beat butter and sugar at medium speed with an electric mixer until creamy; add eggs, beating well.
- Add pineapple with juice and cream, mixing well. Add bread cubes, stirring well. Pour mixture into a greased 2-quart baking dish.
- Bake at 350° for 1 hour, covering with aluminum foil after 45 minutes to prevent over browning if necessary.

Serves 8

Hot Baked Chicken Salad

4	cups cubed cooked chicken	1	cup slivered almonds
2	cups thinly sliced celery	2	cups (8 ounces) shredded cheddar cheese
¼	cup diced onion		
2	cups mayonnaise	1	cup finely crushed potato chips

- Combine chicken, celery, onion, mayonnaise, and almonds, stirring well.
- Spread mixture into a 9 x 13 x 2-inch baking dish and top with cheese and crushed potato chips.
- Bake at 450° for 10 to 15 minutes or until thoroughly heated. Serve immediately.

Serves 6 to 8

Sausage and Apple Ring

Serve with fruit, eggs, and coffee cake for a special breakfast.

2	pounds mild or hot bulk sausage	½	cup milk
1½	cups cracker crumbs	¼	cup minced onion
2	large eggs, lightly beaten	1	cup finely chopped apple

- Combine all ingredients and shape into a ring. Place in a shallow pan or iron skillet.
- Bake at 350° for 1 hour and 15 minutes.

Serves 8

This can be frozen, if desired. Thaw and bake as directed.

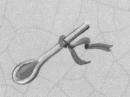

Crystal Gayle

Born Brenda Gail Webb in Paintsville, Kentucky in 1951, Crystal Gayle is a famous country and pop song singer and sister of Loretta Lynn, country music's "coal miner's daughter". **Loretta Lynn** wrote her sister's first song and gave her the stage name Crystal after a hamburger chain by the same name. In 1977, Gayle was the Country Music Association's female vocalist of the year. She went on to win four Academy of Country Music Awards and three Grammy Awards.

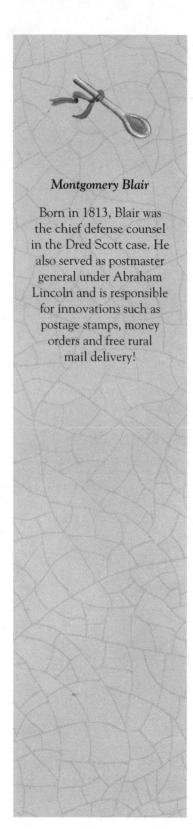

Montgomery Blair

Born in 1813, Blair was the chief defense counsel in the Dred Scott case. He also served as postmaster general under Abraham Lincoln and is responsible for innovations such as postage stamps, money orders and free rural mail delivery!

Breakfast Burritos

2	large flour tortillas	1	cup (4 ounces) shredded Monterey Jack cheese
2	tablespoons vegetable oil, divided		
3	large eggs	8	bacon slices, cooked and crumbled
½	teaspoon salt		Salsa
¼	teaspoon pepper		

- Cook tortillas, 1 at a time, in 1 tablespoon hot oil in a skillet over medium heat 15 seconds on each side or until tender. Remove from skillet and drain on paper towels.
- Whisk together eggs, salt, and pepper. Cook eggs in remaining 1 tablespoon hot oil in skillet over medium heat until set.
- Sprinkle cheese evenly down the center of each tortilla; top evenly with eggs and bacon. Roll up and serve with salsa.

Makes 2 burritos

Sausage and Potato Breakfast Lasagna

Satisfy a hungry breakfast or brunch crowd with this scrumptiously rich dish . . . the potatoes are a delicious substitute for the noodles in a traditional lasagna.

1	pound Italian sausage	2	cloves garlic, minced
2	cups peeled and thinly sliced mushrooms	2	tablespoons butter
4	cups peeled and thinly sliced potatoes	2	tablespoons flour
1	beaten egg	¼	teaspoon ground nutmeg
1½	cups ricotta or cottage cheese	½	cup whole milk
½	cup Parmesan cheese	1	teaspoon salt
1	(10-ounce) package frozen chopped spinach	¼	teaspoon white pepper
1	medium onion, chopped	2	cups shredded mozzarella cheese

- Cook sausage and mushrooms in a skillet over medium heat until meat is brown. Crumble and drain meat.
- Cook potatoes in boiling water for 5 minutes, drain, set aside (they will be undercooked). Stir together egg, ricotta, Parmesan and spinach, set aside.
- Cook onion and garlic in hot butter until tender but not brown. Stir in flour and nutmeg. Add milk all at once and cook until thickened and bubbly.
- Layer half of the potatoes in a greased 13 x 9 x 2-inch baking dish. Top with half of the spinach filling, half of the meat mixture, half of the sauce and half of the cheese. Repeat layers. Reserving the remaining 1 cup cheese.
- Cover and bake at 350° for 40 to 45 minutes until potatoes are tender. Uncover, sprinkle with remaining cheese and bake an additional 10 minutes until cheese is melted and golden. Let stand 10 to 15 minutes before serving.

Serves 6 to 8

Breads

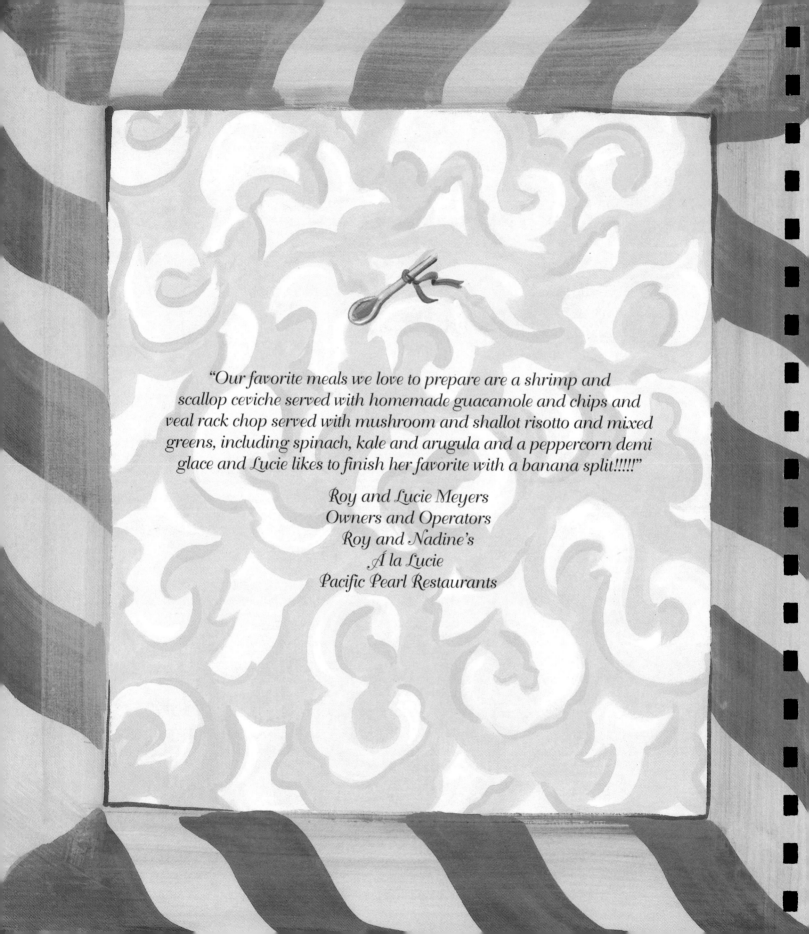

"Our favorite meals we love to prepare are a shrimp and scallop ceviche served with homemade guacamole and chips and veal rack chop served with mushroom and shallot risotto and mixed greens, including spinach, kale and arugula and a peppercorn demi glace and Lucie likes to finish her favorite with a banana split!!!!!"

Roy and Lucie Meyers
Owners and Operators
Roy and Nadine's
Á la Lucie
Pacific Pearl Restaurants

Mini Glazed Almond Loaves

½ cup butter, softened
1 cup sugar
2 large eggs
1¾ cups all-purpose flour
1 teaspoon baking powder
½ teaspoon salt
½ cup milk
½ teaspoon almond extract
3 tablespoons slivered almonds
 Almond Glaze

- Beat butter at medium speed with an electric mixer until creamy; add sugar, beating until light and fluffy. Add eggs, 1 at a time, beating well after each addition.
- Sift together flour, baking powder, and salt.
- Add flour mixture to butter mixture alternately with milk and almond extract, beating well after each addition.
- Pour batter into 2 lightly greased miniature loaf pans, filling three-fourths full. Sprinkle with almonds.
- Bake at 350° for 50 minutes (do not overbake).
- Cool slightly on wire racks. Remove loaves from pans and drizzle with Almond Glaze.

Almond Glaze
¼ cup powdered sugar
½-1 tablespoons cream
½ teaspoon almond extract

- Whisk together all ingredients until smooth.

Makes 2 miniature loaves

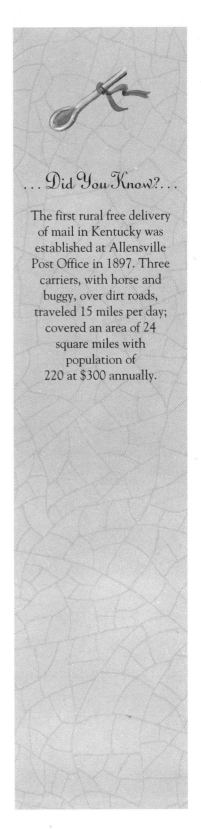

Miniature Pecan Muffins

Children love these!

2 large eggs, lightly beaten
1 cup firmly packed brown sugar
⅓ cup butter, melted
1 teaspoon vanilla extract
½ cup all-purpose flour
1 cup chopped pecans

- Combine eggs, brown sugar, butter, and vanilla in a large bowl, stirring well. Add flour and nuts, stirring well.
- Spoon batter into miniature muffin pan cups lightly coated with vegetable cooking spray.
- Bake at 350° for 12 to 15 minutes.

Makes 3 dozen muffins

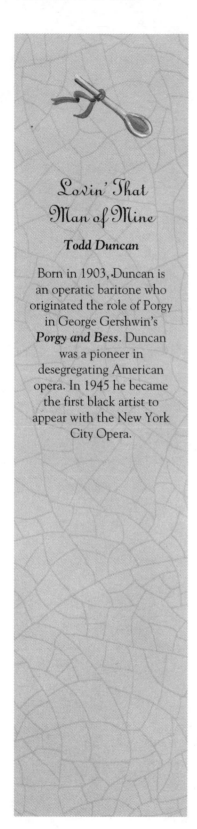

Harvest Pumpkin Bread

This wonderfully spicy bread makes a fabulous fall treat!

3⅓ cups all-purpose flour	2 teaspoons ground cloves
2 teaspoons baking soda	1 cup vegetable oil
½ teaspoon baking powder	½ cup dry sherry
1½ teaspoons salt	½ cup water
3 cups sugar	4 large eggs
2 teaspoons ground cinnamon	2 cups canned pumpkin
2 teaspoons ground nutmeg	1 cup chopped pecans

- Combine flour, baking soda, baking powder, salt, sugar, cinnamon, nutmeg, and cloves in a large bowl; set aside.

- Beat oil, sherry, ½ cup water, eggs, and pumpkin in a separate bowl at medium speed with an electric mixer until well blended.

- Gradually add flour mixture to pumpkin mixture, beating well.

- Stir in pecans. Pour batter into 6 lightly greased loaf pans.

- Bake at 350° for 50 to 60 minutes.

- Cool slightly on wire racks. Remove from pans and wrap in aluminum foil while still warm.

Makes 6 miniature loaves

Banana-Chocolate Chip Muffins

1¾ cups all-purpose flour	1 large egg
1 tablespoon baking powder	¼ cup vegetable oil
½ teaspoon salt	¼ cup milk
½ cup sugar	3 medium bananas, mashed
½ cup semisweet chocolate morsels	½ cup walnuts (optional)

- Combine flour, baking powder, salt, sugar, and chocolate morsels in a large bowl, making a well in center.

- Beat egg at medium speed with a hand held mixer until frothy; add oil milk, and banana, beating well. Pour mixture into well of dry ingredients and stir just until moistened, adding more milk if needed. (Batter will be lumpy.) Stir in walnuts, if desired.

- Spoon batter into greased muffin pan cups, filling three-fourths full.

- Bake at 400° for 20 minutes.

Makes 1 dozen muffins

Blueberry Buckle with Cinnamon Streusel

Easy and delicious! Try substituting raspberries or blackberries for a different taste.

¾ cup sugar
¼ cup shortening
1 large egg
2 cups all-purpose flour
2½ teaspoons baking powder

¾ teaspoon salt
¾ cup milk
2 cups blueberries, well drained
Cinnamon Streusel

- Beat sugar and shortening at medium speed with an electric mixer until creamy; add egg, beating well.

- Combine flour, baking powder, and salt.

- Add flour mixture to sugar mixture alternately with milk, beating well after each addition. Gently fold in blueberries.

- Spread batter into a greased 8-inch round or square pan. Sprinkle Cinnamon Streusel over top.

- Bake at 375° for 45 to 50 minutes.

Cinnamon Streusel

½ cup sugar
⅓ cup all-purpose flour

½ teaspoon ground cinnamon
¼ cup butter, softened

- Combine all ingredients, stirring until crumbly.

Serves 8 to 12

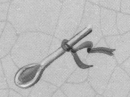

Simon Flexner

Born in Louisville, Kentucky in 1863. Flexner was a pathologist that is known for his serum against meningitis. His serum helped to significantly reduce the mortality rate from 75% to 25%. He was awarded the distinguished Cameron Prize for his achievement.

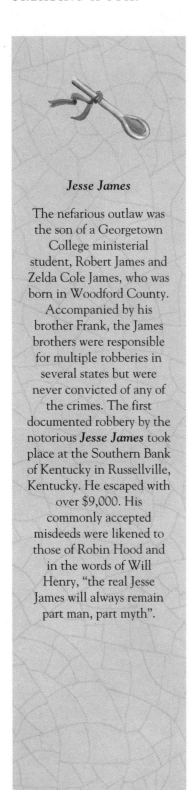

Mini French Breakfast Puffs

Everyone's favorite . . . they're a snap to make!

⅓	cup shortening	½	teaspoon ground nutmeg
½	cup sugar	½	cup milk
1	large egg	1	cup sugar
1½	cups all-purpose flour	2	teaspoons ground cinnamon
1½	teaspoons baking powder	1	cup butter, melted
½	teaspoon salt		

- Beat shortening and ½ cup sugar at medium speed with an electric mixer until creamy; add egg, beating well.
- Combine flour, baking powder, salt, and nutmeg.
- Add flour mixture to sugar mixture alternately with milk, beating well after each addition. Spoon batter into lightly greased miniature muffin pan cups.
- Bake at 350° for 20 to 25 minutes.
- Combine sugar and cinnamon in a shallow dish.
- Remove puffs from pans and dip in butter. Dredge in cinnamon mixture.

Makes 24 to 30 miniature puffs

Pineapple-Zucchini Bread

Incredibly moist! The pineapple gives this traditional zucchini bread its tropical twist!

3	large eggs	3	cups all-purpose flour
2	cups sugar	2	teaspoons baking soda
1	cup vegetable oil	½	teaspoon baking powder
2½	teaspoons vanilla extract	1	teaspoon salt
2	cups coarsely shredded unpeeled zucchini	1½	teaspoons ground cinnamon
1	(8¼-ounce) can crushed pineapple, drained	¾	teaspoon ground nutmeg
		1	cup finely chopped walnuts

- Preheat oven to 350°.
- Beat eggs at medium speed with an electric mixer until frothy; add sugar, oil, and vanilla, beating until thick and foamy. Stir in zucchini and pineapple.
- Combine flour, baking soda, baking powder, salt, cinnamon, nutmeg, and walnuts; add to zucchini mixture, stirring just until moistened.
- Spoon batter into 2 lightly greased 5 x 9 x 3-inch or 4 (3 x 5 x 2-inch) loaf pans.
- Bake at 350° for 50 to 60 minutes.

Makes 2 large or 4 small loaves

Orange-Cranberry Bread

*Makes a beautiful bread that will win you
points with friends and family should you decide to share!*

1	cup sugar	2	large eggs
2½	cups all-purpose flour	¾	cup fresh orange juice
2	teaspoons baking powder	½	cup mayonnaise
½	teaspoon baking soda	1½	cups chopped fresh cranberries
¼	teaspoon salt	2	tablespoons sugar
¾	cup chopped nuts	½	teaspoon grated orange zest
2	teaspoons grated orange zest		

- Combine sugar, flour, baking powder, baking soda, and salt in a large bowl, stirring well. Stir in nuts and 2 teaspoons orange zest.

- Combine eggs, orange juice, and mayonnaise, stirring well. Add to dry ingredients, stirring just until moistened.

- Fold in cranberries and spoon into a greased and floured 5 x 9 x 3-inch loaf pan.

- Combine 2 tablespoons sugar and ½ teaspoon orange zest; sprinkle over top of loaf.

- Bake at 350° for 50 minutes. Cover with aluminum foil and bake an additional 10 minutes.

Makes 1 loaf

Strawberry-Nut Bread

This is an excellent "quick bread!"

3	cups all-purpose flour	4	large eggs, lightly beaten
2	cups sugar	1¼	cups vegetable oil
1	teaspoon baking soda	2	(10-ounce) packages frozen strawberries, thawed and chopped (juice reserved)
1	teaspoon salt		
2	teaspoons ground cinnamon	1-1¼	cups chopped pecans

- Combine flour, sugar, baking soda, salt, and cinnamon in a large bowl, making a well in the center of the mixture.

- Combine eggs, oil, strawberries, juice from berries, and pecans in a separate bowl, mixing well. Pour strawberry mixture into center of flour mixture, stirring just until moistened.

- Pour batter into 6 small or 2 large greased and floured loaf pans.

- Bake at 350° for 45 to 55 minutes.

Makes 6 small or 2 large loaves

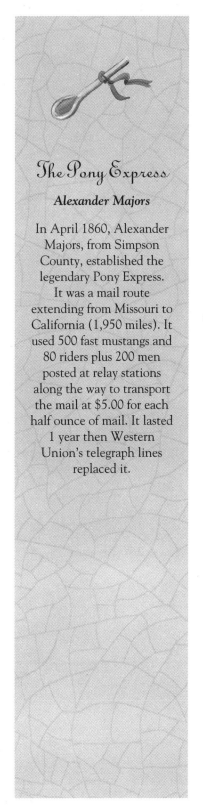

The Pony Express

Alexander Majors

In April 1860, Alexander Majors, from Simpson County, established the legendary Pony Express. It was a mail route extending from Missouri to California (1,950 miles). It used 500 fast mustangs and 80 riders plus 200 men posted at relay stations along the way to transport the mail at $5.00 for each half ounce of mail. It lasted 1 year then Western Union's telegraph lines replaced it.

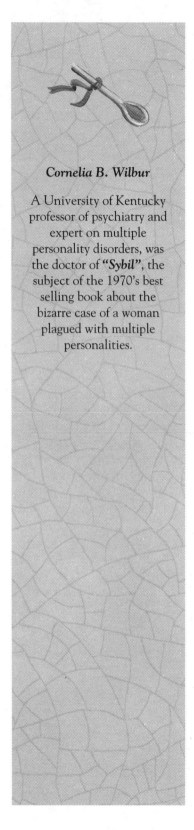

Cornelia B. Wilbur

A University of Kentucky professor of psychiatry and expert on multiple personality disorders, was the doctor of *"Sybil"*, the subject of the 1970's best selling book about the bizarre case of a woman plagued with multiple personalities.

Poppy Seed Muffins with Raspberries

These traditional muffins take on extra flavor with the addition of fresh raspberries!

2¼ cups cake flour
1 teaspoon baking soda
½ teaspoon baking powder
½ cup unsalted butter, softened
⅔ cup sugar
1 tablespoon vanilla extract
5 egg yolks

1 cup sour cream
¼ cup poppy seeds
3 egg whites
¼ teaspoon cream of tartar
½ cup sugar
3 cups fresh raspberries

- Sift together flour, baking soda, and baking powder.

- Beat butter and ⅔ cup sugar at medium speed with an electric mixer until creamy; add vanilla, beating well. Add egg yolks, 1 at a time, beating well after each addition, 3 minutes or until light, fluffy, and pale yellow.

- Add sour cream and poppy seeds to butter mixture, beating well. Add flour mixture, beating well.

- Beat egg whites and cream of tartar in a separate bowl with clean beaters at medium speed until foamy. Gradually beat in remaining ½ cup sugar until stiff peaks form. Gradually fold egg whites into batter.

- Fold in raspberries. Spoon batter into buttered and floured miniature muffin pan cups.

- Bake at 350° for 20 minutes or until golden brown.

Makes 2 dozen miniature muffins

Sweet Potato-Cinnamon Swirl Bread

This is a lovely bread that makes great toast . . . it tastes like cinnamon bread!
A favorite of the Niemi grandchildren. Grandpa Niemi stays quite busy trying to
keep them supplied with this wonderful treat!

1¼	cups water	1	cup water
1	cup cubed peeled sweet potato	⅓	cup sugar
2	(¼-ounce) envelopes active dry yeast	3	tablespoons margarine
		2	teaspoons salt
¼	cup warm water	6¼-7	cups all-purpose flour
1	teaspoon sugar		Walnut Filling
4	tablespoons dry buttermilk		

- Boil 1¼ cups water and sweet potato in a saucepan until tender. Drain sweet potato, reserving water; mash sweet potato. Add enough water to sweet potato water to measure 1¾ cup.

- Combine yeast, ¼ cup warm water, and 1 teaspoon sugar in a large bowl, stirring to dissolve.

- Combine dry buttermilk powder and 1 cup water, stirring well.

- Combine sweet potato, 1¾ cup sweet potato water, buttermilk, sugar, margarine, and salt in a bowl, stirring to dissolve. Gradually add to yeast mixture.

- Gradually stir in flour to make a soft dough; turn dough out a lightly floured surface. Knead 5 to 8 minutes or until smooth and elastic. Place in a greased bowl, turning to grease top.

- Cover and let rise in a warm place (85°), free from drafts, 1 hour or until doubled in bulk.

- Punch dough down and divide into 3 portions. Roll each portion into a 10 x 15-inch rectangle.

- Brush half of each rectangle with water and sprinkle each with one-third of Walnut Filling. Fold over to make a 10 x 7½-inch rectangle. Roll up, jelly roll fashion, starting with a short side; seal edges.

- Place each roll in a greased 4 x 8-inch loaf pan. Let rise in a warm place, free from drafts, 30 minutes.

- Bake at 375° for 30 minutes.

Walnut Filling

½	cup sugar	2½	teaspoons ground cinnamon
½	cup chopped toasted walnuts		

- Combine all ingredients.

Makes 3 loaves

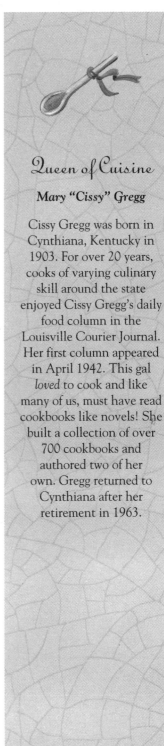

Queen of Cuisine

Mary "Cissy" Gregg

Cissy Gregg was born in Cynthiana, Kentucky in 1903. For over 20 years, cooks of varying culinary skill around the state enjoyed Cissy Gregg's daily food column in the Louisville Courier Journal. Her first column appeared in April 1942. This gal *loved* to cook and like many of us, must have read cookbooks like novels! She built a collection of over 700 cookbooks and authored two of her own. Gregg returned to Cynthiana after her retirement in 1963.

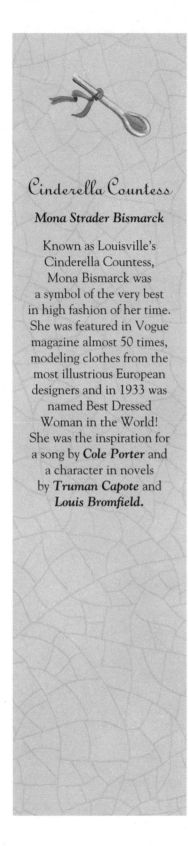

Glazed Pecan-Cinnamon Rolls

Takes a little bit of time, but the results are well worth it!
They are delicious and pretty to look at. You will make them again and again!

1	cup milk	3	large eggs
⅓	cup butter	¾	cup chopped pecans
⅓	cup sugar	½	cup golden raisins (optional)
½	teaspoon salt	1	tablespoon half-and-half or light
5	cups all-purpose flour		cream
1	(¼-ounce) envelope active dry		Brown Sugar Filling
	yeast		Sugar Glaze

- Cook milk, butter, sugar, and salt in a saucepan over medium heat, stirring constantly, until butter is almost melted.

- Combine 2¼ cups flour and yeast in a large bowl; add milk mixture and eggs and beat at low speed with an electric mixer 30 seconds, scraping down sides constantly. Beat at high speed 3 minutes. Stir in remaining flour to make a soft dough.

- Turn dough out on a lightly floured surface and knead in flour until smooth and elastic. Shape into a ball and place in a greased bowl, turning to grease top.

- Cover dough and let rise in a warm place (85°), free from drafts, 1 hour or until doubled in size.

- Punch dough down and turn out on a lightly floured surface. Cover and let rise 10 minutes. Roll dough into a 12-inch square.

- Sprinkle Brown Sugar Filling over dough; top with pecans and, if desired, raisins. Roll up, jelly roll fashion, and pinch edges to seal.

- Cut roll into 8 (1½-inch) slices. Arrange, cut side up, in a greased 9 x 13 x 2-inch or 12-inch deep-dish pizza pan. Cover loosely with plastic wrap. Let rise in a warm place, free from drafts, 45 minutes or until almost doubled in size.

- Brush rolls with half-and-half and bake at 375° for 20 to 25 minutes or until lightly browned. Cover loosely with aluminum foil and bake 5 to 10 more minutes.

- Remove from oven and brush again with half-and-half. Let cool on a wire rack 1 to 3 minutes. Invert onto wire rack. Invert again on a serving platter. Drizzle with Sugar Glaze.

Brown Sugar Filling

¾	cup firmly packed brown sugar	1	tablespoon ground cinnamon
¼	cup all-purpose flour	½	cup butter, cut into pieces

- Combine sugar, flour, and cinnamon in a small bowl; cut in butter with a fork until crumbly.

Glazed Pecan-Cinnamon Rolls continued

Sugar Glaze

1¼ cups sifted powdered sugar	½ teaspoon vanilla extract
1 teaspoon corn syrup	Half-and-half

- Combine powdered sugar, corn syrup, and vanilla; add enough half-and-half to make a drizzling consistency.

Makes 8 rolls

My Grandma's Mini Orange Loaves

Very unique! A delightful bread for breakfast or
brunch and an exceptionally delicious accompaniment for chicken salad!

2-2½ cups coarsely chopped orange peel (1-inch pieces)	1 large egg
	½ cup milk
2 cups water	3 cups all-purpose flour
1½ cups sugar	2½ teaspoons baking powder
1 tablespoon butter	¼ teaspoon salt

- Bring orange peel and 2 cups water to a boil, covered, in a saucepan; boil 20 minutes. Add sugar and boil 5 minutes, adding ½ to 1 cup water if needed.

- Drain peel, reserving liquid. Add enough water to liquid to measure 1½ cups.

- Process ¾ cup orange liquid, peel, and butter on low speed in a blender 30 seconds or until thickened with bits of orange peel. Pour into a large bowl.

- Process remaining ¾ cup orange liquid in blender to clean sides; stir into peel mixture. Let cool.

- Stir egg and milk into cooled zest mixture; add flour, baking powder, and salt, stirring well. Pour batter into 4 (3 x 5 x 2-inch) loaf pans lightly coated with vegetable cooking spray. Place loaf pans on a baking sheet or jelly-roll pan. Let stand at room temperature 20 minutes.

- Bake at 325° for 40 to 50 minutes. Let cool.

Makes 4 miniature loaves

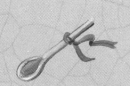

All Aboard . . . !

Casey Jones

Born John Luther Jones in Fulton County, Kentucky in 1864, Jones was a famous railroad engineer who got his nickname "Casey" from his hometown of Cayce, Kentucky. He was the engineer of the famous "Cannonball", the country's fastest passenger train. On April 29, 1900 after he had finished his run, Jones was asked and agreed to fill in for his relay engineer who was ill, continuing on to Mississippi. Close to the end of the run, cars from a freight train stalled on the main track leaving Jones faced with an impending crash. Jones' fireman jumped to safety and Jones was able to slow the train enough to save the lives of all his passengers. Jones was the only fatality. He is immortalized in the ballad "Casey Jones".

Banana-Nut Muffins with Coconut-Pecan Streusel

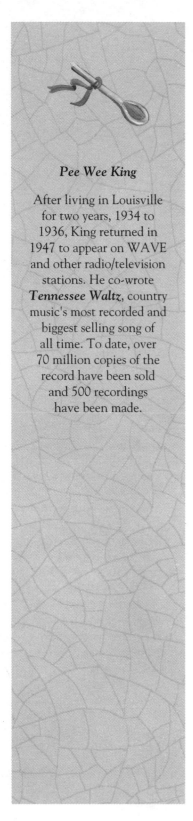

*The coconut streusel gives these otherwise
ordinary muffins their unique flavor. Boy are they good!*

1½ cups all-purpose flour
1   tablespoon baking powder
½   teaspoon salt
½   cup wheat germ
⅓   cup sugar

1¼ cups mashed banana
½   cup milk
¼   cup vegetable oil
1   large egg, lightly beaten
    Coconut-Pecan Streusel

- Combine flour, baking powder, salt, wheat germ, and sugar in a large bowl, making a well in center.

- Combine banana, milk, oil, and egg; add to dry ingredients, stirring just until moistened.

- Spoon 3 tablespoons batter into each lightly greased foil-lined muffin pan cup.

- Bake at 400° for 15 to 20 minutes or until lightly browned.

- Remove from oven and sprinkle 1 teaspoon Coconut-Pecan Streusel over each muffin. Bake an additional 5 minutes.

- Remove from pans immediately.

Coconut-Pecan Streusel

⅓   cup flaked coconut
⅓   cup chopped pecans

2   tablespoons honey
2   tablespoons butter, melted

- Combine all ingredients, stirring well.

Makes about 15 muffins

Herbed Parmesan Bread

A wonderful accompaniment for a bowl of hot soup or salad!

2½ cups all-purpose flour	1 cup grated Parmesan cheese
½ teaspoon baking soda	½ cup fresh parsley, minced
2 teaspoons baking powder	¼ cup shortening
1¼ teaspoons salt	2 tablespoons sugar
⅛ teaspoon cayenne pepper	2 large eggs, lightly beaten
1 teaspoon ground sage	1¼ cups buttermilk
1 teaspoon ground black pepper	½ teaspoon Worcestershire sauce

- Preheat oven to 350°.

- Combine flour, baking soda, baking powder, salt, cayenne pepper, sage, black pepper, Parmesan, and parsley.

- Beat shortening, sugar, and eggs at medium speed with an electric mixer until well blended; add buttermilk and Worcestershire sauce, beating well.

- Stir in flour mixture just until moistened.

- Pour batter evenly into 3 greased 3 x 5 x 2-inch loaf pans.

- Bake at 350° for 40 to 45 minutes. Serve warm with whipped butter.

Makes 3 miniature loaves

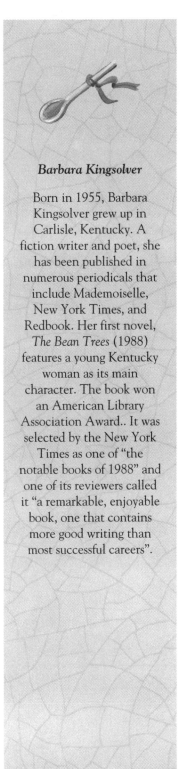

Barbara Kingsolver

Born in 1955, Barbara Kingsolver grew up in Carlisle, Kentucky. A fiction writer and poet, she has been published in numerous periodicals that include Mademoiselle, New York Times, and Redbook. Her first novel, *The Bean Trees* (1988) features a young Kentucky woman as its main character. The book won an American Library Association Award.. It was selected by the New York Times as one of "the notable books of 1988" and one of its reviewers called it "a remarkable, enjoyable book, one that contains more good writing than most successful careers".

Southwestern-Style Spoon Bread

1 cup sweetened yellow cornmeal	1 (16-ounce) can cream-style corn
½ teaspoon baking soda	1 (4.5-ounce) can chopped green chiles
1 teaspoon salt	
¾ cup milk	2 cups (8 ounces) shredded Monterey Jack cheese
⅓ cup vegetable oil	
2 large eggs, lightly beaten	

- Combine cornmeal, baking soda, and salt in a medium bowl; add milk and oil, stirring well. Add eggs and corn, stirring well.

- Spoon half of batter into a greased 9-inch square baking dish. Sprinkle half each of chiles and cheese over batter. Repeat layers with remaining batter, chiles, and cheese.

- Bake at 350° for 45 minutes or until a wooden pick inserted in center comes out clean.

Serves 6

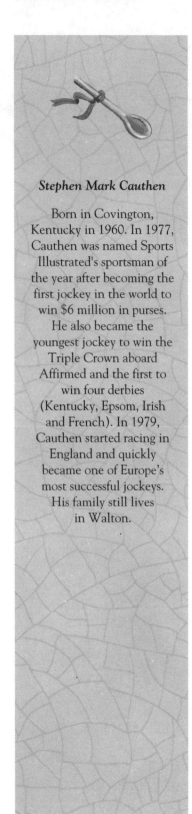

Stephen Mark Cauthen

Born in Covington, Kentucky in 1960. In 1977, Cauthen was named Sports Illustrated's sportsman of the year after becoming the first jockey in the world to win $6 million in purses. He also became the youngest jockey to win the Triple Crown aboard Affirmed and the first to win four derbies (Kentucky, Epsom, Irish and French). In 1979, Cauthen started racing in England and quickly became one of Europe's most successful jockeys. His family still lives in Walton.

Poppy Seed Loaves with Almond Citrus Glaze

Melts in your mouth when fresh from the oven

3	cups all-purpose flour	1½	cups milk
1½	teaspoons baking powder	1½	teaspoons vanilla extract
½	teaspoon salt	1½	teaspoons almond extract
3	large eggs	1½	teaspoons butter flavoring
1½	cups vegetable oil	1½	tablespoons poppy seeds
2¼	cups sugar		Almond Citrus Glaze

- Combine flour, baking powder, and salt in a large bowl.

- Combine eggs, oil, sugar, milk, vanilla, almond extract, butter flavoring, and poppy seeds, stirring well. Add to dry ingredients, stirring just until moistened.

- Pour batter into 4 lightly greased 3 x 5 x 2-inch loaf pans.

- Bake at 350° for 1 hour.

- Remove from oven and drizzle with Almond Citrus Glaze.

Almond Citrus Glaze

¼	cup orange juice	½	teaspoon almond extract
¾	cup powdered sugar	½	teaspoon butter flavoring
½	teaspoon vanilla extract		

- Whisk together all ingredients.

Makes 4 small loaves

Quick and Easy Beer Bread

Incredibly easy and absolutely delicious! This bread has the aroma of a yeast bread and smells heavenly while its baking! So easy and so good!

3	cups self-rising flour	1	(12-ounce) can beer, at room temperature
3	tablespoons sugar	⅓	cup butter, melted

- Combine first 3 ingredients, stirring just until blended. (Do not overmix.)

- Pour batter into a lightly greased 5 x 9 x 3-inch loaf pan. Pour melted butter over top.

- Bake at 350° for 40 to 50 minutes or until golden.

Makes 1 loaf

Pumpkin-Chocolate Chip Muffins

Chocolate chips give a boost of flavor to this traditional muffin. A great fall recipe.

½	cup sliced almonds	½	teaspoon ground cloves
1⅔	cups all-purpose flour	½	teaspoon ground nutmeg
1	teaspoon baking soda	2	large eggs
¼	teaspoon baking powder	1	cup canned plain pumpkin
¼	teaspoon salt	½	cup butter, melted
1	cup sugar	1	cup semisweet chocolate morsels
1	teaspoon ground cinnamon		

- Bake almonds on a baking sheet at 350° for 5 minutes or until toasted; set aside.

- Combine flour, baking soda, baking powder, salt, sugar, cinnamon, cloves, and nutmeg in a large bowl.

- Whisk together eggs, pumpkin, and butter in a separate bowl; add chocolate morsels and almonds, stirring well.

- Fold pumpkin mixture into flour mixture just until dry ingredients are moistened. Spoon batter into greased or foil-lined muffin pan cups.

- Bake at 350° for 20 to 25 minutes.

Makes 1 dozen regular or 4 dozen miniature muffins

English Muffin Bread

Wonderful toasted and served with whipped butter and your favorite jam!

2	cups 2% low-fat milk	2	(¼-ounce) envelopes active dry yeast
½	cup water		
6	cups bread flour	1	tablespoon sugar
½	teaspoon baking soda		Cornmeal
2	teaspoons salt		

- Cook milk and ½ cup water in a saucepan over medium-low heat until warm (115° to 120°).

- Process 3 cups flour, baking soda, salt, yeast, and sugar in a food processor until blended. Add warm milk and process until smooth. Transfer to a large bowl and gradually stir in remaining flour to make a stiff dough. (Batter should only be slightly sticky.)

- Sprinkle cornmeal into 2 (4 x 8 x 2-inch) loaf pans; pour evenly into pans. Sprinkle cornmeal over top. Cover and let rise in a warm place (85°), free from drafts, 45 minutes.

- Bake at 400° for 25 minutes. Remove from pans immediately and let cool.

Makes 2 loaves

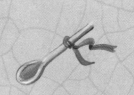

Bybee Pottery
Cornelison Family

The Cornelison Family of Bybee, Madison County, Kentucky has continuously operated Bybee Pottery since the early 1800's. It is one of, if not the, oldest pottery businesses in the country. For over a century, the same central log building has been used for both production and sales of the pottery. Clay deposits from the surrounding area of Bybee continue to supply the business with its source of raw materials.

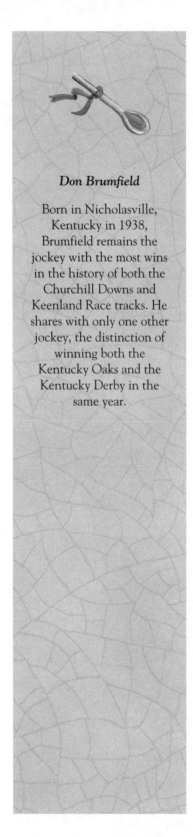

Don Brumfield

Born in Nicholasville, Kentucky in 1938, Brumfield remains the jockey with the most wins in the history of both the Churchill Downs and Keenland Race tracks. He shares with only one other jockey, the distinction of winning both the Kentucky Oaks and the Kentucky Derby in the same year.

Finnish Braid Bread

1	cup milk	½	teaspoon ground cardamom
½	cup butter	2	large eggs
½	cup sugar	1	tablespoon grated orange zest
1	teaspoon salt	⅓	cup fresh orange juice
5-5⅓	cups all-purpose flour	1	egg yolk
2	(¼-ounce) envelopes active dry yeast	1	tablespoon milk

- Cook milk, butter, sugar, and salt in a saucepan over medium-low heat, stirring constantly, until warm (115° to 120°) and butter is almost melted.

- Combine 2 cups flour, yeast, and cardamom in a large bowl. Add milk mixture, whole eggs, orange zest, and juice to flour mixture and beat at low speed with an electric mixer 30 seconds, scraping sides of bowl constantly. Beat at high speed 3 minutes. Stir in enough remaining flour to make a soft dough.

- Turn dough out on a lightly floured surface and knead 5 to 8 minutes. Place in a greased bowl, turning to grease top. Cover and let rise in a warm place (85°), free from drafts, 1 hour or until doubled in bulk.

- Punch dough down and divide in half. Divide each half into 3 portions and shape each portion into a ball. Cover and let rise 10 minutes.

- Roll each ball into a 16-inch rope. Line up 3 ropes 1 inch a greased baking sheets. Braid each loosely beginning in the middle and working toward the ends. Pinch ends together and tuck under. Cover braids and let rise 30 minutes.

- Whisk together egg yolk and 1 tablespoon milk; brush over braids.

- Bake at 350° for 25 to 30 minutes, covering loosely with aluminum foil after 20 minutes to prevent over browning.

Makes 2 loaves

Crusty French Bread

3½ cups light gluten flour
1⅓ cups water

1 tablespoon active dry yeast
1 tablespoon salt

- Combine all ingredients and knead 10 minutes. Cover and let rise in a warm place (85°), free from drafts, 40 to 60 minutes.

- Knead dough 30 seconds and let rise 2 to 3 hours.

- Shape dough into logs, stretching as you fold over 3 times; press down flat. Place in French bread pans. Let rise 1 hour.

- Bake at 450° for 10 minutes. Reduce oven temperature to 400° and bake 10 minutes.

Makes 1 loaf

Mrs. Ashbrook's Yeast Rolls

These are divine!

1½ teaspoons salt
1 cup shortening
1 cup sugar
1 cup boiling water
2 large eggs, lightly beaten

2 (¼-ounce) envelopes active dry yeast
1 cup warm water
6 cups all-purpose flour (5½ cups sifted flour)

- Combine salt, shortening, and sugar and add 1 cup boiling water; beat at medium speed with an electric mixer until smooth. Add eggs, beating well.

- Combine yeast and 1 cup warm water, stirring to dissolve.

- Add flour to egg mixture alternately with yeast mixture, mix by hand after each addition. Chill overnight.

- Knead dough with flour. Pinch off amount needed. Roll into balls, dip in butter. Three small balls will make a beautiful cloverleaf roll. Place in buttered roll pans. Refrigerate. Set out at room temperature and allow to rise until doubled in bulk, about 2 hours.

- Bake at 375° for 20 minutes.

Makes 3 dozen

For remainder of dough cover and refrigerate for 7 days.

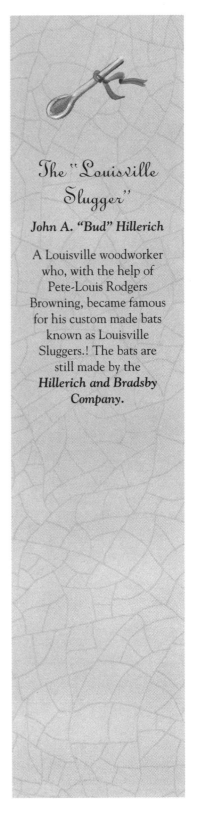

The "Louisville Slugger"

John A. "Bud" Hillerich

A Louisville woodworker who, with the help of Pete-Louis Rodgers Browning, became famous for his custom made bats known as Louisville Sluggers.! The bats are still made by the **Hillerich and Bradsby Company.**

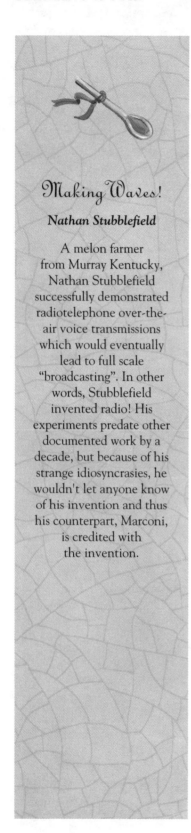

Alabama Biscuits

A wonderful recipe for those who can't make "yeast" rolls

2½ cups all-purpose flour
½ teaspoon baking soda
½ teaspoon salt
¼ cup sugar
6 tablespoons shortening

1 (¼-ounce) envelope active dry yeast
1 cup buttermilk, at room temperature
½ cup butter, melted

- Sift together flour, baking soda, salt, and sugar in a large bowl; cut in shortening with a fork or pastry blender until flaky.

- Combine yeast and buttermilk, stirring to dissolve; add to flour mixture, stirring well.

- Turn dough out on a lightly floured surface and knead 30 times. Roll out to ¼-inch thickness. Cut 1 biscuit with a round cookie cutter; dip in butter and place on a lightly greased baking sheet. Top with another biscuit and brush top with butter. Repeat procedure with remaining dough.

- Bake at 400° for 25 to 30 minutes or until golden.

Makes 12 to 15 biscuits

Rosemary Biscuits

The rosemary makes these biscuits a nice accompaniment to beef or pork tenderloin.

4 cups biscuit mix
2 teaspoons dried rosemary
¼ teaspoon pepper

1¼ cups plus 2 tablespoons milk
6 tablespoons butter, melted

- Combine biscuit mix, rosemary, and pepper in a large bowl; add enough milk to moisten, stirring just until moistened.

- Turn dough out on a lightly floured surface and knead 5 to 6 times. Roll to ½-inch thickness and cut with a 2-inch round cookie cutter. Place biscuits on lightly greased baking sheets.

- Bake at 450° for 6 to 8 minutes or until golden. Remove from oven and brush tops with melted butter.

Makes 1 dozen biscuits

Orange Dinner Rolls

Beautiful and tasty-a delightful addition to any dinner

1	(¼-ounce) envelope active dry yeast	5½	cups all-purpose flour, divided
¼	cup warm water	2	large eggs
1	cup scalded milk	¼	cup fresh orange juice
½	cup shortening	2	tablespoons grated orange zest
⅓	cup sugar		Orange Glaze
1	teaspoon salt		

- Combine yeast and ¼ cup warm water, stirring to dissolve.

- Combine milk, shortening, sugar, and salt in a large bowl and let cool to lukewarm. Stir in 2 cups sifted flour; add eggs, stirring well. Stir in yeast mixture.

- Add orange juice and enough remaining flour to make a soft dough. Cover and let rise 10 minutes.

- Knead dough on a lightly floured surface 8 to 10 minutes or until smooth and elastic. Place in a greased bowl, turning to grease top. Cover and let rise in a warm place (85°), free from drafts, 2 hours or until doubled in bulk.

- Punch dough down and let rise 10 minutes. Roll dough out a lightly floured surface; cut into strips and roll each strip into a cigar shape. Tie each strip in a knot and place on greased baking sheets. Cover and let rise in a warm place 45 minutes or until doubled in bulk.

- Bake at 400° for 12 minutes or until golden. Brush hot rolls with Orange Glaze.

Orange Glaze

1	teaspoon grated orange zest	1	cup powdered sugar, sifted
2	tablespoons fresh orange juice		

- Combine all ingredients, stirring until smooth.

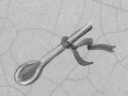

Fee Fi Fo Fum...!

Martin VanBuren Bates

Born in Whitesburg, Kentucky in 1845, Martin Bates is known as the "Giant of Letcher County". Bates reached a maximum height of almost eight feet and weighed approximately 475 pounds. In 1865 he started touring in exhibitions in the United States and Canada. While in New Jersey making plans for a European tour, Bates met, fell in love with and married **Anna Hanen Swan, the "Giantess of Nova Scotia"**. Swan matched him in height! The two toured together for several years. They had two children, neither surviving after birth. Their son is reported to be the largest human baby ever born weighing in at twenty three and three-fourths pounds and measuring 30 inches long!

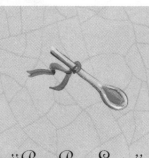

Miniature Parmesan-Basil Biscuits

These miniatures are great with steaming bowls of soup!

2	cups biscuit mix	2	teaspoons dried basil
¼	cup grated Parmesan cheese	⅔	cup milk
2	teaspoons chopped fresh chives		

- Combine biscuit mix, Parmesan, chives, and basil in a large bowl; add milk, stirring just until moistened.
- Drop dough by teaspoonfuls into miniature muffin pan cups lightly coated with vegetable cooking spray.
- Bake at 400° for 10 to 12 minutes or until golden brown. Serve warm.

Makes 18 to 24

Ultimate Biscuits

Delicious! Wonderful served with homemade jams and apple butter

1½	cups plus 3 tablespoons all-purpose flour	½	teaspoon salt
1	tablespoon baking powder	¼	cup unsalted butter, cut into pieces
1	tablespoon sugar	¼	cup shortening
		½	cup milk

- Sift together flour, baking powder, sugar, and salt in a large bowl; cut in butter and shortening with a fork or pastry blender until mixture resembles coarse cornmeal. Add milk, stirring just until moistened.
- Turn dough out on a lightly floured surface and knead. Roll to ½-inch thickness. Cut with a 2-inch round cookie cutter and place on ungreased baking sheets.
- Bake at 375° for 14 to 15 minutes. Serve hot.

Makes 14 biscuits

Salads

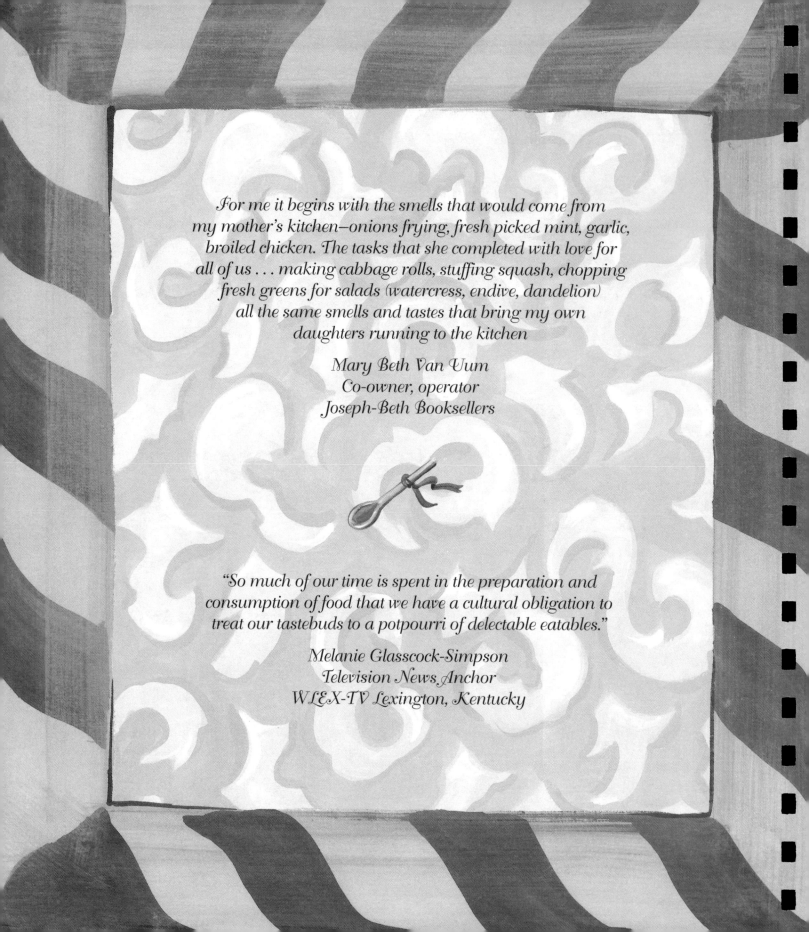

*For me it begins with the smells that would come from
my mother's kitchen—onions frying, fresh picked mint, garlic,
broiled chicken. The tasks that she completed with love for
all of us . . . making cabbage rolls, stuffing squash, chopping
fresh greens for salads (watercress, endive, dandelion)
all the same smells and tastes that bring my own
daughters running to the kitchen*

Mary Beth Van Uum
Co-owner, operator
Joseph-Beth Booksellers

*"So much of our time is spent in the preparation and
consumption of food that we have a cultural obligation to
treat our tastebuds to a potpourri of delectable eatables."*

Melanie Glasscock-Simpson
Television News Anchor
WLEX-TV Lexington, Kentucky

Uptown Bluegrass Salad

Always receives rave reviews!

1 pound bacon, cooked and crumbled	1 large avocado, cut into bite-size
2 heads romaine lettuce, torn into	pieces
bite-size pieces	6 ounces freshly grated Parmesan
1 (14-ounce) can artichoke hearts,	cheese
drained and chopped	Spicy Mustard Dressing

- Combine bacon, lettuce, artichokes, avocado, and Parmesan in a large bowl; add Spicy Mustard Dressing, tossing to coat. Serve immediately.

Spicy Mustard Dressing

⅓ cup chopped onion	½ teaspoon salt
3 tablespoons cider vinegar	¼ teaspoon freshly ground pepper
2 teaspoons spicy brown mustard	¾ cup olive oil
½ teaspoon sugar	

- Process onion and vinegar in a food processor until pureed; transfer to a medium bowl. Whisk in mustard, sugar, salt, and pepper.

- Gradually whisk in oil in a slow, steady stream; whisk until thickened.

Serves 10 to 12

Granny Smith and Blue Cheese Salad

The timeless combination of fruit and cheese melds beautifully to form this savory salad.

1 head green leaf lettuce, torn into	4 ounces blue cheese, crumbled
bite-size pieces	½ bag sea salt bagel chips, broken into
3 Granny Smith apples, peeled and	pieces
chopped	Poppy Seed Dressing

- Place lettuce in a large serving bowl; add apple, cheese, and bagel chip pieces. Add Poppy Seed Dressing, tossing to coat. Serve immediately.

Poppy Seed Dressing

½ cup sugar	1½ teaspoons minced onion
¼ cup cider vinegar	¼ teaspoon Worcestershire sauce
½ cup vegetable oil	¼ teaspoon paprika
1 tablespoon poppy seeds	

- Whisk together all ingredients.

Serves 6 to 8

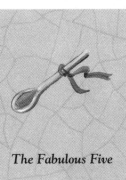

The Fabulous Five

The University of Kentucky basketball team regarded as the greatest in UK history. The 1947-48 team was known as the "Fabulous Five". Members of the five included Kenny Rollins, Ralph Beard, Wallace "WahWah" Jones, Cliff Barker and Alex Groza. The team won The SEC championship, the NCAA National championship, was ranked first in the nation and seven of its players were members of the 1948 Olympic championship team.

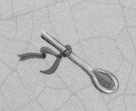

For The Love of Children

Phyllis Cronin

The Lexington community views the list of her volunteer activities as impressive. As founding president of the Ronald McDonald House of the Bluegrass, her tireless, charitable work continues to touch the lives of many Kentuckians, particularly children and their families. Phyllis led the collaborative effort of the Fayette County Medical Society and the Fayette County Medical Auxiliary, to fund, construct and erect the $1 million house. Complete with furnishings, the house was debt free when it opened its doors in 1984. The demand for the facility was so great that an expansion was needed and subsequently completed six years ago. The Ronald McDonald House of the Bluegrass, located in Lexington, continues to service the families of children from around the

Mediterranean Salad
with Balsamic Basil Vinaigrette

*This traditional Greek salad makes a beautiful
presentation and is a wonderful complement to grilled beef or lamb.*

8	cups torn romaine lettuce (about 2 heads)	½	cup sliced pimiento-stuffed or ripe olives
1	large purple onion, shredded	1	pound bacon, cooked and crumbled
2-3	ripe tomatoes, seeded and chopped	1-1½	cups feta cheese, crumbled Balsamic Basil Vinaigrette

- Layer romaine, onion, tomato, olives, bacon, and feta cheese in a large bowl; serve with Balsamic Basil Vinaigrette.

Balsamic Basil Vinaigrette

¼	cup olive oil	½	teaspoon Dijon mustard
1½	tablespoons balsamic vinegar	½	teaspoon salt
1	tablespoon chopped fresh basil	¼	teaspoon pepper

- Whisk together all ingredients in a nonmetallic bowl. Cover and chill until ready to serve.
- Shake dressing or whisk well before serving.

Serves 8

Jackson Salad

Simply the best!

1	(14-ounce) can artichoke hearts, drained and diced	2	garlic cloves, pressed
1	(14-ounce) can hearts of palm, drained and diced	1	ounce fresh lemon juice
		3	ounces vegetable oil
¼	cup finely chopped green onions	4	ounces crumbled blue cheese
2	tablespoons finely chopped fresh parsley		Salt and pepper to taste
½	cup crumbled cooked bacon	1½	heads romaine lettuce, torn into bite-size pieces

- Combine finely chopped artichokes, hearts of palm, green onions, parsley, bacon, garlic, lemon juice, oil, blue cheese, salt, and pepper in a large bowl, stirring well. Cover and chill until ready to serve.
- Toss with romaine and serve immediately.

Makes 6 to 8 large servings

The artichokes and hearts of palm must be finely chopped!

Mixed Greens with Feta and Dried Cranberries

The colors in this vibrant salad will enhance the festive mood at any holiday gathering.

6-8 cups mixed greens or green leaf
    lettuce, torn into bite-size pieces
½ cup dried cranberries

1 cup chopped toasted walnuts
1 cup feta cheese, crumbled
    Vinaigrette

- Combine lettuce, dried cranberries, walnuts, and feta cheese in a large bowl; add Vinaigrette, tossing to coat. Serve immediately.

Vinaigrette

½ cup olive oil
¼ cup cider vinegar
¼ cup sugar
½ medium onion, chopped

½ teaspoon paprika
¼ teaspoon dry mustard
⅛ teaspoon pepper
¼ teaspoon celery salt

- Whisk together all ingredients.

Serves 6 to 8

Romaine, Grapefruit, and Avocados with Red Wine Vinaigrette

Tangy grapefruit and velvety slices of avocado come together in this simple but engaging salad.

2 heads romaine lettuce, torn into
    bite-size pieces
2 avocados, sliced

2 cups fresh grapefruit sections
¼-½ cup sliced ripe olives
    Red Wine Vinaigrette

- Combine romaine, avocados, grapefruit, and olives in a large bowl; add Red Wine Vinaigrette, tossing to coat. Serve immediately.

Red Wine Vinaigrette

½ cup olive oil
¼ cup red wine vinegar
¼ cup sugar
½ teaspoon salt

½ teaspoon celery seeds
½ teaspoon dry mustard
½ purple onion, grated

- Whisk together all ingredients.

Serves 8 to 10

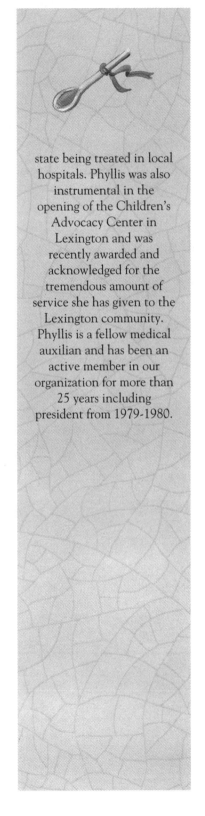

state being treated in local hospitals. Phyllis was also instrumental in the opening of the Children's Advocacy Center in Lexington and was recently awarded and acknowledged for the tremendous amount of service she has given to the Lexington community. Phyllis is a fellow medical auxilian and has been an active member in our organization for more than 25 years including president from 1979-1980.

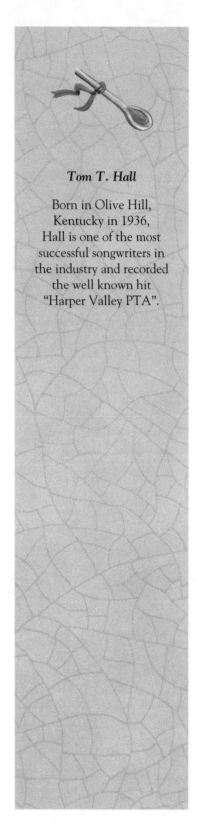

Tom T. Hall

Born in Olive Hill, Kentucky in 1936, Hall is one of the most successful songwriters in the industry and recorded the well known hit "Harper Valley PTA".

Bibb and Endive with Tarragon-Dijon Vinaigrette

2 heads Bibb lettuce
1 head Belgian endive
1 (14-ounce) can artichoke hearts, quartered or chopped

½ cup toasted walnuts or almonds
Tarragon-Dijon Vinaigrette

• Combine Bibb lettuce, Belgian endive, artichokes, and nuts in a large bowl; add Tarragon-Dijon Vinaigrette, tossing to coat. Serve immediately.

Tarragon-Dijon Vinaigrette
1 garlic clove, minced
1 teaspoon salt
½ teaspoon ground white pepper
½ teaspoon dry mustard
1 teaspoon Dijon mustard

2 tablespoons olive oil
2 tablespoons tarragon vinegar
¼ cup vegetable oil
Juice of 1 lemon

• Whisk together all ingredients; chill several hours or overnight.

Serves 6 to 8

Fresh Orange-Tarragon Salad

1 head romaine lettuce, torn into bite-size pieces
1-2 avocados, chopped
1 tablespoon chopped fresh parsley

4 green onions, sliced
2 oranges, sliced and cut up
¼ cup slivered almonds, toasted
Tarragon Vinaigrette

• Combine romaine, avocado, parsley, green onions, orange, and toasted almonds in a large bowl; add Tarragon Vinaigrette, tossing to coat. Serve immediately.

Tarragon Vinaigrette
½ cup vegetable oil
2 tablespoons tarragon vinegar
2 tablespoons sugar

¼ teaspoon hot sauce
⅛ teaspoon salt
⅛ teaspoon pepper

• Combine all ingredients in a jar; cover tightly and shake vigorously.

Serves 8

Mandarin Orange Salad with Caramelized Almonds

Sweet and crunchy bits of caramelized almonds give this popular salad added flavor.

½ cup slivered almonds
2 tablespoons plus 2 teaspoons sugar
1 head romaine lettuce or ½ head romaine and ½ head Bibb lettuce
1 cup chopped celery
½ cup chopped green onions
1 (11-ounce) can mandarin oranges, drained
Parslied Vinaigrette

- Cook almonds and sugar in a skillet over medium heat until sugar is dissolved and almonds are coated. Transfer to wax paper and let cool. Break cooled almonds apart.

- Combine lettuce, celery, and green onions in a medium bowl. Add mandarin oranges and Parslied Vinaigrette, tossing to coat. Add almonds, tossing well. Serve immediately.

Parslied Vinaigrette

¼ cup vegetable oil
2 tablespoons cider vinegar
2 tablespoons sugar
2 tablespoons minced fresh parsley
½ teaspoon salt
¼ teaspoon pepper

- Whisk together all ingredients; cover and chill at least 1 hour.

Serves 6 to 8

Cottage Greens

Easy and delicious! People who don't like cottage cheese love this salad!

10 ounces fresh spinach, torn into bite-size pieces
1 head romaine lettuce, torn into bite-size pieces
1 pound bacon, cooked crisp and crumbled
1 cup cottage cheese
Cottage Vinaigrette

- Combine spinach, romaine, bacon, and cottage cheese in a large bowl; add Cottage Vinaigrette, tossing to coat. Serve immediately.

Cottage Vinaigrette

¼ cup sugar
⅓ cup cider or white vinegar
½ cup vegetable oil
1 teaspoon salt
1½ teaspoons dry mustard
3-4 green onions, chopped

- Whisk together all ingredients; cover and chill at least 6 hours.

Serves 6 to 8

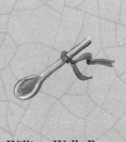

William Wells Brown

William Wells Brown was the country's first African American to publish a novel, the first to publish a drama and the first to publish a travel book. His novel, **Clotel,** or **The President's Daughter,** was a fictional account of Thomas Jefferson's alleged long term affair with his slave mistress and the children he fathered by her. It was considered too controversial for publication in the United States and was released only after all references to Jefferson were removed.

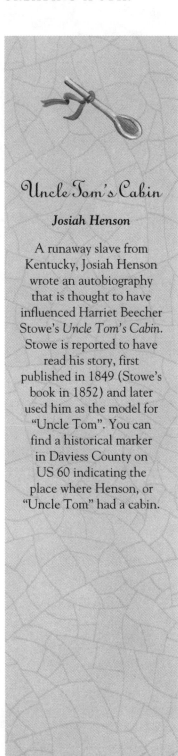

Mesclun with Shaved Reggiano and Left Bank Dressing

Mesclun is not a variety of green, but rather refers to a mixture of edible greens, herb leaves, and flowers. The idea is to balance between the stronger, more pungent types and the more mellowed, delicate types . . . the assortment is up to you!

6-8 cups mesclun, torn into bite-size pieces	1 cup shaved Parmigiano-Reggiano cheese
	Left Bank Dressing

- Toss together mesclun and Left Bank Dressing; top with shaved cheese.

Left Bank Dressing

⅓ cup red wine vinegar	1 cup olive oil
1 teaspoon salt	2 tablespoons chopped fresh basil or favorite herbs
1 tablespoon Dijon mustard	Cracked black pepper to taste
1½ tablespoons chopped shallots	

- Process all ingredients in a blender until creamy. Pour into a glass jar; screw on lid and chill up to 10 days.

- Bring dressing to room temperature before serving.

Caesar Salad with Homemade Sourdough Croutons

1 garlic clove, pressed	Ground pepper
1½ teaspoons salt	½ cup olive oil
½ teaspoon prepared mustard	2 heads romaine lettuce, torn into bite-size pieces
¼ cup lemon juice	¼ cup freshly grated Parmesan cheese
5 anchovy fillets, mashed	½ cup Homemade Sourdough Croutons (see recipe on page 97)
1 tablespoon mayonnaise	
1 teaspoon Worcestershire sauce	
1 egg boiled in water 10 seconds	

- Whisk together garlic, salt, mustard, lemon juice, anchovies, mayonnaise, Worcestershire sauce, egg, and pepper in a bowl; gradually whisk in oil until creamy.

- Combine lettuce and dressing, tossing to coat. Sprinkle with cheese and croutons, tossing well.

Serves 4

Store-bought croutons can be substituted.

Spinach, Strawberries, and Toasted Sesame Seed Salad

A beautiful salad, worthy of company!

2 bunches or 2 (10-ounce) bags fresh spinach, torn into bite-size pieces

2 pints fresh strawberries, sliced
Poppy Seed Dressing

- Combine spinach and strawberries in a large bowl; add Poppy Seed Dressing, tossing to coat. Serve immediately.

Poppy Seed Dressing

2   tablespoons sesame seeds
½   cup sugar
¼   cup apple cider vinegar
½   cup vegetable oil

1   tablespoon poppy seeds
1½   teaspoons minced onion
¼   teaspoon Worcestershire sauce
¼   teaspoon paprika

- Broil sesame seeds on a baking sheet 1 to 2 minutes or until toasted (watch carefully, sesame seeds will burn easily). Or stir constantly over medium heat in a skillet until lightly browned.

- Whisk together sugar, vinegar, oil, poppy seeds, onion, Worcestershire sauce, and paprika; add sesame seeds, whisking well.

Serves 8 to 12

Homemade Sourdough Croutons

6-8 tablespoons butter
8   cups cubed sourdough bread
     (preferably homemade)
2   tablespoons dried oregano

2   tablespoons dried basil
2   tablespoons dried Italian seasoning
1   teaspoon garlic salt
1   teaspoon onion salt

- Melt butter in a large skillet over medium heat; add cubed bread, oregano, basil, Italian seasoning, garlic salt, and onion salt and sauté until golden. Transfer croutons to a roasting pan.

- Bake at 350° until crispy.

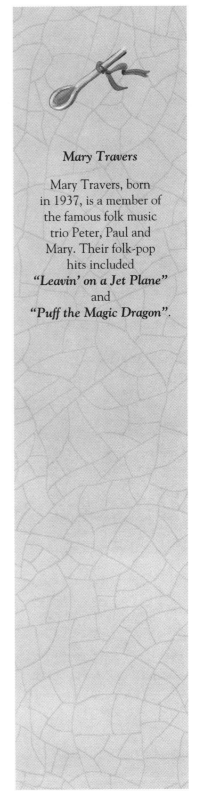

Mary Travers

Mary Travers, born in 1937, is a member of the famous folk music trio Peter, Paul and Mary. Their folk-pop hits included *"Leavin' on a Jet Plane"* and *"Puff the Magic Dragon"*.

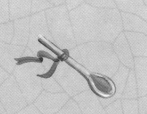

Sugar Cubes for All!

Glenn U. Dorroh, M.D.

Born in White Sulphur, Kentucky in 1901, he left a thriving practice in Midway, Kentucky to join the military in 1933. After WWII he was instrumental in establishing the 810th Convalescent Center in Lexington, and was the Company Commander of the unit. He retired from the military as a Colonel in 1959.

Although he returned to private practice in Lexington in 1946, he remained involved in public medicine much of his life.

During the *polio* outbreak in the early 1960's, Dr. Dorroh was instrumental in organizing and carrying out a mass vaccination program in Lexington, initially purchasing the supply of vaccine with his own funds to expedite the process.

Dr. Dorroh was chairman of the local Board of Health for 16 years. During his tenure a comprehensive maternity and infant program was

Sugar's Cobb Salad

One of the most coveted recipes in town!

2 skinned and boned chicken breasts, poached and diced	1 head romaine lettuce
¼ teaspoon lemon juice	½ head iceberg lettuce
¼ teaspoon olive oil	6 bacon slices, cooked crisp and crumbled
Salt and pepper to taste	2 tomatoes, chopped
3 hard-cooked eggs, chopped	1 avocado, chopped
2 tablespoons minced fresh chives	1 cup Blue Cheese Vinaigrette or Italian dressing
2 ounces crumbled blue cheese	

- Toss together chicken, lemon juice, olive oil, salt, and pepper; cover and chill.

- Place egg in a bowl and season with salt and pepper; add chives and blue cheese and toss.

- Break up lettuces in a large bowl; place chicken in a row down the center of the bowl. Top with bacon.

- Place half of tomato on each side of chicken. Place half of egg mixture on each side of tomato. Place half of avocado on each side of egg mixture.

- Chill salad until ready to serve, if desired. Serve with Blue Cheese Vinaigrette or Italian dressing.

Salad can also be prepared by combining all ingredients except dressing in a large bowl. Toss with Blue Cheese Vinaigrette or Italian dressing. Serve immediately.

Serves 6 to 8

Blue Cheese Vinaigrette

1 garlic clove, minced	⅓ cup blue cheese, crumbled
½ teaspoon salt	1 teaspoon chopped parsley
⅓ cup cider or red wine vinegar	Salt and pepper to taste
1 tablespoon lemon juice	⅔ cup olive oil

- Combine garlic and ½ teaspoon salt to make a paste.

- Add vinegar, lemon juice, blue cheese, parsley, salt, and pepper, mixing well. Whisk in oil in a slow, steady stream.

Dried Bing Cherry and Gorgonzola Salad

This savvy salad sets the stage for an impressive and memorable dinner.

1 head red leaf lettuce, torn into
   bite-size pieces
1 head green leaf lettuce, torn into
   bite-size pieces
1 cup toasted pecans, chopped

1 (6-ounce) package dried Bing
   cherries
4-6 tablespoons crumbled Gorgonzola
   cheese
   Raspberry Vinaigrette

- Arrange lettuces on individual serving plates; top evenly with toasted pecans, cherries, and cheese. Drizzle Raspberry Vinaigrette over each serving.

Raspberry Vinaigrette
1 cup raspberry vinegar
1 cup olive oil

½ cup sugar

- Whisk together all ingredients.

Serves 4

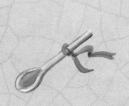

Sautéed Cabbage and Apples with Goat Cheese

*Goat cheese produces more flavor when warm and creamy,
making it the perfect choice for this warm salad.*

½ cup chopped walnuts
1 teaspoon walnut oil
1 purple onion, chopped
2 tablespoons bacon drippings
   or olive oil
1 garlic clove, pressed
1 red cabbage, cored and chopped

2 tablespoons balsamic vinegar
1 tablespoon chopped fresh or
   ½ teaspoon dried sage
1 red apple, cored and chopped
   Salt and pepper to taste
1 goat cheese log, cut into thick slices

- Sauté walnuts in hot walnut oil in a skillet 3 to 5 minutes or until toasted.

- Cook onion in hot bacon drippings in a saucepan over medium heat 1 minute; add garlic and cabbage and cook 2 minutes. Add vinegar, sage, and apple and cook 1 minute. Season with salt and pepper.

- Serve on individual plates; top each serving with a goat cheese slice. Sprinkle evenly with walnuts.

Serves 4 to 6

adopted, a family planning program was instituted, water pollution controls were strengthened, a neighborhood children's clinic and senior day-care centers were established, and low cost rabies immunization clinics were begun. He received the Distinguished Service Award from the Kentucky Medical Association for his contributions to the health of Kentucky's citizens. The *Fayette County Health Department* building is named in his honor. His wife, Ella Pearl Neal Dorroh, was one of the founding members of the Fayette County Medical Auxiliary in 1948. His granddaughter, Debra Ashbrook Adkins, is an active member in our organization and served as president from 1998-1999.

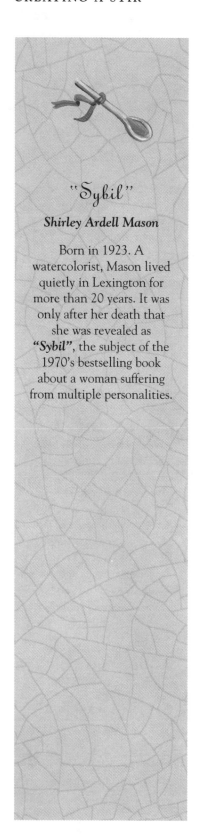

"Sybil"

Shirley Ardell Mason

Born in 1923. A watercolorist, Mason lived quietly in Lexington for more than 20 years. It was only after her death that she was revealed as *"Sybil"*, the subject of the 1970's bestselling book about a woman suffering from multiple personalities.

Spinach Salad

2 (10-ounce) packages fresh spinach
4 hard-cooked eggs, sliced

8 bacon slices, cooked and crumbled
Spinach Salad Dressing

- Combine spinach, eggs, and bacon in a large bowl. Toss with Spinach Salad Dressing, coating evenly.

Spinach Salad Dressing

1 cup vegetable oil
6 tablespoons red wine vinegar
¼ cup sour cream
1½ teaspoons salt
½ teaspoon dry mustard

2 tablespoons sugar
2 garlic cloves, minced
2 teaspoons minced fresh parsley
Coarsely ground pepper

- Whisk together all ingredients; cover and chill at least 6 hours.

Serves 8

Warm Roasted Pear and Blue Cheese Salad

A fabulous mélange of flavors . . . it doesn't get much better than this!

3 cups cornbread, cut into 1-inch cubes
3 medium pears, cored and quartered lengthwise
8 bacon slices
6 tablespoons white balsamic vinegar

2 tablespoons olive oil
6 cups leaf lettuce, torn into bite-size pieces
8 ounces blue cheese, crumbled
Freshly ground black pepper

- Place cornbread cubes in a shallow roasting pan and bake at 400° for 20 minutes or until lightly browned, stirring often. Set aside.

- Bake pears in a greased shallow roasting pan at 400° for 25 minutes or until tender. Let pears cool slightly; cut into ¼-inch slices.

- Cook bacon in a skillet over medium heat until crisp. Remove bacon from skillet, reserving 2 tablespoons drippings in skillet. Crumble bacon and set aside.

- Whisk vinegar and oil into bacon drippings over medium heat; bring to a boil, stirring occasionally.

- Toss lettuce, pear slices, cornbread croutons, and bacon in a large bowl. Add hot dressing, tossing evenly to coat.

- Divide salad evenly among 6 serving plates; sprinkle with blue cheese and cracked pepper. Serve warm.

Serves 6

Blue Cheese Dressing

*This is a thick dressing that doubles nicely
as a dip for fresh veggies and fiery hot buffalo wings!*

4	ounces blue cheese, crumbled	1-2	tablespoons lemon juice
1	cup mayonnaise	1	teaspoon sugar
½	cup sour cream	3	tablespoons chopped green onions
1-2	tablespoons wine vinegar		

• Combine all ingredients, stirring well. Cover and chill overnight.

Honey-Mustard Dressing

¼	cup vinegar	6	ounces brown mustard
¼	cup pureed onion	1-1½	cups mayonnaise
¼	cup sugar	1-1¼	cups buttermilk
1	cup honey		

• Combine all ingredients, stirring well; cover and chill 30 minutes.

Summer Corn Salad

30	ounces corn kernels, drained	1	tablespoon ground cumin
30	ounces black beans, rinsed	1	teaspoon chili powder
2	red bell peppers, chopped	1	teaspoon curry powder
1	medium onion, chopped	1	small bunch fresh cilantro, chopped
⅓-½	cup cider vinegar		Hot sauce to taste
	Juice of 4 limes		

• Combine all ingredients in a large bowl, stirring well. Cover and chill 8 hours or overnight.

Daniel Taradesh

Born in 1913,
Daniel Taradesh is an
Academy Award winning
screenwriter and director
best known for his work on
"From Here to Eternity".

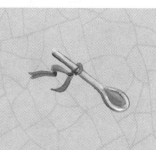

Mrs. Wells' Tomato Aspic

An award-winning recipe

4	cups vegetable juice	1	cup sliced celery
¼	cup minced onion	3	tablespoons lemon juice
¼	cup celery leaves	2½	envelopes unflavored gelatin
2	teaspoons sugar	1½	cups quartered artichoke hearts
1	teaspoon garlic salt	1	medium avocado, thinly sliced
2	bay leaves	1	small onion, chopped
4	whole cloves	½	cup sliced pimiento-stuffed olives
	Hot sauce to taste		

- Cook vegetable juice, onion, celery leaves, sugar, salt, bay leaves, cloves, hot sauce, and celery in a large saucepan over medium-high heat 5 minutes. Pour mixture through a wire-mesh strainer into a bowl, reserving liquid; stir lemon juice into reserved liquid.

- Combine gelatin and 1 cup juice mixture, stirring until dissolved; add to remaining juice mixture, stirring well.

- Layer artichokes, avocado, onion, and olives in the bottom of a mold coated with vegetable cooking spray. Pour juice into mold and chill at least 6 hours or until set. Store mold in refrigerator up to 1 week.

- Serve aspic on watercress or Bibb lettuce; dollop each serving with mayonnaise.

Potato Salad Olé

Southwestern spices give this potato salad a kick!

2	large tomatoes, chopped	1	teaspoon chili powder
2	green onions, chopped	1	teaspoon ground cumin
½	cup salsa	2	pounds red potatoes, cooked
1	cup mayonnaise	1	large bell pepper, chopped
3	tablespoons lime juice	½	teaspoon salt

- Combine tomato, green onions, and salsa; set aside ⅓ cup mixture.

- Combine mayonnaise, lime juice, chili powder, cumin, potato, bell pepper, and salt in a large bowl; stir in remaining tomato mixture. Cover and chill.

- Serve salad on a lettuce-lined platter; top with reserved ⅓ cup tomato mixture.

Serves 6 to 8

Salmon and Potato Salad

2	tablespoons water	½	teaspoon pepper
½	teaspoon grated lemon zest	1	(16-ounce) skinned salmon fillet
2	tablespoons fresh lemon juice	8	small red potatoes, quartered
2	tablespoons mayonnaise	2	(½-inch) onion slices
1	tablespoon capers	½	teaspoon dried dill
¼	teaspoon salt	⅓	cup minced celery

- Combine 2 tablespoons water, lemon zest, lemon juice, mayonnaise, capers, and salt in a small bowl, stirring well; set aside.
- Sprinkle pepper over salmon and place salmon, potato quarters, and onion in a steamer basket coated with vegetable cooking spray over boiling water. Sprinkle with dill; cover and steam 15 minutes or until potato is tender and fish flakes with a fork.
- Break salmon into chunks.
- Combine salmon, potato, onion, and celery in a large bowl; add mayonnaise mixture, tossing gently to coat.

Makes 4 (1-cup) servings

Santa Fe Salad Bowl

This hearty taco salad is a summertime favorite!

1	pound ground round	2	avocados, chopped
1	(1¼-ounce) envelope taco seasoning mix	2	tomatoes, chopped
1	(15-ounce) can light or dark red kidney beans, drained and rinsed	4	green onions, chopped
1	head green leaf lettuce, torn into bite-size pieces	1	(2.25-ounce) can sliced ripe olives Shredded cheddar cheese
	Corn chips or nacho-flavored chips	1	(8-ounce) bottle sweet and spicy French dressing

- Brown ground round in a skillet over medium heat, stirring until it crumbles and is no longer pink; drain.
- Combine beef, taco seasoning, and kidney beans, stirring well.
- Place lettuce in a serving bowl; top with nacho chips, meat mixture, avocado, tomato, green onions, and olives. Top with shredded cheese. To serve, add dressing, tossing to coat.

Serves 6 to 8

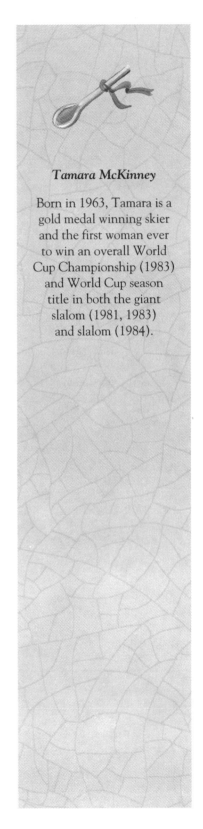

Tamara McKinney

Born in 1963, Tamara is a gold medal winning skier and the first woman ever to win an overall World Cup Championship (1983) and World Cup season title in both the giant slalom (1981, 1983) and slalom (1984).

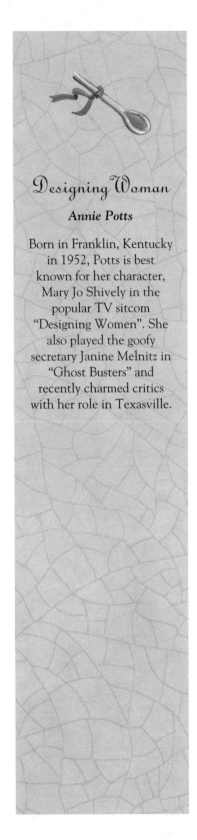

Designing Woman

Annie Potts

Born in Franklin, Kentucky in 1952, Potts is best known for her character, Mary Jo Shively in the popular TV sitcom "Designing Women". She also played the goofy secretary Janine Melnitz in "Ghost Busters" and recently charmed critics with her role in Texasville.

Summer Shrimp and Orzo Salad

Add crusty bread and this chilled, wonderfully light summer pasta becomes a main dish.

⅓ cup red wine vinegar
1 teaspoon dried basil
1 teaspoon olive oil
½ teaspoon salt
½ teaspoon dried oregano
¼ teaspoon pepper
1 cup cooked orzo

2 cups diced seeded tomato
1 cup frozen green peas, thawed
½ cup finely chopped purple onion
¼ cup chopped fresh parsley
1 pound medium-size fresh shrimp, boiled, peeled, and deveined or 1 bag cocktail shrimp

- Whisk together vinegar, basil, oil, salt, oregano, and pepper in a large bowl; add orzo, tomato, peas, onion, parsley, and shrimp, tossing well. Cover and chill.

Makes 4 (1½-cup) servings

Curried Shrimp and Artichoke Salad

1 tablespoon butter or margarine
1 (8-ounce) package chicken Rice-A-Roni
1 (6-ounce) jar marinated artichoke hearts
1½ pounds medium-size fresh shrimp, cooked, peeled, deveined, and chopped

2 green onions, chopped
8 pitted ripe olives, sliced
Curried Dressing
Lemon slices, fresh parsley sprigs for garnish

- Melt butter in a skillet over medium heat; add rice, reserving seasoning packet, and cook until browned. Cook rice according to package directions.
- Drain artichoke hearts, reserving marinade for dressing; chop artichoke hearts.
- Combine rice, artichoke hearts, shrimp, green onions, and ripe olives in a large bowl; add half of dressing, tossing to coat. Cover and chill overnight.
- Add remaining dressing when ready to serve; garnish with lemon slices and fresh parsley sprigs.

Curried Dressing

⅓ cup mayonnaise
½ teaspoon curry powder

Reserved Rice-A-Roni seasoning packet
Reserved artichoke heart marinade

- Combine all ingredients in a bowl, stirring well.

Serves 8

Grape and Walnut Chicken Salad

Ranch dressing seasons this salad making it tantalizingly different!

4	chicken breasts, cooked and diced	1	cup mayonnaise
2	cups seedless red grape halves	1	cup sour cream
2	cups sliced celery	3	tablespoons dry Ranch dressing mix
1	cup walnut pieces		

- Combine chicken, grapes, celery, and walnuts in a large bowl.
- Combine mayonnaise, sour cream, and dressing mix; add to chicken mixture, tossing gently to coat.

Serves 6 to 8

Roasted Dove Salad

6	roasted dove	¼	cup walnut oil
6	bacon slices	2	tablespoons unsalted butter
1	cup dry white wine	½	cup walnuts
1	tablespoon vinegar	1	head escarole
⅛	teaspoon salt	2	heads Bibb lettuce
	Ground pepper to taste		Juice of 1 lemon
¼	teaspoon Dijon mustard		

- Wrap each dove in a bacon slice; secure with kitchen string and place in a small roasting pan. Pour white wine over top.
- Bake at 400° for 20 to 30 minutes. Let cool.
- Skin and bone doves, reserving drippings in pan; chop meat into slivers.
- Add vinegar, salt, pepper, mustard, and walnut oil to drippings in pan; cook over low heat, whisking to blend.
- Melt butter in a small skillet over medium heat; add walnuts and sauté until browned.
- Combine dove meat, walnuts, lettuces, and vinegar mixture in a large bowl, tossing to coat; squeeze lemon juice over top and season to taste.

Makes 2 main dish or 4 side dish servings

Walnut oil is important to the recipe. It can be found in local gourmet or specialty food shops.

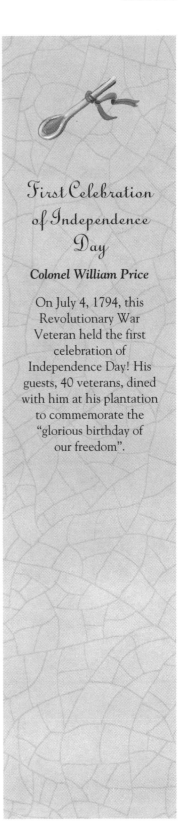

First Celebration of Independence Day

Colonel William Price

On July 4, 1794, this Revolutionary War Veteran held the first celebration of Independence Day! His guests, 40 veterans, dined with him at his plantation to commemorate the "glorious birthday of our freedom".

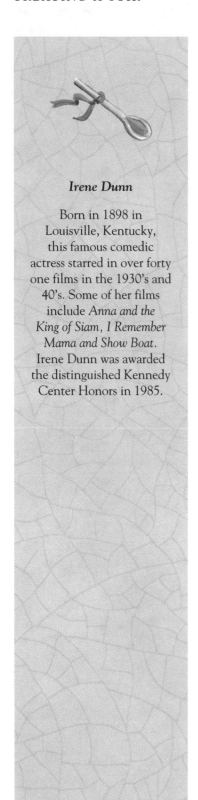

Irene Dunn

Born in 1898 in Louisville, Kentucky, this famous comedic actress starred in over forty one films in the 1930's and 40's. Some of her films include *Anna and the King of Siam, I Remember Mama and Show Boat.* Irene Dunn was awarded the distinguished Kennedy Center Honors in 1985.

Luncheon Chicken Salad

The whipping cream gives this chicken salad an exceptional flavor.

2½ cups diced cooked chicken breasts (4 breasts)	2 tablespoons chopped fresh parsley
1 cup diced celery	¼ teaspoon salt
1 cup sliced green grapes	¾ cup mayonnaise
¾ cup almonds, toasted	½ cup whipping cream, whipped

• Combine all ingredients in a large bowl, tossing to coat. Serve on lettuce-lined plates with sliced avocado and fresh summer tomato or seasonal fruit.

Orzo Salad with Asian Citrus Dressing

Tantalizing!

1 pound orzo	2 cups sunflower seed kernels, toasted
1½ tablespoons sesame oil	Asian Citrus Dressing
4-5 carrots, cut into thin strips using a potato peeler	3 tablespoons chopped fresh parsley
3 cups raisins	2-3 tablespoons chopped green onions

• Cook orzo in boiling water to cover in a saucepan 8 minutes; drain and rinse with cold water.

• Combine orzo and oil, tossing gently. Spoon half of orzo into a large glass bowl. Top with half each of carrot, raisins, and sunflower seeds. Repeat layers once.

• Pour three-fourths of Asian Citrus Dressing over top and let seep in.

• Combine parsley and green onions; sprinkle over salad. Pour remaining dressing over top.

Asian Citrus Dressing

¾ cup corn oil	1 teaspoon pepper
½ cup rice vinegar	1 teaspoon minced fresh ginger
¾ teaspoon salt	1½ teaspoons soy sauce
1 tablespoon sugar	¾ teaspoon minced garlic
2 tablespoons grated orange zest	¼ teaspoon crushed red pepper

• Process all ingredients in a blender until smooth.

Serves 10 to 12

Italian Chicken and Pasta Salad

*This plentiful salad serves nicely as a main dish and is certain
to become one of your most popular and most requested recipes!*

4   cups farfalle pasta, cooked
1   large onion, chopped
1   large green bell pepper, chopped
1   (14-ounce) can artichoke hearts,
      chopped
1   (4.25-ounce) can sliced ripe olives
1½ cups (6 ounces) shredded
      mozzarella cheese

¾   cup freshly grated Parmesan cheese
3-4 skinned and boned chicken breasts,
      cooked and cut into bite-size
      pieces
1   teaspoon garlic powder
      Salt and pepper to taste
16 ounces Italian dressing, divided

• Combine pasta, onion, bell pepper, artichokes, olives, mozzarella, and Parmesan
  cheese, chicken, garlic powder, salt, and pepper in a large bowl; add half of the
  dressing, tossing to coat. Cover and chill several hours or overnight. Toss with
  remaining 8 ounces of dressing before serving.

Serves 10

Caesar Tortellini with Peppers and Artichokes

2-3 (9-ounce) packages refrigerated
      cheese-filled tortellini, cooked
1   red bell pepper, chopped
1   green bell pepper, chopped
1   yellow bell pepper, chopped
1   (14-ounce) can artichoke hearts,
      drained

½   cup sliced ripe olives
1   cucumber, peeled and chopped
16 ounces Caesar dressing
6   ounces freshly grated Parmesan
      cheese

• Combine tortellini, bell peppers, artichokes, olives, and cucumber in a large bowl,
  tossing well. Add half of dressing, tossing to coat.

• Cover salad and chill 2 to 3 hours. Toss with remaining dressing, if needed, before
  serving. Sprinkle Parmesan over top and toss again.

Serves 10 to 12

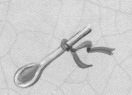

Field of Greens!

John B. Bibb

In 1856, this retired lawyer
and amateur horticulturist
built Gray Gables, (now
the Bibb-Burnley house)
on Wapping Street in
Frankfort, Kentucky.
Sometime after 1865, in a
large garden and
greenhouse at the back of
the house, Bibb developed
a new variety of lettuce.
Originally called limestone
lettuce, it was later named
after Bibb. Bibb lettuce has
a compact head and leaves
of single serving size. Bibb
did not market the new
lettuce but often gave it
away. It was grown by
regional farmers who had
received seeds from Bibb.
The Grenewein
greenhouse in Louisville
began to widely market the
lettuce in 1919.

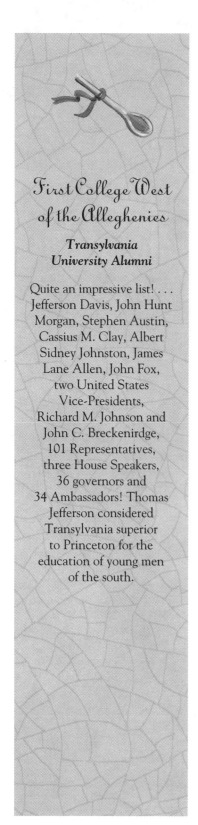

Chicken and Vegetable Fettuccine Salad

Serve with your favorite quick bread for a satisfying lunch or light supper.

2	cups cubed cooked chicken breasts		¼	cup sliced fresh mushrooms
4	ounces fettuccine, cooked		1	cup frozen peas, thawed
¼	cup olive oil		½	cup slivered almonds, toasted
½	cup grated Parmesan cheese		½	cup chopped broccoli (optional)
¼	teaspoon garlic powder		½	cup chopped or sliced carrot
¼	cup chopped celery			(optional)
¼	cup chopped green bell pepper			Herbed Red Wine Vinaigrette
¼	cup sliced green onions			

- Toss together chicken, fettuccine, and oil in a large bowl; let cool. Add cheese and garlic powder, tossing well. Cover and chill 1 hour or overnight.

- Add celery, bell pepper, green onions, mushrooms, peas, almonds, and, if desired, chopped broccoli and carrot to pasta mixture. Pour Vinaigrette over top and toss to coat.

Herbed Red Wine Vinaigrette

¼	cup red wine vinegar		1	teaspoon Worcestershire sauce
⅛	teaspoon ground pepper		1½	tablespoons Dijon mustard
¼	teaspoon salt			Juice of ¼ lemon
¾	teaspoon dried tarragon		¼	cup olive oil
½	teaspoon dried basil		¼	cup water
½	teaspoon dried oregano			

- Combine vinegar, pepper, salt, tarragon, basil, oregano, Worcestershire sauce, mustard, lemon juice, and oil in a jar; cover tightly and shake vigorously. Add ¼ cup water; cover and shake vigorously again.

Serves 6 to 8

Tossed Bow-Ties and Tortellini

2 cups fresh snow pea pods
2 cups broccoli florets
2½ cups cherry tomato halves
2 cups fresh mushrooms, sliced
1 (7.75-ounce) can whole pitted ripe
   olives, drained

1 (9-ounce) package refrigerated
   cheese-filled tortellini, cooked
3 ounces bow-tie pasta, cooked
1 tablespoon grated Parmesan cheese
   Italian Vinaigrette
   Freshly grated Parmesan cheese

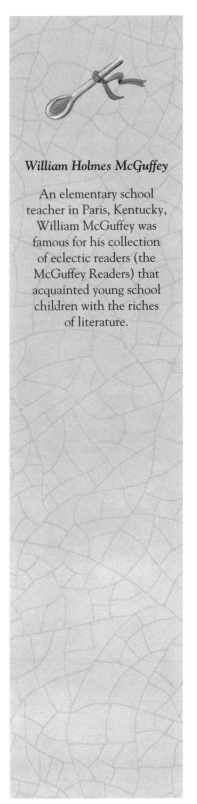

William Holmes McGuffey

An elementary school teacher in Paris, Kentucky, William McGuffey was famous for his collection of eclectic readers (the McGuffey Readers) that acquainted young school children with the riches of literature.

- Bring water to a boil in a saucepan; add snow peas and boil 1 minute. Remove with a slotted spoon.

- Add broccoli to boiling water; boil 1 minute and drain.

- Combine snow peas, broccoli, cherry tomato halves, mushrooms, and olives in a large bowl; add cooked pasta and 1 tablespoon Parmesan cheese. Pour Italian Vinaigrette over top and toss to coat.

- Cover salad and chill several hours. Garnish with additional Parmesan cheese.

Serves 6 to 8

Italian Vinaigrette

½ cup sliced green onions
⅓ cup red wine vinegar
⅓ cup vegetable oil
2 tablespoons chopped fresh parsley
2 garlic cloves, minced
2 teaspoons dried whole basil

1 teaspoon salt
½ teaspoon pepper
½ teaspoon sugar
½ teaspoon dried whole oregano
1½ teaspoons Dijon mustard
1 teaspoon dried whole dill weed

- Combine all ingredients in a jar; cover tightly and shake vigorously.

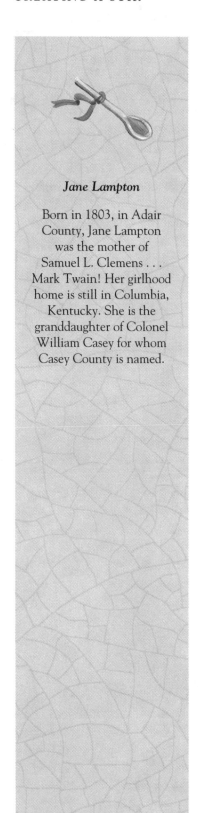

Jane Lampton

Born in 1803, in Adair County, Jane Lampton was the mother of Samuel L. Clemens . . . Mark Twain! Her girlhood home is still in Columbia, Kentucky. She is the granddaughter of Colonel William Casey for whom Casey County is named.

Bow-Tie Pasta with Feta and Sun-Dried Tomatoes

Absolutely delicious! The perfect addition to any summer meal-Chefs Kellie and Michael Stoddart, The Kitchen at Chevy Chase.

1	pound bow-tie pasta, cooked	1	tablespoon chopped fresh parsley
¼	cup sun-dried tomatoes, rehydrated	1	tablespoon chopped fresh oregano
½	cup feta cheese, diced into ¼-inch pieces	¼	cup red wine vinegar
¼	cup shredded Romano cheese	½	cup olive oil
1	tablespoon chopped fresh basil		Salt and pepper to taste

• Combine all ingredients in a large bowl, tossing well. Cover and chill 1 hour.

You can add ½ teaspoon dried crushed red pepper for a spicier salad or grilled chicken strips for an entrée.

Serves 6 to 8

San Juan Couscous Salad

Fabulous! Tastes even better the next day!

2	packages plain couscous	3	cups seeded chopped tomato, drained
2	cups olive oil		
3	cups fresh basil, coarsely chopped	2-3	cups pistachios, very coarsely chopped
4	garlic cloves, minced		
1	cup chopped onion	3	cups shredded Parmesan cheese
	Salt and cracked pepper to taste		

• Cook couscous according to package directions using slightly less water than recommended (it should be dry); cool and fluff.

• Combine oil, basil, garlic, onion, salt, and pepper in a bowl; let stand at room temperature 1 hour. Stir in tomato.

• Combine tomato mixture and couscous in a large bowl, stirring well. Add pistachios and Parmesan cheese and season with salt and pepper. Cover and chill overnight.

• Serve salad at room temperature.

Serves 8 to 10

This recipe was created on a sailboat in the San Juan Islands off the coast of Washington State.

Adjust quantities of ingredients to taste.

Wild Rice and Feta Salad

*This "confettied" rice boasts an exciting mixture
of colors and flavors . . . a delicious side for grilled food.*

6 ounces feta cheese, crumbled
½ cup chopped green bell pepper
½ cup chopped yellow bell pepper
½ cup chopped onion
1 cup toasted pine nuts, coarsely chopped
2 ounces diced pimiento, drained

4 ounces chopped ripe olives
1 (7-ounce) package long-grain and wild rice mix, cooked
⅓ cup olive oil
2 tablespoons tarragon wine vinegar
Dash of pepper

- Combine feta cheese, bell peppers, onion, pine nuts, pimiento, and olives in a large bowl; add cooled cooked rice, stirring well.

- Whisk together oil, vinegar, and pepper; pour over rice mixture, tossing gently to coat. Cover and chill up to 24 hours.

Serves 6 to 8

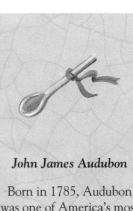

John James Audubon

Born in 1785, Audubon was one of America's most famous ornithologists. He was the writer and illustrator of *The Birds of America*. Audubon traversed the wooded area of Henderson, Kentucky finding, observing and painting birds in their natural habitat. Audubon's wife, Lucy, supported the family financially while he pursued his subject. Audubon State Park is named for him.

Havarti and Italian Rice Salad

*When the party moves outside, don't forget to add this classic
Italian rice salad to your menu. It's a wonderful dish for summer entertaining*

3 cups cooked rice (1½ cups uncooked)
½ cup chopped green onions
⅓ cup chopped fresh parsley
⅓ cup chopped fresh basil
½ cucumber, diced
1 brick Havarti cheese, diced
½ cup olives, chopped

½ cup capers
½ cup extra-virgin olive oil
Salt and pepper to taste
2 small tomatoes, diced
Chopped fresh dill (optional)
Chopped fresh oregano (optional)
Chopped fresh garlic chives (optional)

- Combine rice, green onions, parsley, basil, cucumber, cheese, olives, capers, oil, salt, pepper, tomato, and, if desired, dill, oregano, and garlic chives in a large bowl, stirring well. Cover and chill 2 to 3 hours.

Serves 6 to 8

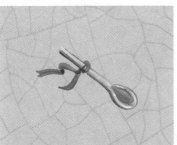

Bangkok Chicken and Capellini Salad

Exotic and hearty! Served chilled or at room temperature,
this salad is perfect for picnics or tail-gating parties!

8	ounces dried capellini		2	cups cooked chicken, cut into thin strips or bite-size pieces
8	green onions, white part only, thinly sliced		½	cup fresh cilantro leaves and chopped peanuts for garnish
¾	cup shredded or thinly sliced carrot			
¾	cup cucumber, cut into thin strips			

- Break pasta strands in half and cook according to directions. Rinse with cold water and drain well.

- Pour into a large bowl and toss with dressing. Add carrots, cucumber and chicken stirps. Toss to combine.

- Refrigerate 1 hour before serving.

- Garnish with fresh cilantro and chopped peanuts.

Dressing

½	cup chunky peanut butter		¼-½	teaspoon red pepper flakes
4	tablespoons soy sauce		4	tablespoons rice wine vinegar
2	teaspoons Dijon mustard		4	teaspoons sesame oil

- Combine all ingredients and stir until thick and creamy.

Serves 4 to 6

Soups, Stews & Sauces

"When I was ten years old, I received a diary for Christmas. I wrote in this diary sporadically for about six years. Many years later, I found the diary and reread the whole thing. The very first entry on January 1, I listed what we had for New Year's dinner: Fried chicken, black-eyed peas and greens. The most amusing thing to me about my diary was that every other entry mentioned what was for dinner and had commentary about it."

"Often we send menu suggestions to clients months in advance. One particular weekend, we had dinner parties on a Friday and Saturday night for two different customers. Over many months, these two customers had picked the same entrée I remember to be a Shrimp, Tasso Ham and Fettuccine dish. I didn't realize the coincidence until the week of the parties, however, I never thought there might be a problem. It turned out that both parties were honoring the same young couple who had just been engaged and the crowd was identical. On the second night when I saw the same crowd coming in the door, I was horrified. Dr. and Mrs. James Gay had been the hosts on Friday night and being the perfect gentleman that he is, he poked his head in the kitchen and said, "Its even better the second time!" After that, I made it a priority to find out a little more about the guest lists at parties we cater."

Chef Harriet Dupree
Dupree Catering, Inc.
Lexington, Kentucky

Tortellini Soup

Quick, easy, and delicious!

1	tablespoon butter or margarine	1	(10-ounce) package frozen chopped spinach, thawed and well drained
4	garlic cloves, crushed		
3	(14.5-ounce) cans chicken broth	1	(14.5-ounce) can stewed tomatoes, undrained
1	(12-ounce) package refrigerated fresh or frozen cheese-filled tortellini	1	(14.5-ounce) can red beans, rinsed and drained

- Melt butter in a large saucepan over medium-high heat; add garlic and sauté, stirring occasionally, 1 to 2 minutes.

- Add broth and tortellini and bring to a boil. Reduce heat and simmer 10 minutes.

- Stir in spinach, tomatoes, and beans and simmer 5 minutes.

Serves 8

Oyster-Artichoke Soup

Pamper guests with this elegant appetizer soup; it's luscious!

1	quart oysters	1½	(14-ounce) cans artichoke hearts, coarsely chopped
1	cup butter		
½	cup chopped onion	1	cup cream
½	cup chopped celery	½	teaspoon salt
1	teaspoon minced garlic	1	teaspoon ground white pepper
2	tablespoons minced fresh parsley	½	teaspoon cayenne pepper
2	tablespoons all-purpose flour	½	teaspoon dried thyme
2	cups chicken broth		

- Drain oysters, reserving liquid. Mince three-fourths of oysters; set all aside.

- Melt butter in a saucepan over medium heat; add onion, celery, garlic, and parsley and sauté 10 minutes or until soft. Whisk in flour and cook 1 minute.

- Add broth, artichoke hearts, cream, salt, white pepper, cayenne pepper, and thyme to onion mixture; reduce heat and simmer 10 minutes.

- Just before serving bring soup to a boil; add minced oysters, whole oysters, and reserved liquid. Return to a boil and cook 2 minutes. Serve immediately.

Serves 8

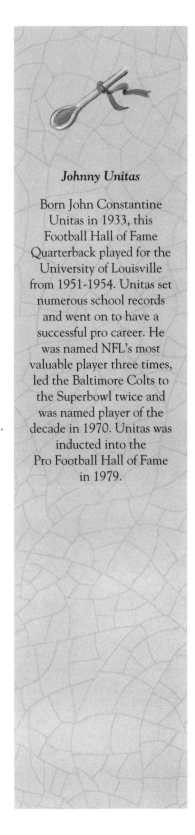

Johnny Unitas

Born John Constantine Unitas in 1933, this Football Hall of Fame Quarterback played for the University of Louisville from 1951-1954. Unitas set numerous school records and went on to have a successful pro career. He was named NFL's most valuable player three times, led the Baltimore Colts to the Superbowl twice and was named player of the decade in 1970. Unitas was inducted into the Pro Football Hall of Fame in 1979.

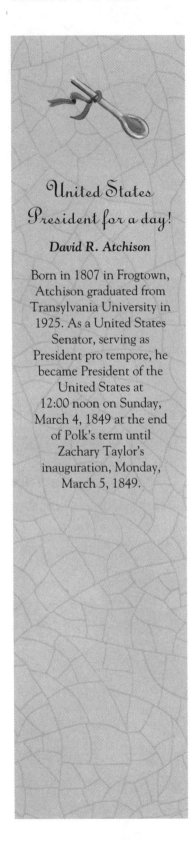

Elijah's Mushroom Provençal Soup

2	tablespoons butter, melted	¼	teaspoon coarsely ground pepper
1	(8-ounce) package fresh mushrooms, sliced	¼	teaspoon garlic salt
½	medium onion, diced	1	teaspoon salt
½	teaspoon dried basil	4	cups beef broth
¼	teaspoon dried oregano	1	(6-ounce) can tomato paste

- Melt butter in a saucepan over medium heat; add mushrooms and onion and sauté until tender. Stir in basil, oregano, pepper, garlic salt, and salt.

- Bring broth to a boil in a large Dutch oven; reduce heat to medium and whisk in tomato paste until blended. Add mushroom mixture and cook until thoroughly heated.

Serves 4

Curried Corn Bisque

This soup is outstanding! The curry beautifully shades the soup's rich creamy texture.

¼	cup butter	½	teaspoon salt
1	large onion, chopped	⅛	teaspoon cayenne pepper
1	cucumber, peeled, seeded, and chopped	2	cups chicken broth
		2	cups half-and-half or light cream
3	cups corn kernels	¼	cup chopped green onions
2	teaspoons curry powder		

- Melt butter in a large saucepan over medium heat; add onion, cucumber, and corn and sauté 15 minutes. Stir in curry powder, salt, and cayenne pepper and cook 30 seconds.

- Add broth; reduce heat and simmer 20 minutes. Process mixture in a blender until pureed. Return to pan and bring to a simmer.

- Stir in half-and-half and simmer until thoroughly heated (do not let boil). Garnish with chopped green onions.

Serves 4 to 6

Spicy Lentil Chili

Scrumptiously thick and spicy-you won't miss the meat in this soup!

2 cups diced carrot	1 teaspoon salt
2 cups diced zucchini	1 bay leaf
2 cups diced unpeeled eggplant	2 (28-ounce) cans diced tomatoes, undrained
1½ cups chopped onion	2½ cups chicken stock or vegetable broth
2-3 tablespoons chopped seeded jalapeño pepper	1½ cups red or brown lentils
1 tablespoon minced garlic	Salt and pepper to taste
3 tablespoons olive oil	Corn tortillas
5 teaspoons dried oregano	Sour cream
1½ tablespoons ground cumin	Chopped fresh cilantro
½ teaspoon cayenne pepper	

- Sauté carrot, zucchini, eggplant, onion, jalapeño pepper, and garlic in hot oil in a large Dutch oven over medium heat 5 minutes or until crisp-tender. Stir in oregano, cumin, cayenne pepper, salt, and bay leaf and cook 30 seconds.

- Add tomatoes, broth, and lentils and bring to a boil. Reduce heat and simmer 40 minutes or until lentils and vegetables are tender. Season with salt and pepper. Discard bay leaf.

- Serve soup with corn tortillas and garnish with sour cream and chopped fresh cilantro.

Serves 8 to 10

Split Pea Soup

2 cups dried split peas (1 pound), rinsed	1 fresh parsley sprig, chopped
2-3 quarts cold water	3 tablespoons butter (optional)
1 ham bone	3 tablespoons all-purpose flour (optional)
1 large onion, chopped	Freshly cracked pepper
3 celery ribs, chopped	

- Bring peas, water, ham bone, onion, celery, and parsley to a boil in a large Dutch oven over medium-high heat. Cover, reduce heat, and simmer 4 to 5 hours or until peas are tender. Skim off excess fat.

- Melt 3 tablespoon butter in a small skillet over medium heat; add flour and cook, stirring constantly, until smooth. Add to pea mixture to thicken, if desired.

- Remove ham bone and cut off meat; add meat to soup.

- Serve soup in bowls or cups and garnish with freshly cracked pepper.

Serves 6

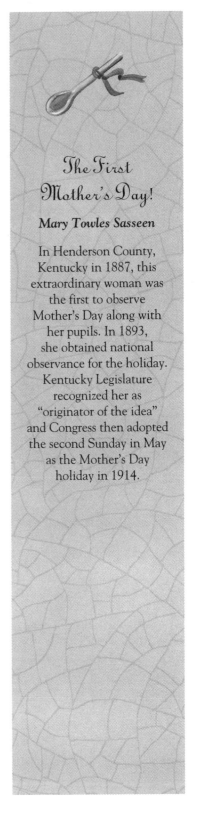

The First Mother's Day!

Mary Towles Sasseen

In Henderson County, Kentucky in 1887, this extraordinary woman was the first to observe Mother's Day along with her pupils. In 1893, she obtained national observance for the holiday. Kentucky Legislature recognized her as "originator of the idea" and Congress then adopted the second Sunday in May as the Mother's Day holiday in 1914.

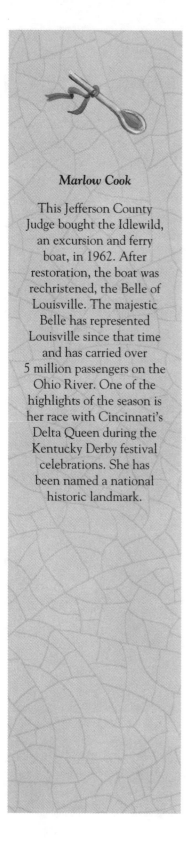

Marlow Cook

This Jefferson County Judge bought the Idlewild, an excursion and ferry boat, in 1962. After restoration, the boat was rechristened, the Belle of Louisville. The majestic Belle has represented Louisville since that time and has carried over 5 million passengers on the Ohio River. One of the highlights of the season is her race with Cincinnati's Delta Queen during the Kentucky Derby festival celebrations. She has been named a national historic landmark.

Rotini and Italian Sausage Soup

2 cups uncooked rotini pasta
1 pound mild or hot Italian sausage, cut into ¼-inch slices
2 onions, chopped
2 garlic cloves, minced
2 tablespoons vegetable oil
1 (28-ounce) can whole tomatoes, undrained
3 tablespoons tomato paste
7 cups beef broth

1 cup dry red wine
2 tablespoons dried basil
2 tablespoons dried oregano
2 medium zucchini, thinly sliced
½ cup chopped fresh parsley
1 (16-ounce) can garbanzo beans, drained
Salt and pepper to taste
Freshly grated Parmesan cheese

- Cook pasta as directed; drain and set aside.

- Cook sausage in a large skillet over medium heat until lightly browned. Transfer to a large Dutch oven using a slotted spoon, reserving drippings in skillet.

- Sauté onion and garlic in hot oil and drippings in skillet until soft; transfer to Dutch oven using a slotted spoon.

- Add tomatoes, tomato paste, beef broth, wine, basil, and oregano to Dutch oven and cook 30 minutes over medium heat, stirring occasionally.

- Add zucchini, parsley, and pasta to soup and cook, stirring occasionally, 10 to 20 minutes. Add garbanzo beans during the last 10 minutes of cooking.

- Season with salt and pepper. Sprinkle each serving with Parmesan cheese and serve with garlic bread.

Serves 6 to 8

Tomato Soup with Gin

This unusual soup sets the stage for a very memorable dinner!

¼ cup diced bacon	2 fresh oregano sprigs
¼ cup olive oil	3 fresh basil leaves
¾ cup chopped onion	2 fresh sage leaves
½ cup chopped carrot	1 quart chicken broth
¼ cup chopped leek (white and tender green parts)	2 tablespoons sugar
	Salt and freshly ground white pepper
3 tablespoons chopped celery	¼ cup whipping cream
7 tablespoons tomato sauce	⅓ cup gin
3 large fresh tomatoes, peeled, seeded, and chopped (about 1½ pounds)	

- Cook bacon in hot oil in a large 4- to 5-quart saucepan over medium heat 4 minutes or until lightly browned. Add onion, carrot, leek, and celery and cook, stirring occasionally, 10 minutes or until soft.

- Stir in tomato sauce; reduce heat and simmer 10 minutes. Add fresh tomato, oregano, basil, and sage; simmer, stirring occasionally, 10 minutes or until mixture resembles a puree.

- Stir in broth, sugar, and salt and pepper. Simmer, stirring occasionally, 10 minutes.

- Process soup in a blender in batches until pureed. Pour through a wire-mesh strainer into pan; bring to a boil, stirring occasionally. Adjust seasonings to taste.

- Beat whipping cream at medium speed with an electric mixer until soft peaks form.

- Stir gin into soup and ladle into serving cups. Top each serving with a dollop of whipped cream and serve immediately.

Serves 6

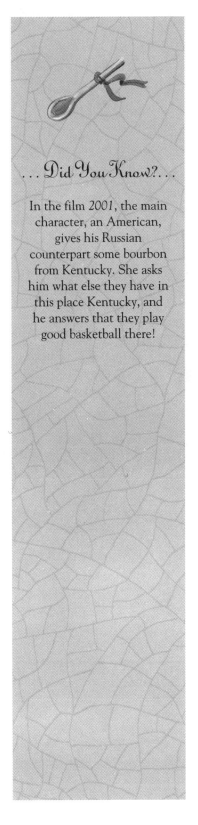

...Did You Know?...

In the film *2001*, the main character, an American, gives his Russian counterpart some bourbon from Kentucky. She asks him what else they have in this place Kentucky, and he answers that they play good basketball there!

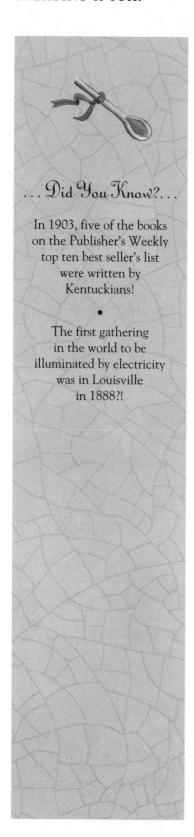

Autumn Sweet Potato - Nut Cream Soup

*This is a must-try! The combination
of flavors is uniquely different and absolutely delicious!*

2	large sweet potatoes or yams, peeled and quartered	1	(6-ounce) can tomato paste
6	cups water	1½-2	teaspoons salt
1	medium onion, chopped	¼	teaspoon garlic powder
1	garlic clove, crushed	¼	teaspoon onion powder
1½	tablespoons olive oil		Cayenne pepper to taste
1	cup creamy peanut butter		Crushed peanuts
1	(10½-ounce) can condensed chicken broth, undiluted		Oyster crackers

- Bring sweet potatoes and 6 cups water to a boil in a large Dutch oven. Cover, simmer 15 to 20 minutes. Drain sweet potato, reserving broth.

- Sauté onion and garlic in hot oil in skillet until tender (do not brown).

- Process sweet potato, onion, and garlic in a food processor until pureed, adding sweet potato broth as needed. Add peanut butter and process until smooth.

- Whisk together pureed mixture, remaining sweet potato broth, chicken broth, and tomato paste in a large Dutch oven; add salt, garlic powder, onion powder, and cayenne pepper and bring to a simmer. Simmer 10 minutes, adding more water or broth as necessary.

- Serve immediately or cover and chill several days. Top each serving with crushed peanuts and serve with crackers.

Serves 6 to 8

Do not use reduced-fat peanut butter.

Carrot and Orange Soup

Easy and rich! Try this colorful soup as a starter for an elegant dinner

¼ cup butter
2 cups diced onion
12 large carrots, grated
4 cups chicken broth
1 cup orange juice
    Salt and pepper to taste

½ teaspoon curry powder
½ teaspoon ground ginger
1 cup half-and-half
    Grated orange zest, chopped fresh
    parsley for garnish

- Melt butter in a Dutch oven over low heat; add onion and carrot and cook 25 minutes or until tender (do not brown). Add broth and simmer 30 minutes.

- Process 2 cups soup at a time in a food processor until pureed; return to Dutch oven.

- Add orange juice, salt, pepper, curry powder, ginger, and half-and-half to Dutch oven and cook until thoroughly heated. Garnish with grated orange zest and chopped fresh parsley.

Serves 6 to 8

Cold Spanish Salad Soup

Brimming with vegetables!

4 medium to large tomatoes,
    quartered
½ medium onion, chopped
½ large cucumber, sliced
½ large green bell pepper, sliced
5 fresh parsley sprigs
1 teaspoon salt
¼ teaspoon pepper
2 garlic cloves, minced

2 tablespoons olive oil
2 tablespoons red wine vinegar
¾ teaspoon Worcestershire sauce
½ cup ice water
½ cup red wine
⅛ teaspoon chopped fresh basil
2 dashes of hot sauce (optional)
    Garnishes: sliced green onion tops,
    croutons, sour cream

- Process all ingredients except for garnishes and, if desired, hot sauce in a food processor 15 seconds or until chopped. (Do not overprocess; vegetables should be crunchy.)

- Serve chilled and garnish with green onions, croutons, and sour cream.

Serves 6

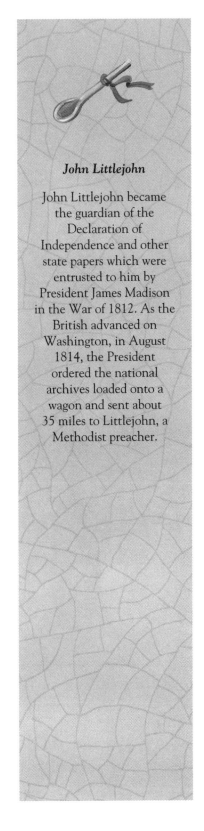

John Littlejohn

John Littlejohn became the guardian of the Declaration of Independence and other state papers which were entrusted to him by President James Madison in the War of 1812. As the British advanced on Washington, in August 1814, the President ordered the national archives loaded onto a wagon and sent about 35 miles to Littlejohn, a Methodist preacher.

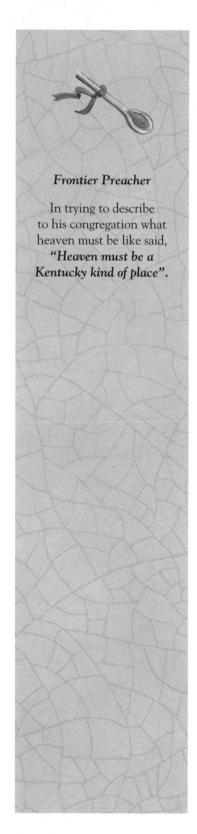

Gazpacho

A great way to enjoy summer's surplus from the garden.

4 cups tomato juice, chilled	Juice of half a lemon
1 small onion, minced	Juice of 1 lime
2 cups fresh or canned diced tomato	1 teaspoon dried tarragon
1 green bell pepper, minced	1 teaspoon dried basil
1 diced cucumber	Dash of ground cumin
2 green onions, chopped	Dash of hot sauce
1 teaspoon honey	1½ tablespoons olive oil
1 garlic clove, crushed	Salt and pepper to taste
2 tablespoons wine vinegar	

- Combine all ingredients in a large bowl. Chill at least 2 hours.

Serves 6

You can puree soup in a food processor if you prefer it less chunky.

Chicken Tortilla Soup

If you like Tex-Mex, this bowl's for you!

4 skinned and boned chicken breasts (about ⅔ pound), cut into bite-size pieces	¼ teaspoon ground cumin
	2 (14.5-ounce) cans chicken broth
	1 cup chunky salsa
½ teaspoon olive oil	1 small can sweet corn kernels
1 cup chopped onion	1 (4½-ounce) can green chiles
Juice of half a lime	Tortilla chips
½ teaspoon crushed garlic	Shredded Monterey Jack cheese
½ teaspoon chili powder	Chopped avocado

- Cook chicken in hot oil in a large saucepan over high heat, stirring occasionally, 2 minutes. Add onion, lime juice, garlic, chili powder, and cumin and cook, stirring occasionally, 2 minutes.

- Stir in broth, salsa, and corn. Cover and bring to a boil. Reduce heat to medium-high and boil 8 to 10 minutes. Let simmer until thickened.

- Place chips in individual serving bowls. Ladle soup over chips and sprinkle with cheese. Garnish with avocado.

Serves 6

Creamy Roasted Red Pepper Soup

3 red bell peppers, cored and halved	3 cups milk
6 tablespoons butter	3 cups chicken broth
¼ cup all-purpose flour	Salt and pepper to taste

- Place bell peppers, cut side down, on a broiler pan. Broil 4 inches from heat (with electric oven door partially open) 10 minutes or until blackened. Place in a zip-top plastic bag; seal and let stand 10 minutes. Discard skin.

- Melt butter in a skillet over medium heat; add flour, stirring until smooth. Gradually stir in milk; reduce heat and simmer until thickened.

- Process bell pepper halves and 2 cups broth in a blender until smooth. Add puree and remaining 1 cup broth to milk mixture.

- Season with salt and pepper and cook until thoroughly heated.

Serves 6

Corn and Roasted Poblano Soup

Poblano peppers turn up the heat in this soup!

2 quarts milk	2 teaspoons salt
2 tablespoons cumin seeds	4 garlic cloves, minced
2 bay leaves	2 teaspoons ground cumin
1 sprig of fresh or ½ teaspoon dried rosemary	8 cups fresh or frozen corn kernels
2 large onions, diced	6 poblano chile peppers, roasted, peeled, seeded, and diced
¼ cup olive oil	1 bunch fresh chives, thinly diced

- Cook milk, cumin seeds, bay leaves, and rosemary in a medium saucepan over low heat until almost simmering (do not boil). Remove from heat and let stand 20 minutes.

- Sauté onion and salt in hot oil in a Dutch oven over medium heat 15 to 20 minutes or until golden. Add garlic and ground cumin and cook, stirring often, 5 minutes.

- Stir corn and diced pepper into onion mixture; reduce heat and simmer 5 minutes. Pour milk mixture through a wire-mesh strainer into corn mixture. Bring to a simmer and cook 15 minutes.

- Process one-third of soup in a food processor until pureed. Return to Dutch oven and cook until thoroughly heated. Sprinkle with chives.

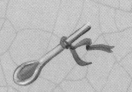

Rescue Attempt is Followed by the World

Floyd Collins

Floyd Collins was born in 1887 in Edmunson County, Kentucky just a few miles away from Mammoth Cave. His attempted rescue from Sand Cave was publicized worldwide and aroused the sympathy of the nation. On January 30, 1925, Collins was trapped in a narrow passage just 150 feet from the entrance of the cave. Rescuers were able to reach him but couldn't reach the rock that had pinned him at the ankles. A rescue shaft and tunnel were not completed in time to save him. He had been exploring for a connection to his family's Crystal Cave which had once been opened for tours.

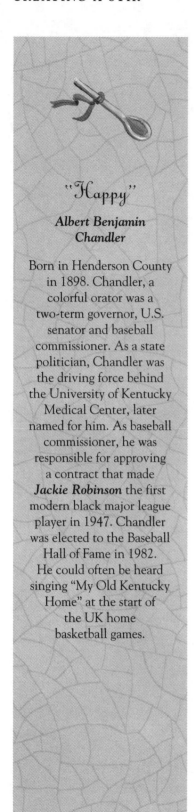

"Happy"

**Albert Benjamin
Chandler**

Born in Henderson County
in 1898. Chandler, a
colorful orator was a
two-term governor, U.S.
senator and baseball
commissioner. As a state
politician, Chandler was
the driving force behind
the University of Kentucky
Medical Center, later
named for him. As baseball
commissioner, he was
responsible for approving
a contract that made
Jackie Robinson the first
modern black major league
player in 1947. Chandler
was elected to the Baseball
Hall of Fame in 1982.
He could often be heard
singing "My Old Kentucky
Home" at the start of
the UK home
basketball games.

Escarole, Sausage, and White Bean Stew

Chase away winter's chill with a bowl of this hearty stew.

8 ounces sweet and/or hot Italian sausage, broken into 1-inch chunks
1 teaspoon olive oil
5 garlic cloves, minced
½ teaspoon dried red pepper flakes
1 head escarole, chopped into 2-inch pieces
3 cups cooked fresh or canned white beans
3 cups chicken broth

¼ cup unsalted butter
½ cup freshly grated Parmesan or Romano blend cheese
2 plum tomatoes, diced
2 tablespoons chopped fresh parsley, divided
   Salt and freshly ground pepper to taste
   Freshly shaved or grated Parmesan cheese

• Cook sausage in 1 teaspoon hot oil in a large deep skillet over medium-high heat 10 minutes or until lightly browned. Add garlic and red pepper flakes and cook 2 minutes.

• Add escarole to skillet and cook 2 minutes or until wilted. Add beans and cook, stirring constantly, 1 minute.

• Add broth to skillet and bring to a boil; add butter, cheese, tomato, and 1 tablespoon parsley and cook until thoroughly heated. Season with salt and pepper.

• Serve soup in heated bowls. Sprinkle each serving evenly with remaining parsley; top with Parmesan cheese.

Serves 4 to 6

Cock-a-Leekie Soup

Serve with a salad and bread for a perfect winter meal.

½ cup butter, divided	¾ cup half-and-half
1½ cups chopped chicken breast	2 cups milk
2 cups chopped leek	1 teaspoon poultry seasoning
3 cups chicken broth	3 tablespoons minced fresh parsley
¾ cup uncooked barley	Salt and pepper to taste
¼ cup all-purpose flour	

- Melt ¼ cup butter in a large saucepan over medium heat; add chicken and cook until done. Transfer chicken to a plate, reserving drippings in pan.

- Add leek to pan and sauté until tender. Stir in broth and barley; reduce heat and simmer 30 minutes or until barley is tender.

- Melt remaining ¼ cup butter in a medium saucepan over medium heat; gradually stir in flour and cook, stirring constantly, 5 minutes.

- Gradually whisk half-and-half and milk into flour mixture; cook, whisking constantly, until thickened. Add poultry seasoning, parsley, and salt and pepper; simmer 20 minutes.

- Add milk mixture and chicken to broth mixture; cook 5 minutes or until thoroughly heating, adding more broth to thin if necessary.

Serves 6 to 8

You may substitute additional broth for half-and-half for a soup not as rich.

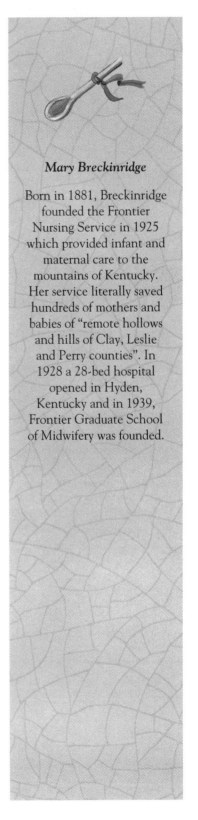

Mary Breckinridge

Born in 1881, Breckinridge founded the Frontier Nursing Service in 1925 which provided infant and maternal care to the mountains of Kentucky. Her service literally saved hundreds of mothers and babies of "remote hollows and hills of Clay, Leslie and Perry counties". In 1928 a 28-bed hospital opened in Hyden, Kentucky and in 1939, Frontier Graduate School of Midwifery was founded.

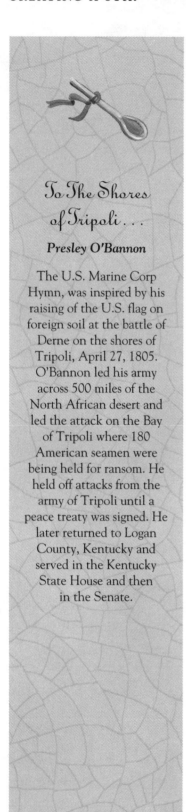

Mixed Bean Soup

The flavor of this soup improves with age! Make ahead!

2	cups mixed dried beans	1	(16-ounce) can diced tomatoes
2	quarts water	1	large onion, chopped
1	ham bone		Juice of 1 lemon
1	pound chopped regular or country ham		Salt and pepper to taste
1	garlic clove, minced		Hot sauce to taste

- Wash beans; soak in water to cover 3 hours or overnight. Drain.

- Bring beans, 2 quarts water, ham bone, ham, garlic, tomatoes, onion, lemon juice, salt, pepper, and hot sauce to a boil in a large Dutch oven; reduce heat and simmer at least 4 hours or all day.

Makes 1½ quarts

You can also cook this soup in a slow cooker.

Broccoli and Cheese Soup

5	cups water, divided	1½	teaspoons salt
2	(10-ounce) packages frozen chopped broccoli, thawed	¾	teaspoon pepper
1	medium onion, chopped	¼	teaspoon ground nutmeg
3	tablespoons butter	1	cup whipping cream
3	tablespoons all-purpose flour	1-1½	cups (4 to 6 ounces) shredded cheddar cheese
1	tablespoon chicken bouillon granules		

- Bring 2 cups water to a boil in a 3-quart saucepan; add broccoli and onion and return to a boil. Cover and boil 10 minutes. Do not drain. Process mixture in a food processor until almost pureed; set aside.

- Melt butter in a saucepan over low heat; add flour and cook, stirring constantly, until smooth and bubbly.

- Stir in remaining 3 cups water and bring to a boil, stirring constantly. Boil, stirring constantly, 1 minute. Add broccoli mixture, bouillon granules, salt, pepper, and nutmeg, stirring well.

- Stir in cream; add cheese, stirring until melted.

Serves 6

Vegetarian Southwestern Chili

A delicious crowd pleaser!

2 cups dried black beans, rinsed	2 tablespoons dried oregano
10 cups water	¼ cup all-purpose flour
1 teaspoon ground black pepper	2½ tablespoons chili powder
½ cup unsalted butter	2½ tablespoons ground cumin
2 medium-size fresh or canned green chile peppers, seeded and chopped	2 tablespoons ground coriander
⅔ cup chopped purple onion	1 teaspoon salt
⅔ cup chopped celery	½ teaspoon sugar
⅔ cup chopped red bell pepper	5 cups chicken broth
1 medium zucchini, sliced crosswise and quartered	2½ cups frozen corn kernels, thawed
1 large leek, chopped	Toppings: shredded cheddar cheese, chopped onion, sour cream, tortilla chips
2 garlic cloves, minced	

- Soak beans in water to cover overnight; drain.

- Bring beans, 10 cups water, and black pepper to a boil in a large Dutch oven; reduce heat and simmer 1 hour and 30 minutes. Drain and transfer beans to a bowl.

- Melt butter in Dutch oven over medium heat; add chiles, onion, celery, bell pepper, zucchini, leek, garlic, and oregano and cook 10 to 15 minutes.

- Reduce heat and stir in flour, chili powder, cumin, coriander, salt, and sugar. Simmer, stirring often, 5 minutes. Add half of broth and simmer, stirring often.

- Process 1½ cups corn and remaining half of broth in a food processor until pureed; add to Dutch oven. Stir in black beans and remaining 1 cup corn. Simmer, stirring often, 15 minutes. (Do not let bottom burn.)

- Serve chili over rice, if desired, with desired toppings.

Serves 6

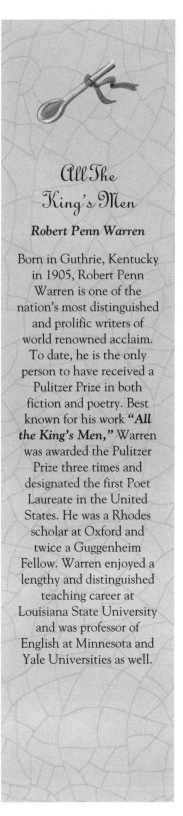

All The King's Men

Robert Penn Warren

Born in Guthrie, Kentucky in 1905, Robert Penn Warren is one of the nation's most distinguished and prolific writers of world renowned acclaim. To date, he is the only person to have received a Pulitzer Prize in both fiction and poetry. Best known for his work **"All the King's Men,"** Warren was awarded the Pulitzer Prize three times and designated the first Poet Laureate in the United States. He was a Rhodes scholar at Oxford and twice a Guggenheim Fellow. Warren enjoyed a lengthy and distinguished teaching career at Louisiana State University and was professor of English at Minnesota and Yale Universities as well.

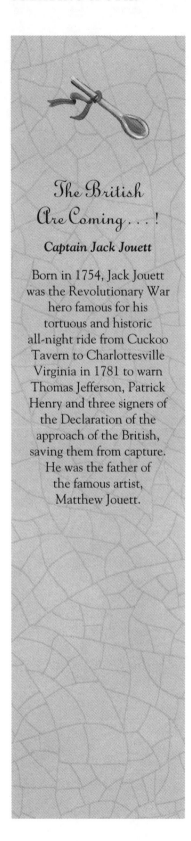

The British Are Coming . . . !

Captain Jack Jouett

Born in 1754, Jack Jouett was the Revolutionary War hero famous for his tortuous and historic all-night ride from Cuckoo Tavern to Charlottesville Virginia in 1781 to warn Thomas Jefferson, Patrick Henry and three signers of the Declaration of the approach of the British, saving them from capture. He was the father of the famous artist, Matthew Jouett.

Spicy Tailgating Chili

Wonderfully thick and spicy. . .especially great for serving a large crowd! Accompanied by a hearty bread or sturdy tortilla chips, this chili is sure to score major points.

¼ cup olive oil	2 tablespoons salt
2½ cups yellow onions, coarsely chopped	2 tablespoons dried basil
1 pound sweet Italian sausage meat, removed from casings	2 tablespoons dried oregano
4 pounds beef chuck, ground	3 pounds canned Italian plum tomatoes, drained
2 teaspoons freshly ground black pepper	¼ cup burgundy wine (or more)
1 (12-ounce) can tomato paste	⅛ cup lemon juice
4½ teaspoons minced fresh garlic	¼ cup chopped fresh dill
6 tablespoons ground cumin seed	¼ cup chopped Italian parsley
8 tablespoons plain chili powder	1-2 (16-ounce) cans dark red kidney beans, drained and rinsed
¼ cup prepared Dijon-style mustard	4 (2½-ounce) cans sliced black olives, drained

- Heat olive oil in a very large soup kettle. Add onions and cook over low heat, covered, until tender and translucent, about 10 minutes.

- Crumble the sausage meat and ground chuck into the kettle and cook over medium-high heat, stirring often, until meats are browned well. Spoon out as much excess fat as possible.

- Over low heat stir in black pepper, tomato paste, garlic, cumin seed, chili powder, mustard, salt, basil and oregano.

- Add drained tomatoes, Burgundy, lemon juice, dill, parsley and drained kidney beans. Stir well and simmer, uncovered, for another 15 minutes.

- Taste and correct seasonings. Add olives, simmer for another 5 minutes to heat through and serve immediately.

- Serve with grated cheddar cheese, sour cream, chopped green onions, if desired.

Serves 15 to 20

Chili powder and cumin can be adjusted to accommodate those who prefer a more mild flavor.

Cold Weather Potato Soup

Perfect after a day of raking leaves!

2	(14½-ounce) cans chicken broth	2½	cups milk
1	cup water	2	cups (8 ounces) shredded sharp cheddar cheese
6	medium potatoes, peeled and cubed		
2	tablespoons butter	8	bacon slices, cooked and crumbled
	Chopped onion to taste		Shredded sharp cheddar cheese
	Salt and pepper to taste		

- Bring broth and 1 cup water to a boil in a Dutch oven; add potato and boil 20 minutes or until tender. Remove from heat.

- Add butter, onion, and salt and pepper to potato mixture. Add milk, stirring to slightly mash potato cubes.

- Cook over low heat; stir in 2 cups cheese and bacon and cook until cheese is melted and soup is thoroughly heated.

- Sprinkle each serving with shredded cheese.

Serves 8

Chicken Chili

Very satisfying . . . a savory ending to a busy day.

8	skinned and boned chicken breasts	1	tablespoon plus 1 teaspoon ground cumin
1	cup diced onion		
1	(4.5-ounce) can diced green chiles	1½	teaspoons dried oregano
4	cups chicken broth	2	teaspoons dried parsley flakes
3-4	(15-ounce) cans great Northern beans	1	tablespoon salt
1	cup salsa		Toppings: shredded Monterey Jack cheese, sour cream, tortilla chips, salsa
1	tablespoon dried crushed red pepper		
2	teaspoons garlic powder		

- Bring chicken and water to cover to a boil in a large Dutch oven; boil 45 to 60 minutes or until done. Drain chicken and cube.

- Cook chicken, onion, chiles, and 4 cups broth in Dutch oven over medium heat, stirring often, until warm. Add beans, salsa, red pepper, garlic powder, cumin, oregano, parsley, and salt; reduce heat and simmer, stirring often, 20 minutes.

- Serve with desired toppings and cornbread.

Serves 8

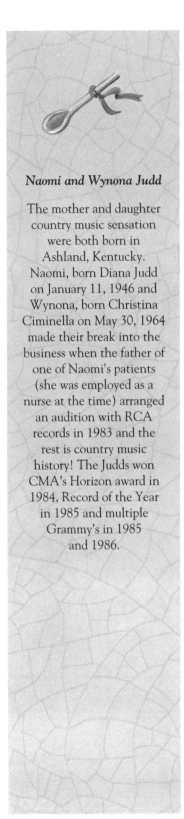

Naomi and Wynona Judd

The mother and daughter country music sensation were both born in Ashland, Kentucky. Naomi, born Diana Judd on January 11, 1946 and Wynona, born Christina Ciminella on May 30, 1964 made their break into the business when the father of one of Naomi's patients (she was employed as a nurse at the time) arranged an audition with RCA records in 1983 and the rest is country music history! The Judds won CMA's Horizon award in 1984, Record of the Year in 1985 and multiple Grammy's in 1985 and 1986.

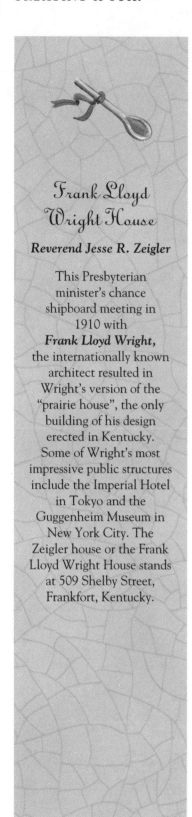

Frank Lloyd
Wright House

Reverend Jesse R. Zeigler

This Presbyterian
minister's chance
shipboard meeting in
1910 with
Frank Lloyd Wright,
the internationally known
architect resulted in
Wright's version of the
"prairie house", the only
building of his design
erected in Kentucky.
Some of Wright's most
impressive public structures
include the Imperial Hotel
in Tokyo and the
Guggenheim Museum in
New York City. The
Zeigler house or the Frank
Lloyd Wright House stands
at 509 Shelby Street,
Frankfort, Kentucky.

Creole-Style Shrimp and Sausage Gumbo

1½ pounds medium-size fresh shrimp	1 teaspoon dried thyme
4½ cups water	1 teaspoon salt
3½ cups ice water	½ teaspoon cayenne
1 (8-ounce) bottle clam juice (1 cup)	2 bay leaves
½ cup vegetable oil	¾ pound smoked andouille or kielbasa sausage
½ cup all-purpose flour	½ cup chopped fresh parsley
2 onions, diced	6 green onions, chopped
1 celery rib, diced	½ teaspoon filé powder
6 garlic cloves, minced	

- Peel shrimp and devein, if desired, reserving shells; set shrimp aside.

- Bring shrimp shells and 4½ cups water to a boil in a large Dutch oven over medium-high heat; reduce heat to medium-low and simmer 20 minutes.

- Pour broth through a wire-mesh strainer into a large bowl, discarding shells. Add clam juice and 3½ cups ice water; set aside.

- Heat oil in Dutch oven over medium-high heat to 200°; reduce heat to medium and gradually stir in flour with a wooden spoon until smooth. Cook, stirring constantly, 20 to 30 minutes or until it develops a nutty aroma and is a deep red brown. (If roux begins to smoke, remove from heat and stir constantly to cool slightly.)

- Add onion, celery, garlic, thyme, salt, and cayenne pepper to roux; cook, stirring often, 8 to 10 minutes. Add 1 quart reserved broth mixture in a slow, steady stream, stirring vigorously. Stir in remaining broth mixture.

- Increase heat to high and bring to a boil. Reduce heat to medium-low and skim foam off surface. Add bay leaves and simmer 30 minutes.

- Stir in sausage and simmer 30 minutes. Add reserved shrimp and simmer 5 minutes or until shrimp turn pink.

- Remove from heat and stir in parsley and green onions. Adjust seasonings to taste; stir in filé powder. Discard bay leaves.

- Let stand at room temperature 5 to 10 minutes. Serve with rice and garlic French bread.

Serves 8

Kentucky Burgoo

Traditional Kentucky fare for a "Day at the Races"

2 pounds pork shank	2 cups corn kernels
2 pounds veal shank	2 red chile peppers
2 pounds beef shank (soup meat)	2 cups diced okra
2 pounds breast of lamb	2 cups lima beans
1 (4-pound) hen	1 cup diced celery
8 quarts water	Chopped fresh thyme to taste
1½ pounds potatoes, cubed	Salt and cayenne pepper to taste
1½ pounds onions, diced	Chopped fresh oregano to taste
1 bunch carrots, chopped	Worcestershire sauce to taste
2 green bell peppers, chopped	Hot sauce to taste
2 cups chopped cabbage	Chopped fresh parsley to taste
1 quart tomato puree	

- Bring pork, veal, beef, lamb, hen, and water to a boil in a large stockpot; reduce heat and simmer until meat is tender and falling off bones. Remove meat from pot. Let cool and chop, discarding bones.
- Combine meat, cubed potato, onion, carrot, bell pepper, cabbage, tomato puree, corn, chile peppers, okra, lima beans, and celery in pot; bring to a simmer. Simmer, stirring often, 4 hours or until thickened (do not let burn on bottom).
- Add chopped fresh thyme, cayenne pepper, oregano, Worcestershire sauce, and hot sauce to mixture. Add parsley when ready to serve.
- Serve with warm homemade bread.

You may substitute game meat, such as dove or duck, if desired. Be sure to balance substitution with water.

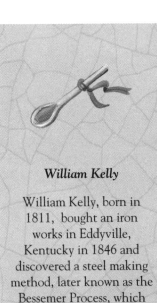

William Kelly

William Kelly, born in 1811, bought an iron works in Eddyville, Kentucky in 1846 and discovered a steel making method, later known as the Bessemer Process, which made it possible for civilization to pass from the Iron Ages to the Steel Age.

Spicy Seafood Cocktail Sauce

Serve with fish, shellfish, or crab cakes.

1 cup mayonnaise	3 tablespoons lemon juice
¼ cup ketchup	1 small onion, finely grated
¼ cup chili sauce	½ cup vegetable oil
1 teaspoon prepared mustard or horseradish mustard	1 teaspoon pepper
1 teaspoon Worcestershire sauce	1 teaspoon paprika
	2 garlic cloves, minced

- Combine all ingredients; cover and chill.

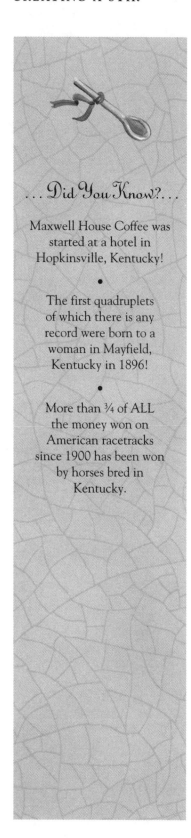

Lentil and Brown Rice Soup

Good for you!

5	cups chicken broth	½	cup chopped celery
3	cups water	3	garlic cloves, minced
1½	cups lentils, rinsed	½	teaspoon dried basil
1	cup long-grain brown rice	½	teaspoon dried oregano
1	(35-ounce) can whole tomatoes, undrained and diced	½	teaspoon dried thyme
		1	bay leaf
3	carrots, halved lengthwise and cut crosswise into ¼-inch pieces	½	cup minced fresh parsley
		2	tablespoons cider vinegar
1	cup chopped onion		Salt and pepper to taste

- Bring broth, 3 cups water, lentils, rice, tomatoes, carrot, onion, celery, garlic, basil, oregano, thyme, and bay leaf to a boil in a large Dutch oven; cover, reduce heat, and simmer, stirring occasionally, 45 to 55 minutes or until lentils and rice are tender. Discard bay leaf.

- Stir in parsley, vinegar, and salt and pepper. Add more broth or water to thin soup, if desired. Cook until thoroughly heated.

Serves 6 to 10

Marchand de Vin Sauce

An elegant sauce-serve over steak.

½	cup butter	1	teaspoon salt
3	tablespoons all-purpose flour	¼	teaspoon ground black pepper
¼	cup minced ham	⅛	teaspoon cayenne pepper
½	cup minced shallots	1	cup beef broth
3	tablespoons minced onion	½	cup dry red wine
4	garlic cloves, minced		

- Melt butter in a heavy saucepan over low heat; gradually stir in flour until smooth. Cook, stirring constantly, until lightly browned.

- Add ham, shallots, onion, and cloves to roux; cook, stirring constantly, 5 minutes. Add salt and peppers.

- Stir in broth and wine and simmer over very low heat 30 minutes.

Serves 8

Jezebel Sauce

1	cup apple jelly	½	teaspoon pepper
5	ounces prepared horseradish	1	cup pineapple preserves
6	ounces prepared mustard		

- Process all ingredients in a food processor or blender until combined.

- Serve sauce with pork or as an appetizer over cream cheese with crackers.

Dr. B's BBQ Sauce

*Use as a baste for the grill, a marinade, or a sauce when
cooking meat in a slow cooker. Great for beef, pork, or chicken.*

2	cups vinegar	2	tablespoons instant minced onion
1	cup ketchup	1½	teaspoons garlic powder
½	cup soy sauce	1-1½	teaspoons hot sauce
1	tablespoon Worcestershire sauce		

- Bring all ingredients to a boil in a saucepan over medium heat, whisking often (do not let burn on bottom). Cover and chill at least 24 hours.

- Store in refrigerator for months.

Henry Bain Sauce

This recipe was created by the head waiter at the Pendennis Club.

1	(12-ounce) bottle chili sauce	1	(1-pound 1-ounce) jar mango chutney, finely chopped or pureed
1	(14-ounce) bottle ketchup		Hot sauce to taste
1	(11-ounce) bottle A.1. steak sauce		
1	(10-ounce) bottle Worcestershire sauce		

- Combine all ingredients, adjusting hot sauce to taste.

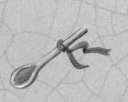

Wing Commander

Wing Commander, another famous four-legged Kentuckian is considered to be the greatest gaited horse the world has ever known. He belonged to Castleton Farms in Lexington, Kentucky.

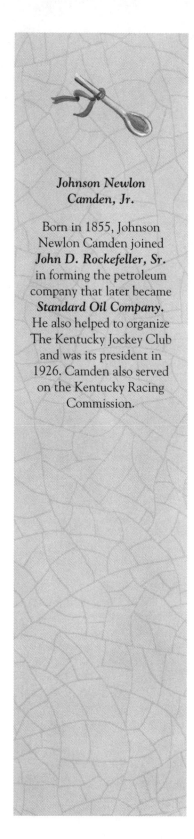

*Johnson Newlon
Camden, Jr.*

Born in 1855, Johnson
Newlon Camden joined
John D. Rockefeller, Sr.
in forming the petroleum
company that later became
Standard Oil Company.
He also helped to organize
The Kentucky Jockey Club
and was its president in
1926. Camden also served
on the Kentucky Racing
Commission.

Pineapple Sauce

Serve with ham or pork.

1	(15-ounce) can crushed pineapple or tidbits	¼	cup firmly packed brown sugar
1	tablespoon cornstarch	½-¾	teaspoon prepared mustard

- Drain pineapple, reserving juice. Add enough water to juice to measure 1 cup. Set pineapple aside.

- Combine cornstarch and juice mixture in a saucepan, stirring until smooth. Add brown sugar and bring to a boil, stirring constantly; boil, stirring constantly, until thickened.

- Stir in mustard and pineapple and cook until thoroughly heated.

Hot Fudge Sauce

Not for the calorie conscious!

6	tablespoons butter	1	cup sugar
1	(1-ounce) unsweetened chocolate square	½	teaspoon salt
⅓	cup milk	½	teaspoon vanilla extract

- Melt butter and chocolate in a saucepan over low heat. Add milk, sugar, and salt and cook, stirring occasionally, 30 minutes or until slightly thickened.

- Remove from heat and let cool. Stir in vanilla.

- Transfer sauce to a glass container and chill. To serve, place in a pan of hot water or microwave at MEDIUM (50% power), stirring often, until warm.

Makes 14 ounces

Decadent Caramel Sauce

Irresistible over ice cream, pound cake, or sautéed fruit

4   cups firmly packed brown sugar   2   cups evaporated milk
2   cups light corn syrup   1   teaspoon vanilla extract
2   tablespoons butter   ½   teaspoon salt

- Cook brown sugar and syrup in a saucepan over medium-high heat, stirring often, 6 minutes or until dissolved. Remove from heat.

- Add butter, stirring until melted. Stir in milk, vanilla, and salt.

- Pour sauce into sterilized jars; screw on lids and chill up to 1 week.

Makes 5 to 6 cups

Cranberry-Wine Relish

Excellent served warm with poultry, pork, or game

3   cups fresh whole cranberries   ¼   cup cold water
1½ cups sugar   1½ tablespoons cornstarch
1¼ cups port wine (we used Paul
    Masson ruby port)

- Bring cranberries, sugar, and port wine to a boil in a large saucepan; boil, stirring occasionally, 5 to 7 minutes or until cranberries pop.

- Combine ¼ cup cold water and cornstarch, stirring until smooth; add to cranberry mixture and return to a boil. Cook, stirring constantly, 1 minute.

- Serve sauce warm.

Serves 12

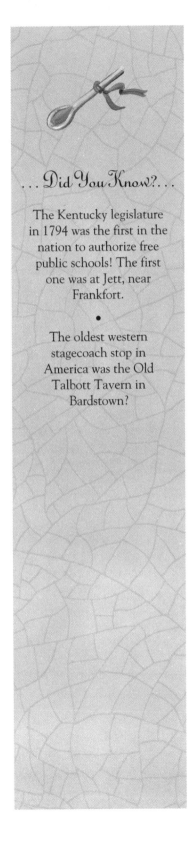

... *Did You Know?* ...

The Kentucky legislature in 1794 was the first in the nation to authorize free public schools! The first one was at Jett, near Frankfort.

•

The oldest western stagecoach stop in America was the Old Talbott Tavern in Bardstown?

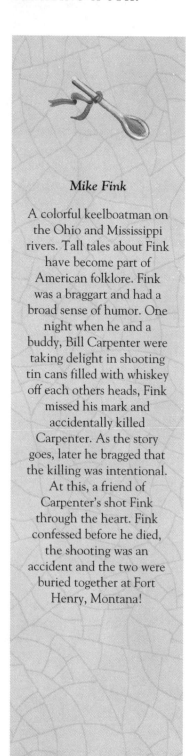

Mike Fink

A colorful keelboatman on the Ohio and Mississippi rivers. Tall tales about Fink have become part of American folklore. Fink was a braggart and had a broad sense of humor. One night when he and a buddy, Bill Carpenter were taking delight in shooting tin cans filled with whiskey off each others heads, Fink missed his mark and accidentally killed Carpenter. As the story goes, later he bragged that the killing was intentional. At this, a friend of Carpenter's shot Fink through the heart. Fink confessed before he died, the shooting was an accident and the two were buried together at Fort Henry, Montana!

Orange-Cranberry Relish

1	(18-ounce) jar orange marmalade	½	cup water, divided
12	ounces fresh whole cranberries	2	tablespoons cornstarch
2	cups sugar		

- Bring marmalade, cranberries, sugar, and ¼ cup water to a boil in a saucepan over medium heat; boil, stirring often, 5 minutes or until cranberries pop.

- Combine remaining ¼ cup water and cornstarch, stirring until smooth; add to cranberry mixture and bring to a boil, stirring constantly. Boil 1 minute.

- Remove relish from heat and let cool. Serve with pork tenderloin.

Cranberry Chutney

Delicious on turkey sandwiches!

4	cups fresh whole cranberries	2	tart apples, peeled and diced
2½	cups sugar	2	pears, peeled and diced
1	cup water	1	small onion, chopped
6	whole cloves	½	cup sliced celery
2	cinnamon sticks	½	cup chopped toasted walnuts
½	teaspoon salt	1	teaspoon grated lemon zest
1	cup golden raisins		

- Bring cranberries, sugar, 1 cup water, cloves, cinnamon, and salt to a boil in a large saucepan; boil, stirring often, 10 minutes. Add raisins, apple, pear, onion, and celery and cook 15 minutes or until thickened.

- Remove from heat and stir in walnuts and lemon zest.

- Pour chutney into hot sterilized jars, filling to ¼ inch from top; wipe jar rims. Cover at once with metal lids and screw on bands. Process in boiling water bath 10 minutes.

Makes 2 quarts

Potatoes, Rice & Beans

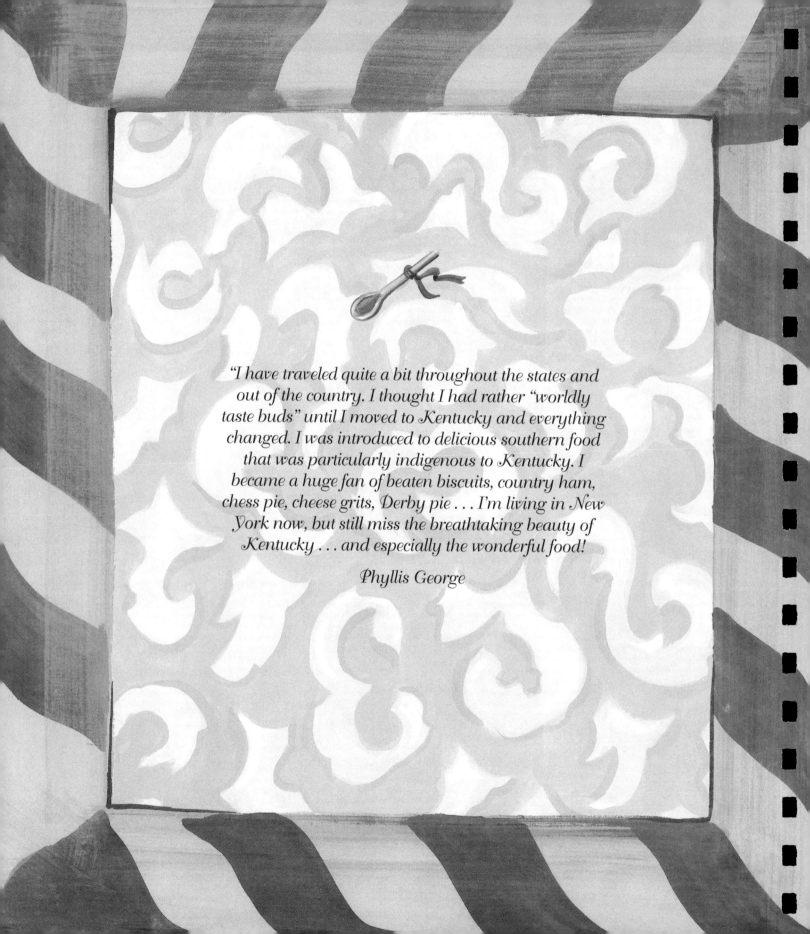

"I have traveled quite a bit throughout the states and out of the country. I thought I had rather "worldly taste buds" until I moved to Kentucky and everything changed. I was introduced to delicious southern food that was particularly indigenous to Kentucky. I became a huge fan of beaten biscuits, country ham, chess pie, cheese grits, Derby pie . . . I'm living in New York now, but still miss the breathtaking beauty of Kentucky . . . and especially the wonderful food!

Phyllis George

Potatoes Boursin

Forget about the leftovers!

5   ounces Boursin cheese with herbs
2   cups whipping cream
3   pounds new potatoes, unpeeled
      and thinly sliced

Salt and pepper to taste
½   tablespoon chopped fresh parsley,
      divided

- Cook cheese and cream in a saucepan over medium heat, stirring constantly, until lumps disappear.
- Arrange half of potato slices in a lightly greased 9 x 13 x 2-inch baking dish, overlapping edges. Sprinkle with salt and pepper and half of parsley.
- Pour half of cheese mixture over potato slices; repeat layers once.
- Bake at 400° for 1 hour or until golden and bubbly.

Serves 8 to 10

Swiss and White Cheddar Scalloped Potatoes

These are fabulous! Wonderfully rich, these potatoes
are guaranteed to win plenty of praise from family and friends.

3   pounds russet potatoes, unpeeled
2   teaspoons salt
1   teaspoon ground white pepper
1   medium onion, chopped
½   cup chopped fresh parsley

1¼ cups (6 ounces) shredded Swiss
      cheese
1¼ cups (6 ounces) shredded white
      cheddar cheese
2   cups half-and-half

- Boil potatoes in water to cover in a large saucepan 30 minutes or just until tender. Drain and let cool. Peel and slice potatoes.
- Arrange half of potato slices in a buttered 9 x 13 x 2-inch baking dish and season with half each of salt and pepper. Top with half each of onion, parsley, and cheeses. Repeat layers once.
- Pour half-and-half over top of mixture.
- Bake, covered, at 350° for 30 minutes. Uncover and bake 45 minutes or until liquid is almost absorbed and top begins to brown. When done, the top should be a pretty golden color all over.
- Remove from oven and let stand at room temperature 15 minutes before serving.

Serves about 12

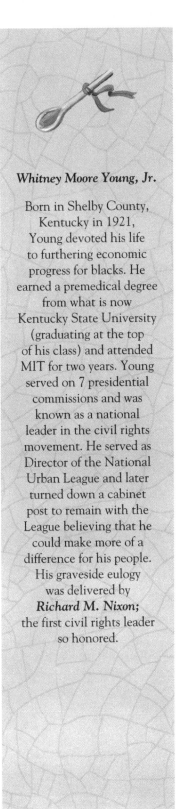

Whitney Moore Young, Jr.

Born in Shelby County, Kentucky in 1921, Young devoted his life to furthering economic progress for blacks. He earned a premedical degree from what is now Kentucky State University (graduating at the top of his class) and attended MIT for two years. Young served on 7 presidential commissions and was known as a national leader in the civil rights movement. He served as Director of the National Urban League and later turned down a cabinet post to remain with the League believing that he could make more of a difference for his people. His graveside eulogy was delivered by *Richard M. Nixon;* the first civil rights leader so honored.

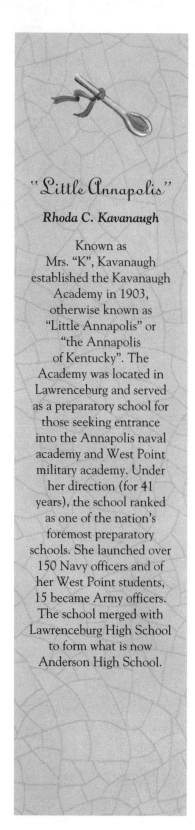

"Little Annapolis"

Rhoda C. Kavanaugh

Known as
Mrs. "K", Kavanaugh
established the Kavanaugh
Academy in 1903,
otherwise known as
"Little Annapolis" or
"the Annapolis
of Kentucky". The
Academy was located in
Lawrenceburg and served
as a preparatory school for
those seeking entrance
into the Annapolis naval
academy and West Point
military academy. Under
her direction (for 41
years), the school ranked
as one of the nation's
foremost preparatory
schools. She launched over
150 Navy officers and of
her West Point students,
15 became Army officers.
The school merged with
Lawrenceburg High School
to form what is now
Anderson High School.

Mashed Potatoes à la Laura

An updated and sophisticated version of the down-home classic . . . soooo good!

9 large baking potatoes, peeled and diced	12 ounces cream cheese, cut into pieces and softened
6 garlic cloves, halved	¾ cup sour cream
½ cup unsalted butter, cut into pieces and softened	¼ cup whipping cream
	Salt and pepper to taste
	Butter, cut into pieces

- Bring potato and garlic to a boil in water to cover in a large saucepan; reduce heat to medium and simmer until tender. Drain and discard garlic.

- Beat potato, butter, and cream cheese at medium speed with an electric mixer until light and fluffy. Add sour cream and whipping cream, beating well. Season with salt and pepper.

- Spoon mixture into a buttered baking dish and dot with butter.

- Bake at 300° for 20 minutes.

Serves 6 to 8

Gratin Dauphinois

Gloriously rich and elegant! Pair these with beef tenderloin for a spectacular meal.

1 garlic clove, halved	½ teaspoon pepper
1 tablespoon butter, softened	⅛ teaspoon freshly grated or ground nutmeg
1 (2½-pound) bag baking potatoes, peeled and thinly sliced	1 cup (4 ounces) grated Gruyère or Fontinella cheese
3 cups half-and-half	
1 teaspoon salt	

- Preheat oven to 350°.

- Rub a 12-inch gratin dish or shallow 3-quart baking dish with garlic; let dry. Coat with softened butter.

- Bring sliced potatoes, half-and-half, salt, pepper, and nutmeg to a boil in a large saucepan over medium heat, stirring constantly; cook, stirring constantly, 5 minutes or until liquid thickens slightly. Pour into prepared dish.

- Press down potato slices to submerge in liquid; sprinkle with cheese.

- Bake at 350° for 45 to 60 minutes or until potato slices are tender and top is golden.

Serves 6 to 8

Roquefort Baked Potatoes

6	baking potatoes	1	cup sour cream
	Vegetable oil	1	tablespoon chopped fresh parsley
½-¾	cup Roquefort cheese, crumbled	1	teaspoon salt

- Rub potatoes with oil.

- Bake at 400° for 1 hour or until tender.

- Combine cheese, sour cream, parsley, and salt in a bowl, stirring well.

- Remove potatoes from oven and cut a slit lengthwise and crosswise in each; press sides to enlarge opening. Fill each "pocket" with cheese mixture.

- Broil 4 inches from heat (with electric oven door partially open) 3 to 5 minutes or until cheese melts and potatoes are thoroughly heated.

Makes 6 potatoes

Southern Potatoes

A great side for summer dishes, outdoor cooking, picnics

6	medium potatoes or 4 baking potatoes, unpeeled	½	cup chopped green onions
¼	cup butter	1	teaspoon salt
2	cups (8 ounces) shredded sharp cheddar cheese	¼	teaspoon pepper
		2	tablespoons butter
1½	cups sour cream, at room temperature		Paprika to taste

- Boil potatoes in water to cover in a large saucepan until tender. Drain and let cool. Peel and coarsely shred.

- Cook ¼ cup butter and cheese in a saucepan over low heat, stirring constantly, until melted. Remove from heat and stir in sour cream, green onions, salt, and pepper.

- Fold shredded potato into cheese sauce (it will be stiff). Spoon mixture into a large greased baking dish. Dot with 2 tablespoons butter and sprinkle with paprika.

- Bake at 350° for 30 minutes.

Serves 8 to 10

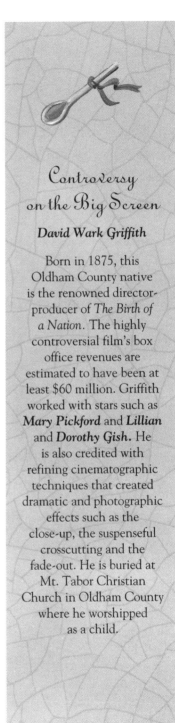

Controversy on the Big Screen
David Wark Griffith

Born in 1875, this Oldham County native is the renowned director-producer of *The Birth of a Nation*. The highly controversial film's box office revenues are estimated to have been at least $60 million. Griffith worked with stars such as **Mary Pickford** and **Lillian** and **Dorothy Gish.** He is also credited with refining cinematographic techniques that created dramatic and photographic effects such as the close-up, the suspenseful crosscutting and the fade-out. He is buried at Mt. Tabor Christian Church in Oldham County where he worshipped as a child.

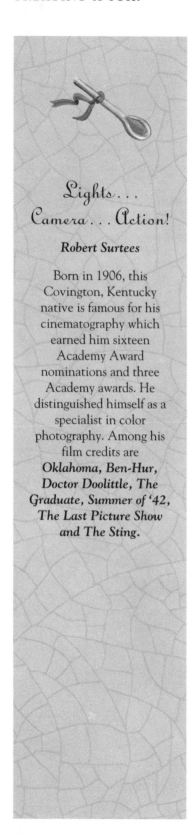

Twice Baked Spinach Potatoes

Omit the spinach for traditional twice baked potatoes-they're tasty either way!

4	baking potatoes	12	ounces sour cream
1	pound bacon, cooked and crumbled	1	teaspoon salt
½	cup chopped green onions	½	teaspoon pepper
1	cup (4 ounces) shredded cheddar cheese	1	(10-ounce) package frozen chopped spinach, cooked and well drained

- Bake potatoes at 400° for 1 hour or until tender. Remove from oven and let cool slightly.
- Cut potatoes in half and scoop out pulp, reserving shells. Combine pulp, bacon, green onions, cheddar cheese, sour cream, salt, pepper, and spinach in a large bowl, stirring well.
- Spoon mixture into shells and place on a baking sheet.
- Bake at 400° for 20 to 30 minutes.

Makes 8

Blue Cheese Tossed Potatoes

Yummy! Blue cheese fans will request them again and again!

3	pounds tiny new potatoes	3-4	ounces crumbled blue cheese
1½	tablespoons butter	¾	teaspoon salt
1½	cups chopped green onions	¼	teaspoon ground white pepper
1	cup plus 2 tablespoons whipping cream	8-10	bacon slices, cooked crisp and crumbled
1½	tablespoons all-purpose flour	3	tablespoons chopped fresh parsley

- Cook potatoes in boiling water to cover in a saucepan 15 minutes or until tender. Drain and quarter.
- Combine potatoes, butter, and green onions in a large bowl, tossing to coat.
- Whisk together whipping cream and flour in a saucepan; stir in cheese. Cook over medium heat, stirring constantly, until thickened. Stir in salt and pepper.
- Pour cheese mixture over potatoes, tossing gently. Sprinkle with bacon and parsley; toss gently and serve immediately.

Serves 8

Swiss Potatoes

1½ cups (6 ounces) shredded Swiss cheese
  Salt to taste
¼ teaspoon pepper
1 tablespoon butter

1 cup whipping cream
½ small onion, chopped
6 medium-size red potatoes, peeled and sliced

- Combine Swiss cheese, salt, pepper, butter, whipping cream, and onion in a bowl, stirring well.
- Layer half of potato slices in a 3-quart baking dish; top with half of sauce. Repeat layers once.
- Bake at 325° for 1 hour to 1 hour and 30 minutes.

Serves 6 to 8

Baked Yams with Lime and Honey

A pleasing addition to any ethnic dish.

3 large yams or sweet potatoes
½ cup water
6 tablespoons honey
¼ cup unsalted butter, softened

Juice of 4 limes
1½ teaspoons salt
½ teaspoon freshly ground black pepper

- Preheat oven to 350°.
- Place yams and ½ cup water in a baking dish.
- Bake at 350° for 1 hour and 30 minutes or until soft. Remove from oven and let cool slightly.
- Peel yams and place in a 2-quart baking dish; add honey, butter, lime juice, salt, and pepper, mashing with a potato masher (a few lumps are okay). Cover with aluminum foil.
- Bake 15 to 20 minutes.

Serves 8

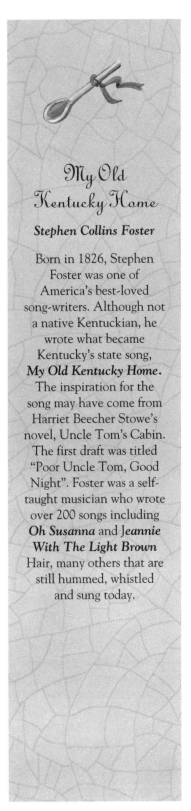

My Old Kentucky Home

Stephen Collins Foster

Born in 1826, Stephen Foster was one of America's best-loved song-writers. Although not a native Kentuckian, he wrote what became Kentucky's state song, **My Old Kentucky Home**. The inspiration for the song may have come from Harriet Beecher Stowe's novel, Uncle Tom's Cabin. The first draft was titled "Poor Uncle Tom, Good Night". Foster was a self-taught musician who wrote over 200 songs including **Oh Susanna** and **Jeannie With The Light Brown Hair**, many others that are still hummed, whistled and sung today.

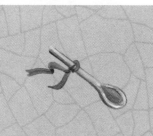

Mary Todd Lincoln

Mary Todd Lincoln, born in Lexington, Kentucky in 1818, was the granddaughter of Levi Todd, founder of Lexington, and the wife of Abraham Lincoln, our sixteenth president. Mary made a profound impact on Lincoln by polishing his social graces, reading books and reviewing them for him; and by researching the historical aspects of slavery so that he might be familiar with current events. She took notes on his speeches and made suggestions which ultimately put him in the White house. By today's standards, Mary would be regarded as bright, talented, ambitious and articulate. Mary's life in the White House was anything but glamorous. Many suspected her of disloyalty to the Union because of her southern upbringing and her haughty manner made her unpopular among government official wives.

Mashed Sweets with Pecan Praline

A nice change from the traditional sweet potato casserole

6	cups mashed sweet potato	½	cup honey
½	cup sour cream	2½	teaspoons ground cinnamon
¾	cup firmly packed brown sugar		Pecan Praline

- Combine sweet potato, sour cream, brown sugar, honey, and cinnamon in a bowl, stirring well. Spoon into a 9 x 13 x 2-inch baking dish.
- Bake at 350° for 20 to 30 minutes.
- Sprinkle with Pecan Praline and serve.

Pecan Praline

1½	cups coarsely chopped pecans	½	cup water
1	cup sugar		

- Place pecans on a baking sheet.
- Bake at 350°, stirring occasionally, 15 minutes or until toasted.
- Cook sugar and ½ cup water in a saucepan over medium heat, stirring until sugar is dissolved; increase heat to high and bring to a boil. Cook, stirring constantly, until mixture is a golden/amber color.
- Stir toasted nuts into sugar mixture and pour onto a lightly greased aluminum foil-lined baking sheet. Let cool completely.
- Chop cooled mixture finely.

Serves 10 to 14

Orange Herbed Rice

A wonderful side for citrus marinated poultry or beef.

2	tablespoons butter	¾	teaspoon dried thyme
⅓	cup chopped onion	1	teaspoon dried parsley
2	cups water	1	cup uncooked long-grain rice
¾	cup orange juice		

- Melt butter in a saucepan over medium heat; add onion and sauté until tender. Add 2 cups water, orange juice, thyme, and parsley and bring to a boil.
- Stir rice into boiling mixture; cover, reduce heat, and simmer 20 to 30 minutes or until liquid is absorbed.

Serves 6

California Rice Casserole

Everyone loves this dish! Preparing it ahead makes it ideal for company.

¼	cup butter	2	teaspoons salt
1	cup chopped onion	1	teaspoon pepper
4	cups cooked white converted rice	2	(4.5-ounce) cans chopped green chiles
1	(16-ounce) container sour cream	3	cups (12 ounces) shredded cheddar cheese
1	cup cottage cheese		
1	bay leaf		

- Melt butter in a skillet over medium heat; add onion and sauté 5 to 10 minutes or until golden.

- Combine onion, cooked rice, sour cream, cottage cheese, bay leaf, salt, and pepper in a large bowl, tossing lightly to blend.

- Layer half of rice mixture in a baking dish; top with chiles and sprinkle with half of cheese. Top with remaining rice mixture.

- Bake at 375° for 25 minutes.

- Sprinkle with remaining cheese and bake 15 more minutes.

Serves 10 to 12

Wild Rice and Prosciutto Dressing

Serve with poultry or pork in place of typical bread dressing.

⅓	cup uncooked wild rice, rinsed	½	cup chopped onion
1¼	cups water	½	cup chopped pecan pieces
⅓	cup brown rice	2	ounces prosciutto, chopped (½ cup)
½	teaspoon chicken bouillon granules	2	tablespoons chopped fresh parsley
1½	cups sliced fresh mushrooms	¼	cup ice water

- Bring wild rice, 1¼ cups water, brown rice, and bouillon granules to a boil in a medium saucepan over medium-high heat; cover, reduce heat, and simmer 45 minutes.

- Add mushrooms and onion; increase heat to medium and cook, covered, 10 minutes, stirring often.

- Stir in pecans, prosciutto, parsley, and ¼ cup ice water; transfer mixture to a 1-quart baking dish.

- Bake, covered, at 370° for 30 minutes.

Serves 8

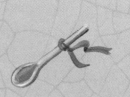

With a Bible in One Hand, and a Hatchet in the Other . . .

Carry Nation

Born in Garrard County, Kentucky in 1846, Nation became a violent crusader against alcohol, her intolerance evolving from her bitter marriage to a drunkard. Nation, always seen with a bible in one hand and an ax in the other, was arrested 30 times for her destructive protests, for disturbing the peace and harassing saloon owners across the United States. She carried her temperance crusade from the level of education to that of action and helped bring on national prohibition in 1919.

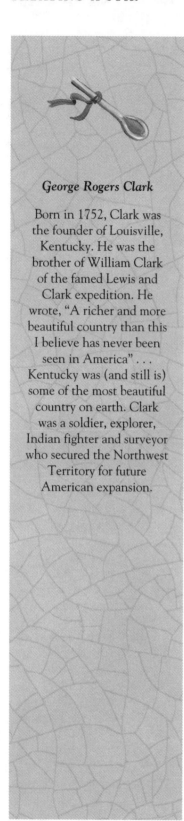

George Rogers Clark

Born in 1752, Clark was the founder of Louisville, Kentucky. He was the brother of William Clark of the famed Lewis and Clark expedition. He wrote, "A richer and more beautiful country than this I believe has never been seen in America" . . . Kentucky was (and still is) some of the most beautiful country on earth. Clark was a soldier, explorer, Indian fighter and surveyor who secured the Northwest Territory for future American expansion.

Exotic Rice

The perfect accompaniment for beef!

½	cup margarine	1	can French onion soup
1	(8-ounce) package fresh mushrooms, sliced	¼	teaspoon curry powder
1	cup uncooked long-grain rice (we used Uncle Ben's)	½	teaspoon salt
		½	teaspoon pepper
1	can sliced water chestnuts, chopped	½	cup slivered almonds (optional)

- Melt margarine in a saucepan over medium heat; add mushrooms and sauté until tender.

- Add rice, water chestnuts, onion soup, curry, salt, pepper, and, if desired, almonds to mushrooms, stirring well. Spoon into a 2-quart baking dish and cover.

- Bake at 350° for 1 hour, stirring after 30 minutes and adding water if needed.

Serves 4 to 6

Coastal-Style Rice

Pretty and flavorful!

2	cups uncooked rice	1½	cups chopped carrot
¼	onion, cut into chunks	4	cups hot water
3	garlic cloves, minced	2	teaspoons salt
½	cup water	1½	cups corn
	Vegetable oil	2	cups coarsely chopped cabbage

- Soak rice in warm water to cover in a saucepan 5 minutes; drain and return to pan.

- Puree onion, garlic, ½ cup water, and a small amount of oil in a blender until transparent; pour off excess oil.

- Add onion mixture, carrot, 4 cups hot water, and salt to rice; bring to a boil.

- Add corn and cabbage to rice mixture and cook, covered, over medium-low heat 20 to 30 minutes or until rice is tender.

Serves 6

Green Rice

An interesting combination of ingredients gives this easy recipe a superb twist!

1	small onion, peeled and quartered	2	cups chicken broth, divided
2	poblano chile peppers, deveined, seeded, and quartered		Salt and pepper to taste
3	garlic cloves	1	cup uncooked long-grain rice, rinsed
1	cup fresh cilantro	2	tablespoons vegetable oil

- Process onion, chile peppers, garlic, cilantro, and 1 cup broth in a blender until pureed; pour through a wire-mesh strainer, discarding solids. Season with salt and pepper.
- Sauté rice in hot oil in a heavy saucepan over medium-low heat, stirring constantly, 2 minutes. Add onion mixture and remaining 1 cup broth.
- Cover and simmer 20 minutes. Remove from heat and let stand, covered, at room temperature 10 minutes before serving.

Serves 4

Three-Bean Bake

2	garlic cloves, chopped	1	(15.5-ounce) can small green lima beans, drained
3	medium onions, chopped		
¼	cup canola oil	1	(15.5-ounce) can red kidney beans, drained
½	cup firmly packed brown sugar		
¼	cup vinegar	1	(15.5-ounce) can pinto beans, drained
½	cup ketchup		
1	teaspoon dry mustard	1	teaspoon salt
		½	teaspoon pepper

- Sauté garlic and onion in hot oil in a large skillet over medium heat until tender (do not brown).
- Add brown sugar, vinegar, ketchup, mustard, lima beans, kidney beans, pinto beans, salt, and pepper to onion mixture, stirring well. Spoon into a 2-quart baking dish.
- Bake at 350° for 45 to 60 minutes, covering with aluminum foil the last 15 minutes if necessary to prevent over browning.

This can also be baked at 300° for 1 to 2 hours for a richer flavor. This recipe can be doubled or tripled.

Serves 8

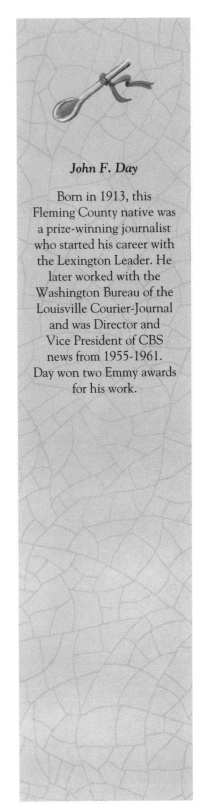

John F. Day

Born in 1913, this Fleming County native was a prize-winning journalist who started his career with the Lexington Leader. He later worked with the Washington Bureau of the Louisville Courier-Journal and was Director and Vice President of CBS news from 1955-1961. Day won two Emmy awards for his work.

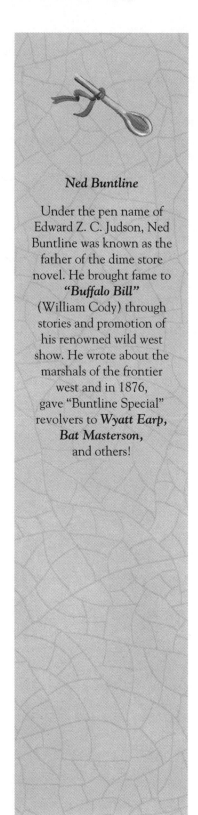

Fresh Tomato and Basil Risotto with Mozzarella

*A salad and crusty bread turns this
tempting side dish into a delightful main course for two.*

1½ cups diced plum tomato
2 tablespoons chopped fresh basil
1 tablespoon olive oil
½ teaspoon salt
1 garlic clove, crushed
42 ounces chicken broth
½ cup finely chopped onion
2 teaspoons olive oil

1½ cups uncooked Arborio rice
⅓ cup dry white wine
½ cup (2 ounces) diced mozzarella
   cheese
½ teaspoon ground pepper
3 tablespoons freshly grated Parmesan
   cheese

- Combine tomato, basil, oil, salt, and garlic in a small bowl; set aside.

- Bring broth to a simmer in a medium saucepan; keep warm over low heat.

- Sauté onion in 2 teaspoons hot oil in a large saucepan over high heat 3 minutes.
  Add rice and cook, stirring constantly, 1 minute.

- Add wine to rice mixture and cook, stirring constantly, until liquid is nearly
  absorbed. Add warm broth, ½ cup at a time, cooking until each portion is absorbed
  before adding more.

- Add tomato mixture to rice mixture, stirring well. Remove from heat and stir in
  mozzarella and pepper.

- Sprinkle with Parmesan cheese and serve.

Serves 4 to 6

Kentucky Bourbon Baked Beans

4 No. 2 cans baked beans
1 tablespoon molasses
¼ teaspoon dry mustard
½ cup chili sauce
½ cup bourbon

⅓ cup strong-brewed coffee
1 small can crushed pineapple
½ cup firmly packed brown sugar
   Bacon slices, cooked crisp

- Combine beans, molasses, mustard, chili sauce, bourbon, and coffee in a baking dish,
  stirring well. Let stand at room temperature 3 hours.

- Bake at 300° for 30 minutes.

- Add pineapple and brown sugar, stirring well. Bake 30 more minutes.

- Top with crisp bacon slices and serve.

Hoppin' John with Country Ham Bits and Shredded White Cheddar

Don't reserve this bountiful dish for New Year's-it's great anytime! White cheddar and country ham add a unique and distinctive flavor to this traditional favorite.

1 (16-ounce) package dried black-eyed peas
1 large onion, coarsely chopped
1 small green bell pepper, coarsely chopped
3 garlic cloves, crushed
½ pound country ham bits
3 tablespoons vegetable oil
2 (14.5-ounce) cans Cajun-style diced tomatoes

2 dashes of dried crushed red pepper
1 teaspoon ground cumin
2 tablespoons chopped fresh chives
2 teaspoons coarsely ground black pepper
1 teaspoon salt
Hot cooked brown rice
Shredded white cheddar cheese

- Sort peas and soak in water to cover overnight; drain, reserving liquid. Set peas and liquid aside.
- Cook onion, bell pepper, garlic, and country ham bits in hot oil in a saucepan over medium heat until onion is translucent. Add diced tomatoes, red pepper, cumin, chives, black pepper, and salt; cover, reduce heat, and simmer, stirring often, 2 hours.
- Add peas and some of reserved liquid; simmer 45 minutes or until peas are tender, adding more reserved liquid if needed.
- Serve over hot cooked brown rice and sprinkle with cheese.

Serves 8 to 10

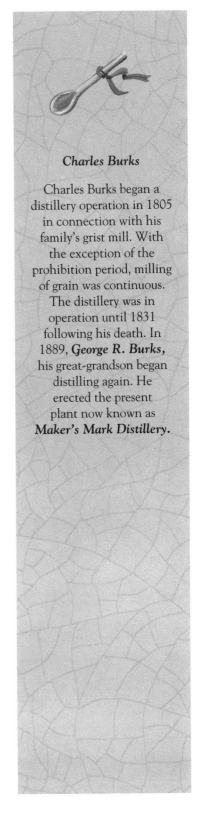

Charles Burks

Charles Burks began a distillery operation in 1805 in connection with his family's grist mill. With the exception of the prohibition period, milling of grain was continuous. The distillery was in operation until 1831 following his death. In 1889, *George R. Burks,* his great-grandson began distilling again. He erected the present plant now known as *Maker's Mark Distillery.*

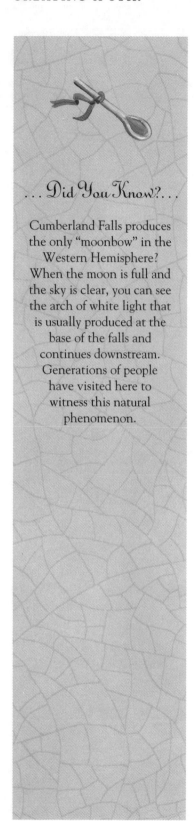

Cajun Red Beans and Andouille Sausage

A Southern staple with many variations. You won't be disappointed with this one!

2	cups dried red beans	1	medium onion, chopped
1	pound andouille sausage	1	cup chopped celery (3 ribs)
8	cups water	1	teaspoon black pepper
1	garlic clove, minced	2	teaspoons Tony Chacheres
½	pound smoked sausage		seasoning

- Sort beans and soak in water to cover in a Dutch oven overnight.

- Simmer andouille sausage in a small amount of water 20 minutes or until cooked.

- Drain beans and add 8 cups water; bring to a boil and add garlic, sausage, onion, celery, black pepper, and seasoning. Return to a boil; reduce heat and simmer 4 hours.

Serves 10

Beef and Mushroom Barley

*A delightful dish with a delicate roasted nut taste-
wonderful to accompany grilled salmon or most meats.*

1	(8-ounce) package fresh mushrooms, sliced	1	(15-ounce) can beef broth
1	large onion	1	tablespoon chopped fresh parsley
	Vegetable oil	1	teaspoon onion salt
1	cup dried barley (not quick cooking)		Ground pepper to taste

- Sauté mushrooms and onion in hot oil in a skillet over medium heat until tender.

- Combine onion mixture, barley, beef broth, parsley, salt, and pepper in a 2-quart baking dish.

- Bake at 350° for 1 hour.

Serves 6

Vegetables

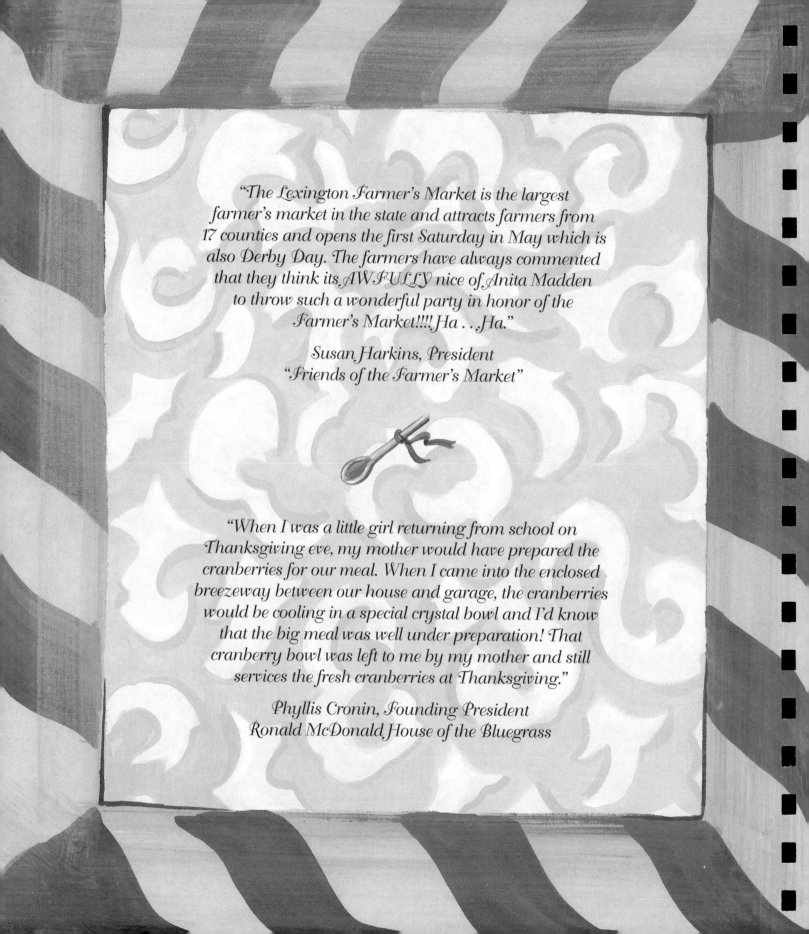

"The Lexington Farmer's Market is the largest farmer's market in the state and attracts farmers from 17 counties and opens the first Saturday in May which is also Derby Day. The farmers have always commented that they think its AWFULLY nice of Anita Madden to throw such a wonderful party in honor of the Farmer's Market!!!! Ha . . . Ha."

Susan Harkins, President
"Friends of the Farmer's Market"

"When I was a little girl returning from school on Thanksgiving eve, my mother would have prepared the cranberries for our meal. When I came into the enclosed breezeway between our house and garage, the cranberries would be cooling in a special crystal bowl and I'd know that the big meal was well under preparation! That cranberry bowl was left to me by my mother and still services the fresh cranberries at Thanksgiving."

Phyllis Cronin, Founding President
Ronald McDonald House of the Bluegrass

Elegant Broccoli and Walnuts

These simple ingredients turn plain broccoli into a showy side dish.

1½-2	pounds fresh broccoli, cut into short spears or florets	1	cup chopped walnuts
1	pound bacon	¾	cup sliced green onions

- Place broccoli in a steamer basket over boiling water; cover and cook 8 to 10 minutes or until crisp-tender. Keep warm.
- Cook bacon in a skillet over medium heat until crisp; drain, reserving 1 tablespoon drippings in skillet. Crumble bacon and set aside.
- Cook walnuts in reserved drippings in skillet over medium heat, stirring constantly, 3 to 5 minutes (do not burn). Add green onions and cook, stirring constantly, 3 minutes.
- Transfer warm broccoli to a serving platter; spoon walnut mixture over top. Sprinkle with bacon.

Serves 4 to 6

Lemon-Carrot Bundles

Guests will be impressed when served these elegant bundles!

2	pounds carrots, cut into 3-inch sticks	7	tablespoons butter
10	green onions, white part trimmed	3½	tablespoons sugar
⅔	cup fresh lemon juice	¾	teaspoon salt

- Place carrot sticks in a steamer basket over boiling water; cover and steam 8 to 10 minutes or until crisp-tender. Rinse immediately with cold water. Pat dry with paper towels and separate into 10 bundles.
- Dip green onion stems in boiling water 30 seconds. Tie 1 around each carrot bundle; double knot and trim green onions as needed.
- Bring lemon juice, butter, sugar, and salt to a boil in a large saucepan; reduce heat and simmer until sugar is dissolved.
- Carefully add carrot bundles to lemon mixture and cook, basting often, just until thoroughly heated.
- Carefully remove bundles with a spatula and serve immediately.

Serves 10

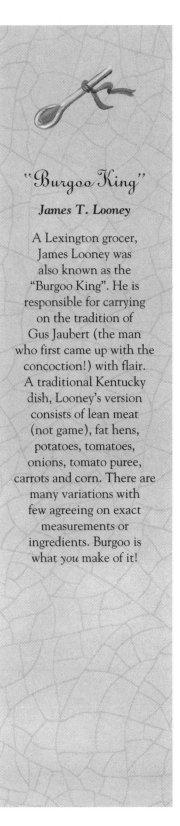

"Burgoo King"

James T. Looney

A Lexington grocer, James Looney was also known as the "Burgoo King". He is responsible for carrying on the tradition of Gus Jaubert (the man who first came up with the concoction!) with flair. A traditional Kentucky dish, Looney's version consists of lean meat (not game), fat hens, potatoes, tomatoes, onions, tomato puree, carrots and corn. There are many variations with few agreeing on exact measurements or ingredients. Burgoo is what *you* make of it!

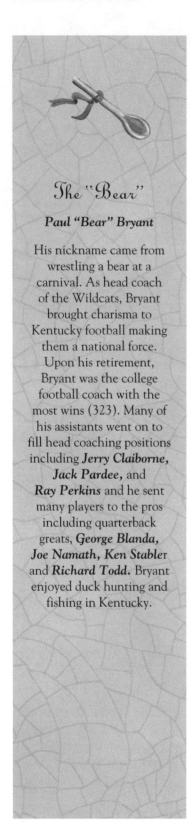

The "Bear"

Paul "Bear" Bryant

His nickname came from wrestling a bear at a carnival. As head coach of the Wildcats, Bryant brought charisma to Kentucky football making them a national force. Upon his retirement, Bryant was the college football coach with the most wins (323). Many of his assistants went on to fill head coaching positions including *Jerry Claiborne, Jack Pardee,* and *Ray Perkins* and he sent many players to the pros including quarterback greats, *George Blanda, Joe Namath, Ken Stabler* and *Richard Todd.* Bryant enjoyed duck hunting and fishing in Kentucky.

Mexican Corn Bake

Olé! This corn bake has pizazz!

1	cup butter	4	(16-ounce) cans shoepeg corn, drained
2	(8-ounce) packages cream cheese	2	cups (8 ounces) shredded cheddar cheese
⅓	cup milk		
2	(4.5-ounce) cans chopped green chiles		

- Melt butter in a saucepan over medium heat; add cream cheese, stirring until melted. Add milk, stirring well.
- Add chiles and corn to cream cheese sauce, stirring well. Pour into a greased 9 x 13 x 2-inch baking dish. Sprinkle with cheese.
- Bake at 350° for 40 to 45 minutes.

Serves 10

Squash Lafayette

A beautiful dish . . . especially nice for a buffet dinner!

2	pounds yellow squash, trimmed and cut into ½-inch slices	1	cup sour cream
¾	cup butter	1	medium onion, chopped
1	(8-ounce) package herb-seasoned stuffing mix, divided	2	carrots, grated
1	(10¾-ounce) can cream of chicken soup, undiluted	1	(2-ounce) jar diced pimiento, drained

- Preheat oven to 350°.
- Boil squash in water to cover in a saucepan 15 to 20 minutes or until tender; drain.
- Melt butter in a large skillet over medium heat; add half of stuffing mix, chicken soup, sour cream, onion, carrot, and pimiento, stirring well. Stir in squash and spoon into a 7 x 11 x 2-inch baking dish.
- Top with remaining stuffing mix and cover with aluminum foil.
- Bake at 350° for 45 minutes or until browned.

Serves 8 to 10

Snow Peas with Shallots and Basil

1 pound fresh snow peas, with strings removed	¼ cup beef bouillon granules
¼ cup butter	Salt and freshly ground pepper to taste
2 tablespoons minced shallots	2 tablespoons chopped fresh basil

- Place snow peas in a steamer basket over boiling water; cover and cook 2 to 3 minutes or until crisp-tender.

- Melt butter in a skillet over medium heat; add shallots and sauté a few minutes. Add bouillon and cook until shallots are tender.

- Increase heat to medium-high and add snow peas to skillet; cook, tossing constantly, 1 minute.

- Season with salt and pepper. Sprinkle with basil and serve.

Serves 4

Zucchini Casserole

This side dish is rich enough to serve in larger portions as a main dish. The combination of peppers, zucchini, and tomatoes with taco seasoning is filling and satisfying.

3 zucchini, cut into ½-inch slices	1½ cups (6 ounces) shredded sharp cheddar cheese
½ onion, cut into rings or strips	
1 green bell pepper, cut into strips	Butter, cut into pieces
1-2 tomatoes, cut into eighths	½ (1¼-ounce) envelope taco seasoning mix
Salt and pepper to taste	
	Buttery round crackers, crushed

- Place zucchini in a greased 7 x 11 x 2-inch baking dish; layer onion, bell pepper, and tomato on top. Season with salt and pepper.

- Sprinkle with cheese and dot with butter. Sprinkle with taco seasoning mix and cover with aluminum foil.

- Bake at 350° for 45 to 60 minutes or until vegetables are tender.

- Sprinkle with crushed crackers to cover and dot with butter. Bake 5 to 10 minutes or until browned.

Serves 6 to 8

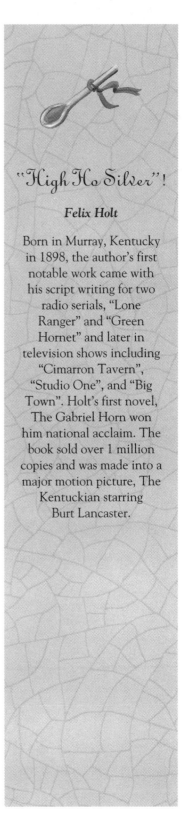

"High Ho Silver"!

Felix Holt

Born in Murray, Kentucky in 1898, the author's first notable work came with his script writing for two radio serials, "Lone Ranger" and "Green Hornet" and later in television shows including "Cimarron Tavern", "Studio One", and "Big Town". Holt's first novel, The Gabriel Horn won him national acclaim. The book sold over 1 million copies and was made into a major motion picture, The Kentuckian starring Burt Lancaster.

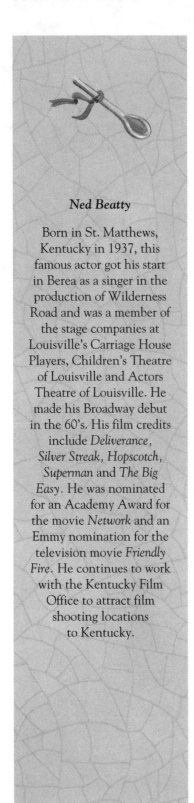

Sautéed Zucchini and Potato Garnish

A new and delicious way to serve zucchini

2 cups red waxy potatoes, cut into ½-inch cubes
2 tablespoons olive oil
1½ cups zucchini, cut into ⅛-inch slices

Salt and pepper to taste
2 teaspoons finely chopped garlic
1 tablespoon chopped fresh chives

- Boil cubed potato in salted water to cover in a saucepan 3 minutes; drain.

- Transfer to a nonstick skillet and cook in hot oil, stirring constantly, until lightly browned. Add zucchini and season with salt and pepper; cook, stirring constantly, a few minutes.

- Add garlic to mixture and cook until zucchini is tender. Sprinkle with chives and serve.

Serves 4

Oriental Green Beans

This alluring side dish always gets rave reviews!

½-1 pound green beans, trimmed
1 tablespoon chopped green onions
2 garlic cloves, minced
3 thinly sliced ginger strips
3 tablespoons sesame oil

1 teaspoon sugar
½ teaspoon salt
2 tablespoons soy sauce
¼ cup water

- Boil green beans in water to cover in a saucepan 3 to 4 minutes; drain. Plunge into cold water and drain.

- Sauté green onions, garlic, and ginger in hot oil in a skillet over high heat 1 minute. Add sugar, salt, and soy sauce and cook, stirring constantly, until sugar is dissolved.

- Add beans and ¼ cup water to skillet; reduce heat to medium and cook 3 minutes.

Serves 4 to 6

Zucchini and Walnuts

Very pretty . . . a splendid summer dish!

¼	cup butter	½	teaspoon lemon juice
½	cup walnut pieces	1	teaspoon salt
2½	cups coarsely shredded zucchini	½	teaspoon pepper

- Melt butter in a skillet over medium heat; add walnuts and cook, stirring constantly, until toasted (do not burn). Transfer to a bowl, reserving drippings in skillet.
- Sauté zucchini in hot drippings 30 to 60 seconds; sprinkle with lemon juice. Remove from heat and add walnuts, tossing well.

Recipe can be doubled and heaped around beef tenderloin on a platter for an elegant display.

Serves 4

Spicy Jalapeño - Broccoli Bake

Broccoli with a zip!

1	(10-ounce) package frozen chopped broccoli, thawed	1	large egg
1	can cream-style corn	½	teaspoon salt
1	teaspoon chopped onion	¼	teaspoon pepper
¼	cup butter	1	cup herb-seasoned stuffing mix (we used Pepperidge Farms)
1-2	jalapeño peppers, seeded and chopped	¼	cup butter, melted
		2	bacon slices, cooked and crumbled.

- Combine broccoli, corn, onion, butter, jalapeño pepper, egg, salt, and pepper; pour into a greased baking dish.
- Combine stuffing mix, melted butter, and bacon; sprinkle over broccoli mixture.
- Bake at 350° for 1 hour.

Serves 4 to 5

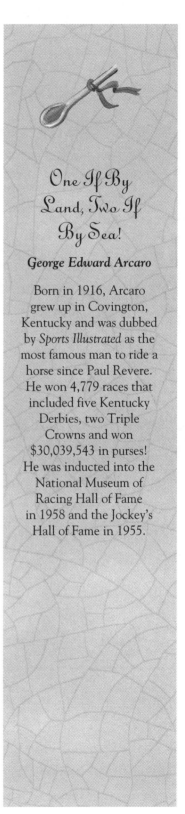

One If By Land, Two If By Sea!

George Edward Arcaro

Born in 1916, Arcaro grew up in Covington, Kentucky and was dubbed by *Sports Illustrated* as the most famous man to ride a horse since Paul Revere. He won 4,779 races that included five Kentucky Derbies, two Triple Crowns and won $30,039,543 in purses! He was inducted into the National Museum of Racing Hall of Fame in 1958 and the Jockey's Hall of Fame in 1955.

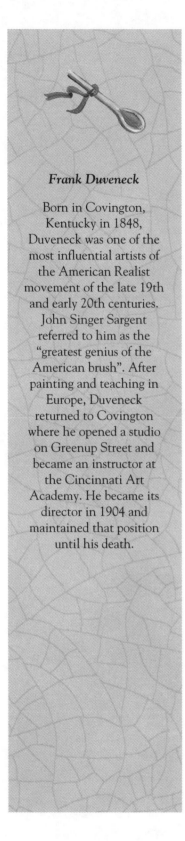

Frank Duveneck

Born in Covington, Kentucky in 1848, Duveneck was one of the most influential artists of the American Realist movement of the late 19th and early 20th centuries. John Singer Sargent referred to him as the "greatest genius of the American brush". After painting and teaching in Europe, Duveneck returned to Covington where he opened a studio on Greenup Street and became an instructor at the Cincinnati Art Academy. He became its director in 1904 and maintained that position until his death.

Sautéed Sesame-Ginger Spinach

1	tablespoon freshly grated ginger		Salt and pepper to taste
2	tablespoons sesame oil	1	tablespoon sesame seeds (optional)
2	(10-ounce) packages fresh spinach, stemmed if desired		

- Sauté ginger in hot oil in a Dutch oven over medium heat 30 seconds. Add 1 package of spinach and toss to coat. Add remaining package of spinach and toss to coat; cook until spinach is wilted.
- Season with salt and pepper and transfer to a serving dish.
- Cook sesame seeds in a nonstick skillet over medium-high heat until golden brown and toasted, if desired. Sprinkle over spinach.

Serves 6

Garlic and Onion Simmered Green Beans

1	large garlic clove, chopped	1	bunch cilantro, chopped
1	medium onion, chopped	1½	cups water
2	tablespoons olive oil		Salt and pepper to taste
1½	pounds green beans		

- Sauté garlic and onion in hot oil in a large saucepan until tender; add cilantro and cook 2 to 3 minutes.
- Add green beans and 1½ cups water; cover and cook until tender. Season with salt and pepper.

Serves 4 to 6

Szechuan Broccoli

Enticing!

6	tablespoons water	1	tablespoon minced fresh ginger
¼	cup sherry	3	garlic cloves, minced
4	teaspoons soy sauce	1	teaspoon sesame oil
2	tablespoons hoisin sauce	2	bunches broccoli, cut into florets
2	teaspoons cornstarch		

- Combine 6 tablespoons water, sherry, soy sauce, hoisin sauce, and cornstarch, stirring well.

- Sauté ginger and garlic in hot oil in a large skillet 1 minute; add broccoli and cook, stirring constantly, 5 to 7 minutes or until crisp-tender. Add sherry mixture and cook, stirring constantly, until coated.

Serves 6 to 8

Broccoli and Cauliflower Gratin

Vegetables are smothered in a creamy cheese sauce, then baked to perfection.

2	tablespoons butter	1	(10-ounce) package frozen broccoli florets, cooked and well drained
1	cup chopped onion		
2	tablespoons all-purpose flour	1	(10-ounce) package frozen cauliflower florets, cooked and well drained
1	teaspoon salt		
1	teaspoon dried basil		
¼	cup chopped fresh chives	½	cup fine, dry breadcrumbs
¼	teaspoon pepper	2	tablespoons butter, melted
1	cup milk	¼	cup grated Parmesan cheese
6	ounces cream cheese		

- Melt butter in a skillet over medium heat; add onion and sauté until tender (do not brown). Add flour, salt, basil, and chives, stirring well.

- Add milk and cook, stirring constantly, until thickened and bubbly. Add cream cheese, stirring until melted.

- Place broccoli and cauliflower in a bowl; add cheese sauce, tossing to coat. Spoon into a 2-quart baking dish.

- Combine breadcrumbs, melted butter, and Parmesan cheese; sprinkle over broccoli mixture.

- Bake at 350° for 30 minutes or until thoroughly heated and crumbs are golden.

Serves 6

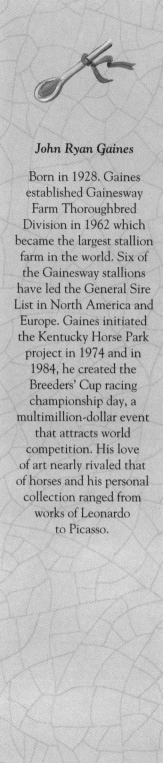

John Ryan Gaines

Born in 1928. Gaines established Gainesway Farm Thoroughbred Division in 1962 which became the largest stallion farm in the world. Six of the Gainesway stallions have led the General Sire List in North America and Europe. Gaines initiated the Kentucky Horse Park project in 1974 and in 1984, he created the Breeders' Cup racing championship day, a multimillion-dollar event that attracts world competition. His love of art nearly rivaled that of horses and his personal collection ranged from works of Leonardo to Picasso.

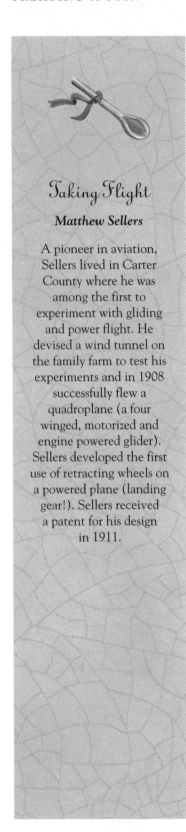

Taking Flight

Matthew Sellers

A pioneer in aviation, Sellers lived in Carter County where he was among the first to experiment with gliding and power flight. He devised a wind tunnel on the family farm to test his experiments and in 1908 successfully flew a quadroplane (a four winged, motorized and engine powered glider). Sellers developed the first use of retracting wheels on a powered plane (landing gear!). Sellers received a patent for his design in 1911.

Mexican Grilled Corn

A spicy grilled version of the American classic!

3 tablespoons butter, melted
1 teaspoon chili powder
½ teaspoon salt
½ teaspoon ground cumin
½ teaspoon garlic powder
6 fresh ears of corn, husked and cleaned

• Combine butter, chili powder, salt, cumin, and garlic powder; brush over corn.
• Wrap corn individually in aluminum foil.
• Grill over medium heat (300° to 350°) 30 to 40 minutes, turning every 10 to 15 minutes.

Makes 6 ears

Sautéed Peas and Limas with Basil

A unique accompaniment to a winter supper.

6 tablespoons butter
1 small onion, chopped
¾ cup milk
1 package frozen baby lima beans
1 package frozen baby green peas
Salt and pepper to taste
1 heaping tablespoon dried sweet basil

• Melt butter in a saucepan over medium heat; add onion and sauté until glazed. Gradually add milk, stirring constantly (do not boil).
• Add lima beans and peas; reduce heat and simmer 30 minutes. Season with salt and pepper and stir in basil.

Serves 8

Herb Crusted Spinach Casserole

3 (10-ounce) packages frozen chopped spinach
1 package dry onion soup mix
2 cups sour cream
½ cup garlic- and herb-seasoned stuffing mix
2 tablespoons melted butter

• Cook spinach until thawed; drain well. Add soup mix and sour cream, stirring well.
• Pour mixture into a greased 1½-quart baking dish.
• Combine stuffing mix and butter; sprinkle over casserole.
• Bake at 325° for 20 to 25 minutes or until top is golden.

Serves 8 to 10

Roasted Vegetables on Couscous

Quick, easy, and healthy to boot!

1	medium eggplant, peeled			Olive oil
1	green bell pepper			Salt and pepper to taste
1	yellow bell pepper		1	(5.8-ounce) package plain or garlic couscous, cooked
1	red bell pepper		1	cup (4 ounces) shredded cheddar cheese
1	medium zucchini		1	cup sliced ripe olives
4	medium tomatoes			
3	medium onions			

- Cut vegetables into bite-size chunks; place in a 9 x 13 x 2-inch pan.

- Drizzle with a small amount of oil and season with salt and pepper.

- Bake at 400° for 35 to 45 minutes or until desired degree of doneness.

- Serve vegetables over hot cooked couscous. Sprinkle with grated cheddar and sliced olives.

Serves 6 to 8

Summer Italian Tomato-Cheese Pie

Easy and delicious . . . tastes almost like pizza!

1	unbaked 9-inch pie crust		2	tablespoons chopped fresh or 1 tablespoon dried basil
1	cup (4 ounces) shredded mozzarella		½	cup mayonnaise
4-6	tomatoes, quartered, sliced in half, and squeezed of all juice		½	cup grated Parmesan cheese Cracked pepper to taste

- Preheat oven to 350°.

- Prick pie crust all over with a fork and bake at 350° for 10 minutes. Remove from oven and let cool.

- Layer ½ cup mozzarella, tomato, basil, and remaining ½ cup mozzarella.

- Combine mayonnaise and Parmesan cheese (mixture will be thick) and spread over top of pie.

- Bake 20 to 30 minutes.

Serves 6

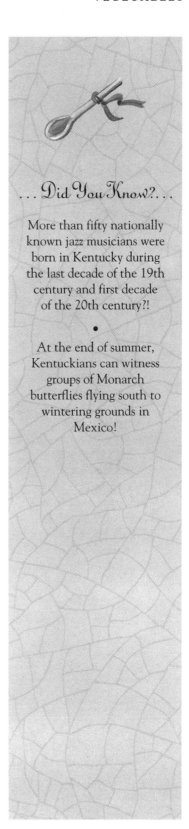

... *Did You Know?* ...

More than fifty nationally known jazz musicians were born in Kentucky during the last decade of the 19th century and first decade of the 20th century?!

•

At the end of summer, Kentuckians can witness groups of Monarch butterflies flying south to wintering grounds in Mexico!

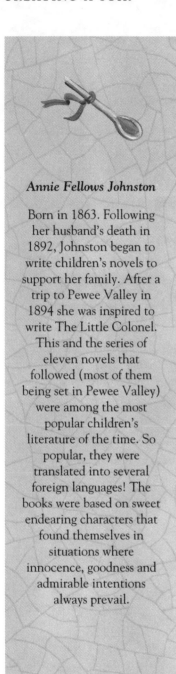

Fresh Tomato and Zucchini Tart

Outstanding!

1 cup coarsely chopped pitted kalamata olives	1 tablespoon finely chopped garlic
3 tablespoons capers, drained	2-3 small zucchini, coarsely shredded (about 1½ cups)
Pastry Shell	Salt and pepper to taste
3 large tomatoes, thinly sliced	Fresh basil leaves for garnish
2 tablespoons olive oil	

- Combine olives and capers; spread over bottom of Pastry Shell. Layer tomato slices in overlapping concentric circles over olive mixture.

- Cook garlic in hot oil in a nonstick skillet over medium-high heat until fragrant; add zucchini and season with salt and pepper. Cook, stirring often, 1 minute or until crisp-tender.

- Spoon zucchini mixture over tomato slices and garnish with fresh basil. Serve at room temperature.

Pastry Shell

4 ounces cream cheese, softened	¼ teaspoon salt
½ cup unsalted butter, softened	1 tablespoon minced fresh chives
1¼ cups all-purpose flour	

- Process cream cheese and butter in a food processor until creamy; add flour and salt and process just until dough forms a ball.

- Sprinkle chives on a work surface and turn dough out on top; knead lightly until chives are well blended. Pat dough into a ½-inch-thick disk. Wrap in plastic wrap and chill 30 minutes or overnight.

- Let dough stand at room temperature 15 minutes. Roll dough into a 14-inch round on a lightly floured surface.

- Fit dough round into an 11-inch fluted tart pan with removable bottom (do not stretch dough to fit). Trim edges, folding excess into sides of pan. Chill 20 minutes.

- Preheat oven to 400°.

- Line prepared crust with aluminum foil and add pastry weights or dried beans.

- Bake at 400° for 15 minutes. Remove weights and foil and bake 10 minutes or until golden.

- Remove from oven and let cool completely on a wire rack. Remove sides of pan and place shell on a serving platter.

Serves 6 to 8

Smothered Okra

4   bacon slices
4   pounds okra, cut into pieces
1½ tablespoons wine vinegar
1½ celery ribs, chopped
1   medium onion, chopped
2   garlic cloves, chopped
1   bell pepper, chopped

1   (16-ounce) can whole tomatoes, coarsely chopped
1   tablespoon Worcestershire sauce
1   teaspoon salt
¼ teaspoon pepper
1   teaspoon accent

- Cook bacon in a skillet over medium heat until crisp; drain, reserving ⅓ cup drippings in pan. Crumble bacon and set aside.
- Cook okra in hot drippings over medium heat; add vinegar, stirring well.
- Reduce heat and add celery, onion, garlic, and bell pepper. Cook 5 minutes.
- Add tomatoes, Worcestershire sauce, salt, pepper, and accent to vegetable mixture, stirring well; simmer, stirring occasionally, 10 minutes. Sprinkle with bacon.

Serves 6

Green Beans with Walnut Dressing

Quick, easy, and impressive! Great for buffets and holidays!

3   quarts water
2   pounds fresh green beans or frozen French cut, trimmed
½ cup finely chopped green onions
⅓ cup olive oil
¼ cup cider vinegar

¼ cup chopped fresh dill
½ teaspoon salt
½ teaspoon pepper
¾ cup coarsely chopped walnuts, toasted

- Bring 3 quarts water to a boil in a Dutch oven; add green beans and cook 10 minutes or until tender. Drain and transfer to a serving bowl.
- Combine green onions, oil, vinegar, dill, salt, and pepper; pour over green beans, tossing gently.
- Sprinkle with walnuts and serve hot or chilled.

Serves 8

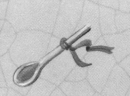

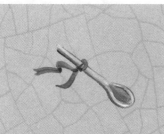

Eat Your Veggies!

Kathy Cary

Restaurateur and owner of Lilly's in Louisville, Kathy Cary was launched into the culinary limelight with her catering business in Washington D.C., serving the likes of **Henry Kissinger** and **Senator Edward Kennedy.** Cary also appeared on the "Today" show to present a cooking series on national television and to cook dinner at the coveted James Beard House in New York City three times. She was also featured in Great Women Chefs. She started a cooking and gardening program in Louisville, "From Seed to Table" at the Cabbage Patch Settlement House which benefits urban at-risk young people. The program nourishes their self esteem as well as an appreciation for fresh vegetables.

Asparagus Bundles with Goat Cheese

24-32	fresh asparagus spears	½	cup fine, dry breadcrumbs
6-8	ounces goat cheese, crumbled	1	tablespoon butter, melted

- Snap off ends of asparagus; cook in boiling water in a saucepan 5 to 8 minutes or until crisp-tender. Drain and plunge into ice water to stop the cooking process. Drain again.

- Place 6 to 8 spears in a bundle on a baking sheet; repeat with remaining asparagus. Top each bundle evenly with goat cheese.

- Combine breadcrumbs and butter; sprinkle evenly over bundles.

- Bake at 475° for 5 minutes or until crumbs are lightly browned.

Serves 4

Leeks Gratinate

Treat family and friends to this classic Italian-style vegetable!

1	tablespoon butter	Salt and pepper to taste
½	cup chopped sweet onion or shallots, trimmed and cut into 3-inch pieces	½ pound pancetta, pan-fried and chopped
½	cup chicken broth	½ cup freshly grated Parmigiano-Reggiano or Parmesan cheese
3	bunches leeks (or 3 leek stalks)	

- Melt butter in a skillet over medium heat; add onion and sauté until tender.

- Add chicken broth to a large skillet ⅛ to ¼ inch deep; add leeks and sauté over medium heat 10 to 15 minutes. Drain and place leeks in a single layer in a baking dish. Season with salt and pepper.

- Layer sautéed onion, pancetta, and cheese over leeks.

- Bake at 350° for 15 to 20 minutes or until lightly browned.

Serves 6 to 8

Herb Roasted Asparagus

A simple but exceptionally delicious way of preparing asparagus.

1	pound asparagus	2	tablespoons minced fresh parsley
2	tablespoons extra-virgin olive oil, divided	2	tablespoons minced fresh chives
	Salt and freshly ground pepper to taste	2	tablespoons minced fresh tarragon

- Preheat oven to 500°.
- Place cleaned and trimmed asparagus in a single layer in a shallow baking dish; drizzle oil lightly over top, tossing to coat.
- Bake at 500° for 10 to 12 minutes. Sprinkle with salt, pepper, remaining oil, parsley, chives, and tarragon, tossing gently to coat.

Serves 4 to 6

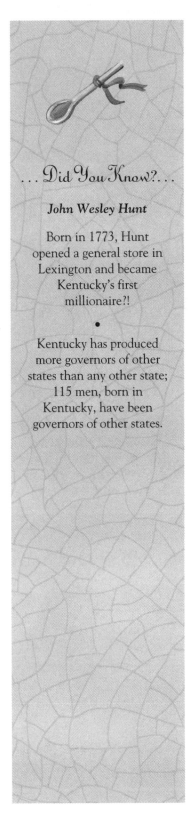

Summer Ripened Tomatoes with Bacon and Gruyère

A delicious way to enjoy summer's sun-kissed treasures!

1	pound bacon, cooked crisp and crumbled	½	cup minced fresh parsley
1	large onion, chopped	2	teaspoons dried basil
8	ounces Gruyère cheese, grated	6	large summer ripened tomatoes, cut into ½ inch slices

- Fry bacon until crisp, reserve ¼ cup drippings.
- Add onion and sauté until soft. Crumble bacon, mix with cheese, parsley and basil.
- Preheat broiler. Place tomatoes on boiler proof platter, overlapping slightly. Top each with bacon mixture. Broil just until cheese is melted and golden.

Serves 8 to 12

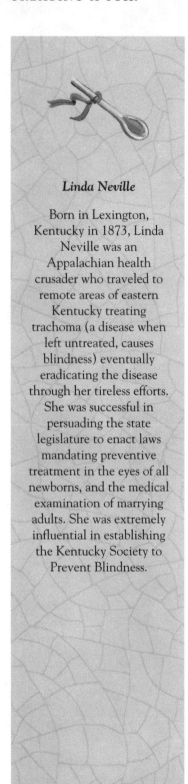

Easy Broccoli-Blue Cheese Bake

The addition of blue cheese adds an interesting twist to this traditional favorite!

2	(10-ounce) packages frozen chopped broccoli, thawed and well drained	½	teaspoon salt
3	tablespoons butter	¼	teaspoon white pepper
3	tablespoons flour	⅓	cup crumbled blue cheese
½	cup half-and-half	½	cup slivered almonds
½	cup milk	¾	cup seasoned stuffing mix
4	ounces cream cheese, softened	2	tablespoons butter, melted

- Melt butter over low heat, add flour and stir until smooth. Gradually add half-and-half and milk, cook stirring constantly until thick and bubbly. Add cream cheese, blue cheese, salt and pepper and stir until melted. Stir in broccoli and almond, tossing lightly.

- Pour broccoli mixture into a buttered 2-quart casserole dish. Bake at 350° for 15 minutes.

- Combine stuffing mix and melted butter, mix well. Sprinkle stuffing mixture over the top and bake an additional 15 minutes until golden and bubbly.

Serves 6 to 8

Summer Fresh Vegetable Medley

Quick and easy to prepare . . . a wonderful way to savor the last of summer's bounty!

4	zucchini, sliced	1½	cups fresh corn
1	medium onion, shredded	¼	cup butter
½	cup chopped green bell pepper		Salt and pepper to taste
2	medium summer ripened tomatoes, thinly sliced	½	teaspoon dill (optional)
		2	cups shredded cheddar cheese

- Melt butter in a large skillet and sauté zucchini, onion, and green pepper for 3 to 5 minutes. Add tomatoes and corn, reduce to medium heat and continue cooking an additional 5 minutes until vegetables are tender.

- Season with dill weed, salt and pepper. Sprinkle with shredded cheese, cover and let simmer for 10 minutes until cheese is melted.

Serves 6 to 8

Pasta

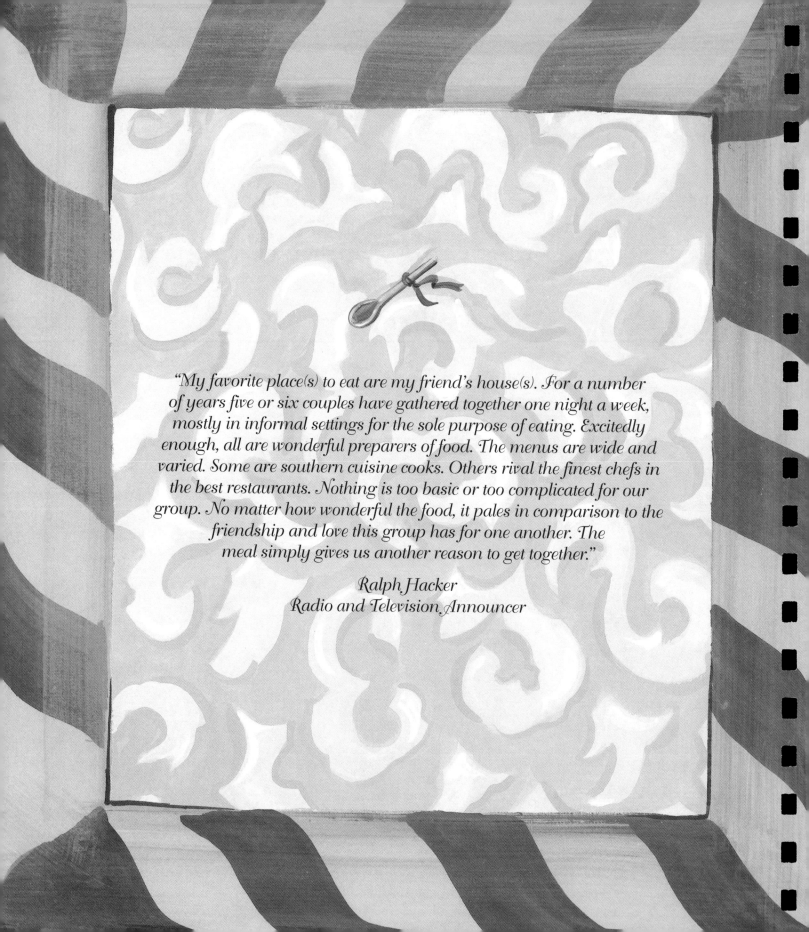

"My favorite place(s) to eat are my friend's house(s). For a number of years five or six couples have gathered together one night a week, mostly in informal settings for the sole purpose of eating. Excitedly enough, all are wonderful preparers of food. The menus are wide and varied. Some are southern cuisine cooks. Others rival the finest chefs in the best restaurants. Nothing is too basic or too complicated for our group. No matter how wonderful the food, it pales in comparison to the friendship and love this group has for one another. The meal simply gives us another reason to get together."

Ralph Hacker
Radio and Television Announcer

Grape, Blue Cheese, and Walnut Pasta

Outstanding-a fabulous mélange of flavors!

8 ounces farfalle pasta, cooked	Salt and pepper to taste
3-4 cups red seedless grapes	1 cup mayonnaise
½ cup chopped green onions	2 tablespoons fresh lemon juice
6 ounces crumbled blue cheese	¾ cup toasted chopped walnuts
1 garlic clove, minced	

- Combine hot cooked pasta, grapes, green onions, blue cheese, garlic, salt, and pepper in a large bowl.

- Combine mayonnaise and lemon juice; add to pasta mixture, stirring well. Cover and chill several hours.

- Add walnuts, tossing well.

Serves 6 to 8

Farfalle with Spinach and Artichokes

Put this flavorful, filling dish on the table in less than 45 minutes!

4 cups thinly sliced onion	1 (14-ounce) can artichoke hearts, drained and chopped
2 tablespoons olive oil	½ cup pine nuts
¾ teaspoon salt	16 ounces farfalle pasta, cooked
1 cup vegetable broth	Freshly grated Parmesan cheese
1-2 packages fresh spinach, washed and chopped	

- Sauté onion in hot oil in a large heavy skillet over medium heat 1 minute. Add salt and cook 5 minutes. Cover, reduce heat, and simmer 20 minutes.

- Add vegetable broth to onion slices and bring to a boil; reduce heat and simmer 5 to 8 minutes. Stir in spinach and cook 1 to 3 minutes.

- Add artichoke hearts and pine nuts, stirring well.

- Combine spinach mixture and hot cooked pasta, tossing well. Sprinkle with Parmesan cheese and serve immediately.

Serves 4 to 6

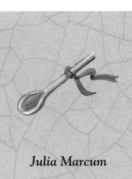

Julia Marcum

Born in 1844, she is the only woman recognized by the United States government as a combatant in the Civil War (she helped her family stave off a Confederate attack) and to have received a military pension for her service. After the war, she returned to teaching school but eventually, her wounds would disable her, leading to her request for pension. She received military honors at her funeral in 1936.

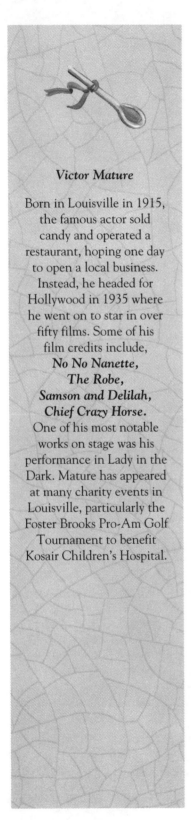

Farfalle with Tarragon Grilled Chicken and Peppers

Great served hot or cold . . . this recipe is always requested!

1¼	cups soy sauce, divided	3	red, yellow, and green bell peppers, halved
½	teaspoon ground ginger		
1¼	cups olive oil, divided	1	pound farfalle pasta, cooked
5	tablespoons dried tarragon, divided	1	bunch green onions, diced
1½	teaspoons paprika, divided	16	ounces crumbled feta cheese
2	teaspoons cracked pepper, divided	1½	teaspoons minced garlic
2	pounds skinned and boned chicken breasts		

- Whisk together 1 cup soy sauce, ginger, ½ cup oil, 2 tablespoons tarragon, ½ teaspoon paprika, and 1 teaspoon pepper.

- Place chicken and bell pepper in a shallow dish; add marinade, tossing to coat. Let stand 30 minutes.

- Drain chicken and bell pepper, reserving marinade.

- Grill chicken and bell pepper over low heat (300°), pouring marinade over top at start of grilling. Grill 10 to 12 minutes on each side. Remove from grill.

- Cut chicken into bite-size pieces and slice bell pepper into strips.

- Combine hot cooked pasta, remaining ¼ cup soy sauce, 1½ teaspoons garlic, 1 teaspoon paprika, 3 tablespoons tarragon, ¾ cup oil, 1 teaspoon cracked pepper, and green onions, tossing well.

- Add grilled chicken and bell pepper, tossing well. Add feta, tossing well.

Serves 8 to 10

Penne with Shiitake and Fresh Ginger

Spicy ginger and the robust flavor of the shiitake passionately meld together in this rich and hearty dish. Just add a salad and crusty French bread for a soul-satisfying meal.

3 purple onions, sliced into half-moon crescents	¼ cup balsamic vinegar
½ cup olive oil, divided	4 pounds fresh shiitake mushrooms, thinly sliced
½ cup firmly packed brown sugar	4 pounds portobella or white mushrooms, thinly sliced
4 cups crushed Italian tomatoes	2 pounds penne pasta, cooked
4 tablespoons ground coriander	1 pound fresh gingerroot, minced
1 tablespoon salt	2 tablespoons soy sauce
1 tablespoon pepper	

- Sauté onion in ¼ cup hot oil in a large saucepan 15 minutes or until caramelized. Add brown sugar and cook several more minutes.

- Add tomatoes, coriander, salt, pepper, and vinegar; cook, stirring often, 30 minutes or until thickened.

- Sauté mushrooms in remaining ¼ cup hot oil over medium heat until slightly crispy; add to tomato mixture.

- Combine hot cooked pasta, minced gingerroot, and soy sauce, tossing to coat well. Add mushroom sauce, tossing well.

Serves 12 to 15

Chef Chris Cox
The Mousetrap
Lexington, Kentucky

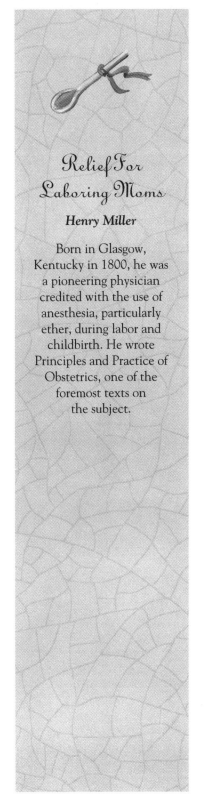

Relief For Laboring Moms

Henry Miller

Born in Glasgow, Kentucky in 1800, he was a pioneering physician credited with the use of anesthesia, particularly ether, during labor and childbirth. He wrote Principles and Practice of Obstetrics, one of the foremost texts on the subject.

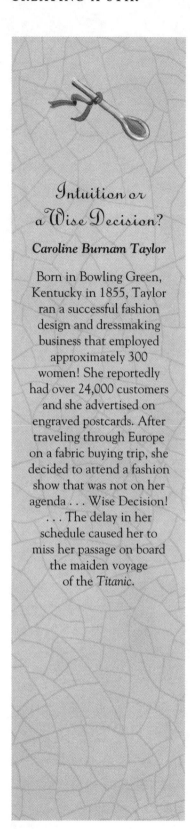

Intuition or a Wise Decision?

Caroline Burnam Taylor

Born in Bowling Green, Kentucky in 1855, Taylor ran a successful fashion design and dressmaking business that employed approximately 300 women! She reportedly had over 24,000 customers and she advertised on engraved postcards. After traveling through Europe on a fabric buying trip, she decided to attend a fashion show that was not on her agenda . . . Wise Decision! . . . The delay in her schedule caused her to miss her passage on board the maiden voyage of the *Titanic*.

Tortellini with Mushrooms and Prosciutto

Add a salad and bread to this rich pasta and you'll have a satisfying meal with very little work!

1 large onion, chopped
6 ounces thinly sliced prosciutto, chopped
2 tablespoons minced garlic
¼ teaspoon dried crushed red pepper
1 teaspoon ground black pepper
3 tablespoons olive oil
1 cup dry white wine
2 cups sliced mushrooms
2 cups chopped red bell pepper
1 cup chopped green onions
1 cup fresh shelled or frozen green peas
1½ cups whipping cream
2 (9-ounce) packages refrigerated cheese-filled tortellini, cooked
½ cup chopped fresh parsley
½ cup chopped fresh basil
1 cup freshly grated Parmesan cheese

• Sauté onion, prosciutto, garlic, red pepper, and black pepper in hot oil in a heavy saucepan over medium heat 10 minutes or until onion is golden brown. Add wine and bring to a boil.

• Add mushrooms, bell pepper, green onions, and green peas; reduce heat and simmer 5 minutes or until liquid is almost evaporated.

• Add cream and bring to a boil; boil 5 minutes or until thickened. Add hot cooked pasta, parsley, basil, and Parmesan; simmer 4 minutes, stirring to coat. Season with salt and pepper to taste.

• Transfer pasta mixture to a large bowl and serve immediately.

Serves 6

Cajun Chicken Fettuccine

This is excellent! A nice balance between the fiery hot Cajun spices of the chicken and the creamy, slightly mellowed flavors of the sauce.

4	skinned and boned chicken breasts	1	tablespoon cornstarch
½-¾	tablespoon Cajun spice	1½	tablespoons water
½	teaspoon cracked black pepper	2	cups half-and-half
1	cup water	¼	teaspoon cayenne pepper
¾	teaspoon salt, divided	¼	teaspoon ground black pepper
1	pound fresh broccoli, cut into pieces	⅓	cup freshly grated Parmesan cheese
¼	cup butter	8	ounces fettuccine, cooked
1-2	garlic cloves, minced		Freshly grated Parmesan cheese

- Sprinkle chicken with Cajun spice and cracked black pepper. Bake at 350° for 30 to 40 minutes. Let cool and cut into strips.

- Bring 1 cup water and ½ teaspoon salt to a boil in a saucepan. Reserve 1 cup broccoli and add remaining broccoli to boiling water; boil 3 to 4 minutes. Drain and rinse with cold water; set aside.

- Melt butter in a skillet over medium heat; add garlic and sauté 1 to 2 minutes. Add reserved uncooked broccoli and sauté 1 to 2 minutes.

- Combine cornstarch and 1½ tablespoons water in a 2-cup glass liquid measuring cup, stirring until smooth; gradually add half-and-half.

- Add cornstarch mixture to garlic mixture; stir in remaining ¼ teaspoon salt, cayenne pepper, ground black pepper and ⅓ cup Parmesan cheese. Bring to a boil.

- Spoon sauce over hot cooked pasta; add chicken and reserved cooked broccoli, tossing to coat. Sprinkle with Parmesan cheese and serve immediately.

Serves 4 to 6

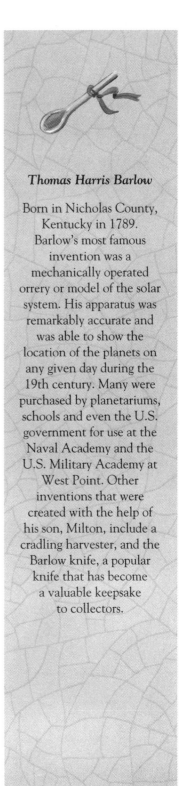

Thomas Harris Barlow

Born in Nicholas County, Kentucky in 1789. Barlow's most famous invention was a mechanically operated orrery or model of the solar system. His apparatus was remarkably accurate and was able to show the location of the planets on any given day during the 19th century. Many were purchased by planetariums, schools and even the U.S. government for use at the Naval Academy and the U.S. Military Academy at West Point. Other inventions that were created with the help of his son, Milton, include a cradling harvester, and the Barlow knife, a popular knife that has become a valuable keepsake to collectors.

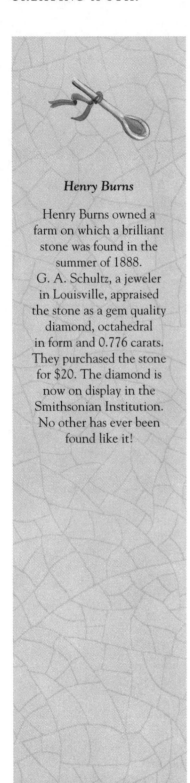

Ziti with Tomatoes, Pesto, and Artichokes

Quick, easy, and delicious!

1	(6-ounce) jar marinated artichoke hearts	½	cup pesto
1	large onion, chopped	12	ounces ziti pasta, cooked
1	garlic clove, minced	⅓	cup freshly grated Parmesan cheese
1	(28-ounce) can diced tomatoes, undrained		Salt and pepper to taste

- Drain artichoke hearts, reserving 3 tablespoons marinade. Set artichoke hearts aside.

- Sauté onion and garlic in 3 tablespoons hot marinade in a skillet over medium heat 7 minutes or until onion is tender.

- Add diced tomatoes and reserved artichoke hearts to skillet; reduce heat and simmer 8 minutes or until thickened. Add pesto and simmer 1 minute.

- Stir in hot cooked pasta and Parmesan cheese; season with salt and pepper.

Serves 4

Orecchiette with Mushrooms, Arugula, Tomatoes, and Brie

Brie brings sophistication to this savvy dish.

2	cups orecchiette	1	pound Italian plum tomatoes, chopped
6	ounces portobella mushrooms, sliced	½	cup dry white wine
2	garlic cloves, minced	2	bunches arugula, stemmed, washed, and drained
2	tablespoons extra-virgin olive oil	¼	pound Brie, cut into small pieces

- Cook pasta in boiling salted water until al dente; drain, reserving ½ cup liquid.

- Sauté mushrooms and garlic in hot oil in a large heavy skillet over medium heat 5 minutes; stir in chopped tomato and cook 2 minutes.

- Add wine and reserved pasta liquid to garlic mixture and bring to a boil; reduce heat and simmer 5 minutes.

- Add hot cooked pasta, arugula, and Brie, tossing until arugula is wilted and cheese is melted.

Serves 2

Penne with Balsamic Dijon Marinated Chicken

An excellent marinade-it makes this dish outstanding!

¾ cup extra-virgin olive oil	5 garlic cloves, crushed
6 tablespoons balsamic vinegar	4½ tablespoons water
1½ teaspoons sugar	6 skinned and boned chicken breasts
3 tablespoons Dijon mustard	16 ounces penne pasta, cooked
¼ teaspoon cayenne pepper	Freshly grated Parmesan cheese

- Combine olive oil, vinegar, sugar, mustard, red pepper, garlic, and water; reserve ½ cup marinade.
- Place chicken in a shallow dish and pour remaining marinade over top; cover and chill at least 2 hours.
- Remove chicken from marinade, discarding marinade. Place chicken on a rack in a roasting pan.
- Broil chicken 4 inches from heat (with electric oven door partially open) until done. Cut chicken into bite-size pieces.
- Combine chicken, reserved ½ cup marinade, and hot cooked pasta, tossing to coat.
- Sprinkle with Parmesan cheese and serve immediately.

Serves 4

Triple-Cheese Penne with Basil

2 garlic cloves, minced	¼ cup dry white wine
2 tablespoons olive oil	⅓-½ cup chopped fresh basil
4 ounces cream cheese	12 ounces penne pasta, cooked
½ cup cottage cheese	Chopped fresh basil for garnish
½ cup grated Parmesan cheese	

- Sauté garlic in hot oil in a skillet over medium-high heat, stirring constantly, 1 to 2 minutes.
- Add cheeses; reduce heat and cook, stirring constantly, until well blended. Add wine and basil and cook, stirring often, 3 to 5 minutes or until thickened.
- Pour sauce over hot cooked pasta, tossing to coat. Garnish with chopped fresh basil.

Serves 4

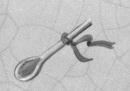

The Father of Bluegrass Music

Bill Monroe

Born near Rosine, Kentucky in 1911, Bill Monroe is known as "the father of bluegrass music". Bluegrass music is a distinct acoustical sound that is formed from a combination of stringed instruments that include the mandolin, guitar, banjo and often times a fiddle, bass and dobro. Monroe put together the ultimate bluegrass band (The Bluegrass Boys) in 1945 which included himself on mandolin, *Lester Flat* on guitar, *Earl Scruggs* on banjo, *Chubby Wise* on fiddle and *Howard Watts* on bass. Other great bluegrass musicians include *Bobby and Sony Osborne, Hylo Brown, Grandpa Jones, Cliff Carlisle, Don Parmley, J.D. Crowe* and *Ricky Skaggs*.

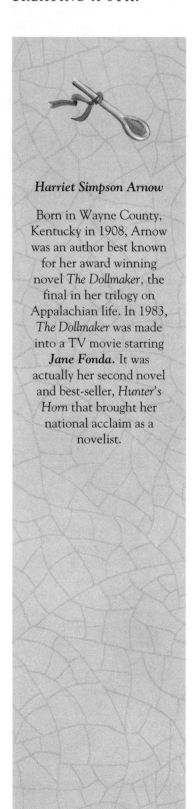

Chicken and Rosemary Pasta

4	skinned and boned chicken breasts, cut into bite-size pieces	1	(14-ounce) can artichoke hearts, drained and chopped
	Salt and pepper to taste	2	fresh rosemary sprigs, chopped
¼	cup butter, melted	½	cup dry white wine
1	small onion, chopped	3	cups whipping cream
2	garlic cloves, minced	¼	cup butter
1	(8-ounce) package fresh mushrooms, sliced	1	package refrigerated fettuccine, cooked
		1	cup freshly grated Parmesan cheese

- Sprinkle chicken with salt and pepper.

- Melt butter in a skillet over medium heat; add chicken and cook 5 minutes or until lightly browned. Transfer chicken to a plate.

- Add onion, garlic, mushrooms, artichoke, and rosemary to skillet and sauté until tender. Drain and transfer to a separate plate.

- Add wine, cream, and ¼ cup butter to skillet; cook, stirring constantly, 10 minutes or until thickened. Add chicken, vegetables, hot cooked pasta, and Parmesan cheese, tossing to coat. Serve immediately.

Serves 6 to 8

Spinach and Gorgonzola Pasta

A must try for blue cheese fans!

5	ounces frozen chopped spinach, cooked and well drained	2	tablespoons freshly grated Parmesan cheese
1½	cups half-and-half	½	teaspoon pepper
6	ounces crumbled Gorgonzola cheese	1	pound penne, fusille, or farfalle pasta, cooked

- Bring spinach and half-and-half to a boil in a large saucepan over high heat. Remove from heat and stir in Gorgonzola, Parmesan, and pepper.

- Cook over low heat, stirring until cheese melts. Add pasta, tossing well.

Serves 8

Creamy Fettuccine with Nutmeg Chicken and Spinach

Rich and satisfying.

4 tablespoons unsalted butter
4 skinned and boned chicken breast
  halves, cut diagonally into
  1- x ½-inch strips
1 pound fresh spinach, stemmed and
  coarsely chopped
¼ teaspoon freshly grated nutmeg

Salt and pepper to taste
1 cup canned Italian plum tomatoes,
  drained and coarsely chopped
1 cup whipping cream or half-and-half
¾ pound fettuccine, cooked
½ cup freshly grated Parmesan cheese
  Freshly grated Parmesan cheese

- Melt butter in a skillet over medium-high heat; add chicken and cook 1 to 2 minutes or until lightly browned. Transfer chicken to a plate.

- Add spinach, nutmeg, and salt and pepper to skillet; cook, stirring occasionally, 2 minutes or until spinach is wilted. Add tomatoes and cook, stirring often, 3 minutes or until thoroughly heated.

- Stir in cream in a slow, steady stream; reduce heat and simmer 4 minutes or until slightly thickened. Season with salt and pepper.

- Add chicken to cream sauce and cook over medium heat until thoroughly heated.

- Combine chicken mixture, hot cooked pasta, and ½ cup Parmesan cheese in a large bowl, tossing to coat. Sprinkle with Parmesan cheese and serve immediately.

Serves 4

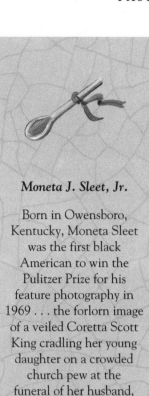

Moneta J. Sleet, Jr.

Born in Owensboro, Kentucky, Moneta Sleet was the first black American to win the Pulitzer Prize for his feature photography in 1969 . . . the forlorn image of a veiled Coretta Scott King cradling her young daughter on a crowded church pew at the funeral of her husband, Dr. Martin Luther King, Jr.

Sun-Dried Tomato and Basil Pasta

3 garlic cloves, minced
2½ (8.5-ounce) jars sun-dried
  tomatoes, drained
6 tablespoons chopped fresh basil
  leaves

1 teaspoon salt
½ teaspoon ground pepper
½ cup olive oil
1-2 pounds cooked pasta
  Freshly grated Parmesan cheese

- Process garlic, tomatoes, basil leaves, salt, pepper, and olive oil in a food processor until a thick paste, adding more oil or warm water to thin if desired.

- Combine tomato mixture and hot cooked pasta, tossing well. Sprinkle with Parmesan cheese.

Serves 8 to 10

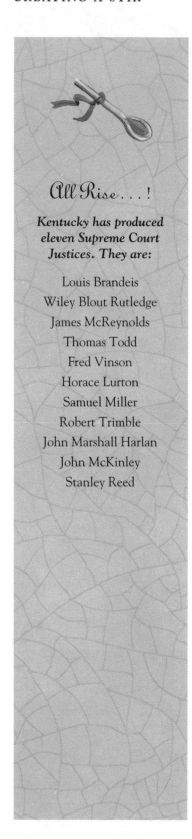

Mediterranean Penne

The exotic flavors of the Mediterranean make this dish incredibly good!

8   ounces penne pasta, cooked
⅔   cup crumbled feta, divided
¼   cup freshly grated Parmesan cheese, divided
1   medium-size purple onion, halved and sliced
2   tablespoons olive oil
1   (14-ounce) can quartered artichoke hearts, rinsed and drained

1   (16-ounce) can crushed tomatoes, undrained
1   (2.25-ounce) can sliced ripe olives, drained
¼   teaspoon salt
½   teaspoon freshly ground pepper
1   teaspoon dried Italian seasoning

- Place pasta in a greased 7 x 11 x 2-inch baking dish; sprinkle with half each of feta and Parmesan cheese.

- Sauté onion in hot oil in a large skillet over medium-high heat until tender; add artichoke hearts and tomatoes and cook 2 to 3 minutes.

- Add olives, salt, pepper, and Italian seasoning to tomato mixture; cover, reduce heat, and simmer 10 minutes.

- Pour sauce over pasta and sprinkle with remaining cheeses.

- Bake at 350° for 20 minutes or until cheese melts.

Serves 4 to 6

Greek Pasta with Tomatoes, Spinach, and White Beans

Short on time? Try this quick fix pasta . . . you'll get big taste in just 20 minutes!

2   (14.5-ounce) cans diced tomatoes with basil, garlic, and oregano
1   (19-ounce) can cannellini or great Northern beans, rinsed and drained

1   (10-ounce) bag fresh spinach, chopped
8   ounces penne pasta, cooked (about 4 cups cooked)
½   cup finely crumbled feta cheese

- Bring tomatoes and beans to a boil in a large nonstick skillet over medium-high heat; reduce heat and simmer 10 minutes.

- Add spinach and cook, stirring occasionally, until spinach wilts.

- Place pasta evenly on 4 serving plates; top each serving with sauce and feta cheese.

Serves 4

For those in a hurry, frozen chopped spinach (cooked and well drained) may be substituted for fresh.

Penne with Chicken, Havarti, Artichokes, and Italian Tomatoes

*Absolutely delicious! Excellent for entertaining-it can
be made ahead and popped into the oven after guests arrive.*

1½ cups chopped onion
1   teaspoon minced garlic
6   tablespoons olive oil, divided
3   (28-ounce) cans Italian plum
    tomatoes, drained
1½ teaspoons dried crushed red pepper
2   teaspoons dried basil
2   cups canned reduced-sodium
    chicken broth

Salt and pepper to taste
1   pound penne pasta, cooked al dente
1   pound cubed poached chicken
2½ cups grated Havarti cheese
⅓   cup sliced pitted kalamata olives
1   (14½-ounce) can artichoke hearts,
    drained and chopped
⅓   cup grated Parmesan cheese
½   cup finely chopped fresh basil

- Sauté onion and garlic in 3 tablespoons hot oil in a large Dutch oven over medium-high heat until opaque.

- Add tomatoes, red pepper, and dried basil and bring to a boil, stirring to break up tomatoes. Add broth and return to a boil; reduce heat and simmer, stirring occasionally, 1 hour and 15 minutes or until mixture thickens to a chunky sauce and is reduced to 6 cups. Season with salt and pepper.

- Preheat oven to 375°.

- Combine hot cooked pasta and remaining 3 tablespoons oil in a large bowl, tossing to coat. Add chicken, tomato sauce, and Havarti cheese, stirring well. Spoon into a 9 x 13 x 2-inch baking dish.

- Sprinkle with olives and Parmesan cheese. Bake at 375° until thoroughly heated. Sprinkle with basil.

Serves 8

*Sauce may be prepared up to 2 days ahead. Cover and chill. Warm over low heat
before continuing.*

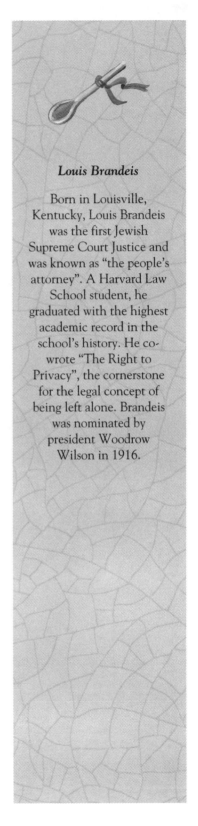

Louis Brandeis

Born in Louisville,
Kentucky, Louis Brandeis
was the first Jewish
Supreme Court Justice and
was known as "the people's
attorney". A Harvard Law
School student, he
graduated with the highest
academic record in the
school's history. He co-
wrote "The Right to
Privacy", the cornerstone
for the legal concept of
being left alone. Brandeis
was nominated by
president Woodrow
Wilson in 1916.

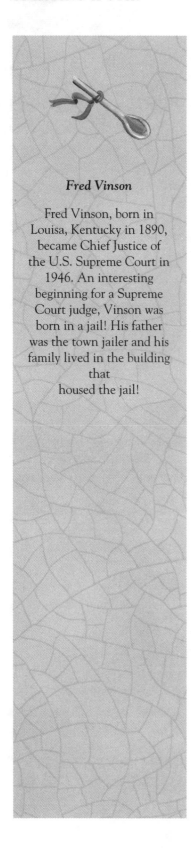

Lemon-Garlic Chicken with Broccoli and Angel Hair Pasta

Very light . . . a nice summer pasta

2	garlic cloves	1½	tablespoons dried marjoram
1	tablespoon olive oil	¼	cup dry white wine
1	pound skinned and boned chicken breasts, cut into bite-size pieces	2	tablespoons olive oil
1	lemon, halved	8	ounces angel hair pasta, cooked
	Salt and pepper to taste	4	cups broccoli florets, cooked crisp-tender

• Sauté garlic cloves in 1 tablespoon hot oil in a skillet over medium heat; discard garlic.

• Squeeze juice from 1 lemon half over chicken; cook in skillet over medium heat until browned. Turn chicken and squeeze remaining lemon half over top. Season with salt and pepper.

• Add marjoram and wine and cook until chicken is done.

• Toss hot cooked pasta in 2 tablespoons oil. Add broccoli and toss well.

• Serve chicken over hot cooked angel hair pasta with broccoli florets.

Shrimp and Asparagus Versailles

An attractive mix of colors creates a beautiful presentation for this dish.

¼	cup butter	2	tablespoons fresh lemon juice
10	ounces 1-inch-long fresh asparagus tips		Salt and freshly ground pepper
1	pound small fresh shrimp, boiled, peeled, and deveined	8	ounces extra wide noodles, cooked
3	tablespoons Dijon mustard	3	tablespoons olive oil
		½	cup freshly grated Parmesan cheese

• Melt butter in a large skillet over medium heat; add asparagus and sauté 4 minutes. Add shrimp and cook until thoroughly heated.

• Add mustard, lemon juice, and salt and pepper, stirring well.

• Combine hot cooked pasta and oil in a large bowl, tossing to coat. Divide pasta evenly onto 4 serving plates. Top each with equal amounts of shrimp mixture and sprinkle with fresh Parmesan.

Serves 4

Country Ham and Pea Tortellini

¼	cup butter		Dash of salt (optional)
¼	cup all-purpose flour	¾	cup frozen peas, thawed
2	cups milk	1	(9-ounce) package refrigerated
1	cup diced country ham		cheese-filled tortellini, cooked

- Melt butter in a saucepan over medium heat; add flour and cook, stirring constantly, until bubbly. Cook, stirring constantly, 1 minute.

- Gradually add milk; cook, stirring constantly, until thickened, adding more milk if needed. Add ham and cook, stirring constantly, several minutes.

- Add salt, if needed. Stir in peas and hot cooked tortellini and cook until thoroughly heated.

Serves 4

Country ham can be purchased sliced and prepackaged in a similar amount.

Walnut-Chicken Fettuccine

½	cup butter, divided	2	garlic cloves, minced
1	cup chopped walnuts	¾	cup half-and-half
4	skinned and boned chicken breast	1	teaspoon salt
	halves, cut into bite-size pieces	½	teaspoon pepper
1	(8-ounce) package fresh	1	cup freshly grated Parmesan cheese
	mushrooms, sliced	¼	cup chopped fresh parsley
1	cup chopped green onions	8	ounces fettuccine, cooked

- Melt ¼ cup butter in a large skillet over medium heat; add walnuts and sauté 3 to 5 minutes or until toasted. Transfer walnuts to a small bowl, reserving drippings in skillet.

- Add chicken to skillet and sauté 7 to 10 minutes or until done. Transfer chicken to a plate, reserving drippings in skillet.

- Add mushrooms, green onions, and garlic to skillet and sauté until tender. Transfer to plate, reserving drippings in skillet.

- Add remaining butter, half-and-half, salt, and pepper to skillet and cook, stirring often, 3 to 5 minutes. Stir in Parmesan cheese and parsley.

- Combine sauce, chicken, vegetables, and hot cooked pasta in a large bowl, tossing to coat. Sprinkle with toasted walnuts and serve immediately.

Serves 4 to 6

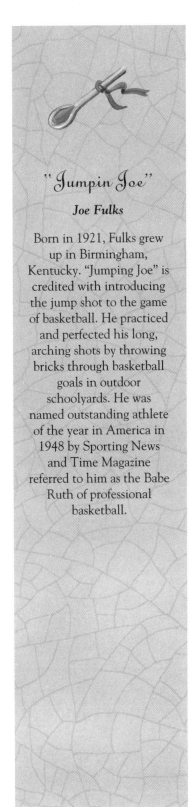

"Jumpin Joe"

Joe Fulks

Born in 1921, Fulks grew up in Birmingham, Kentucky. "Jumping Joe" is credited with introducing the jump shot to the game of basketball. He practiced and perfected his long, arching shots by throwing bricks through basketball goals in outdoor schoolyards. He was named outstanding athlete of the year in America in 1948 by Sporting News and Time Magazine referred to him as the Babe Ruth of professional basketball.

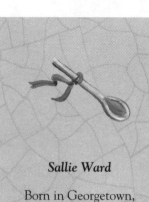

Sallie Ward

Born in Georgetown, Kentucky in 1827, this beautiful, amusing, and egocentric young woman grew up in Louisville where she was very popular and her attendance was in demand at many of the town's social gatherings. She sponsored the first "fancy dress" ball in Kentucky, was a trend setter in her use of cosmetics to embellish her beauty, and introduced opera glasses to the area. She frequently sponsored benefit balls for the poor which endeared her all the more to the city's residents. She gained international prominence as well and was a favorite of *Napoleon III, emperor of France.* So well loved, commercial products bore her name, and racehorses, steamboats and babies were christened in her honor!!

Pasta Peanut Pesto

Deliciously different!

¾	cup salted roasted peanuts	1½	tablespoons chili oil
3	garlic cloves	1	tablespoon molasses
1	cup fresh cilantro leaves	1½	tablespoons soy sauce
1	cup fresh parsley leaves	1½	tablespoons olive oil
5	tablespoons fresh lime juice	1½	teaspoons grated fresh ginger

- Process all ingredients in a food processor until smooth. Chill, if desired.
- Serve over cooked angel hair pasta.

Serves 4

Spicy Black Bean Lasagna

2	(15-ounce) cans black beans, drained and rinsed	12	ounces cottage cheese
½	cup chopped onion	1	(8-ounce) package cream cheese, softened
½	cup chopped green bell pepper	½	cup sour cream
2	garlic cloves, minced	9	lasagna noodles, cooked
2	(15-ounce) cans tomato sauce		Chopped tomato, chopped cilantro
¼	cup chopped fresh cilantro		for garnish

- Preheat oven to 350°.
- Mash 1 can of black beans; set aside.
- Sauté onion, bell pepper, and garlic in a large skillet coated with vegetable cooking spray over medium heat until tender. Add mashed beans, whole beans, tomato sauce, and cilantro and cook until thoroughly heated.
- Combine cottage cheese, cream cheese, and sour cream. Reserve one-third of mixture.
- Layer 3 lasagna noodles, one-third of bean mixture, and half of remaining sour cream mixture in a lightly greased 9 x 13 x 2-inch baking dish. Repeat layers twice ending with bean mixture.
- Bake, covered, at 350° for 40 to 45 minutes.
- Dollop with reserved cream cheese mixture and garnish, if desired.

Serves 8 to 10

Tortellini with Roasted Red Pepper Sauce

3   large red bell peppers
3   shallots, finely chopped
1½ cups chicken broth
1½ cups heavy cream

9   fresh basil leaves, finely chopped
2   (9-ounce) packages refrigerated
     cheese-filled tortellini, cooked

- Broil bell peppers on a baking sheet 4 inches from heat (with electric oven door partially open), turning often, until blackened. Transfer to a zip-top plastic bag; seal and let stand 10 minutes.

- Peel and seed bell peppers. Process in a blender until smooth.

- Cook bell pepper puree and shallots in a skillet over medium heat until shallots are soft. Add broth and bring to a boil; boil until reduced by half.

- Add cream to sauce and bring to a boil; cook until desired thickness. Stir in basil when ready to serve.

- Combine sauce and hot cooked tortellini in a large bowl, tossing to coat.

Serves 8

Pasta with Basil Pesto

*It is worthwhile to make several batches of this recipe in the summer
when basil is abundant. Just freeze in zip-top plastic bags for later use.*

2   cups fresh basil leaves
4   garlic cloves, chopped
1   cup walnuts
1   cup extra-virgin olive oil
1   cup freshly grated Parmesan cheese

¼   cup freshly grated Romano cheese
     Salt and freshly ground pepper to
     taste
2-4 pounds pasta of choice, cooked

- Process basil leaves, garlic, and walnuts in a food processor until blended; with the machine running, add oil in a slow, steady stream.

- Add cheeses, a pinch of salt, and several grindings of pepper; process briefly. Transfer to a bowl and cover until ready to use.

- Toss pesto with hot cooked pasta.

Serves 6 to 10

For a variation add pine nuts and chicken or salmon to pasta.

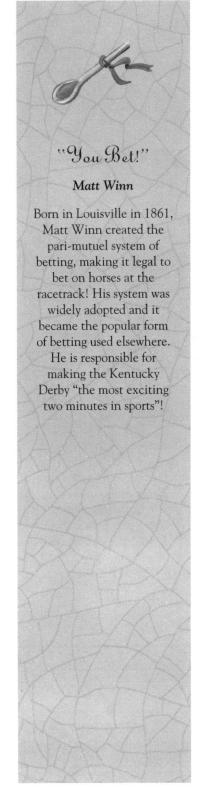

"You Bet!"

Matt Winn

Born in Louisville in 1861, Matt Winn created the pari-mutuel system of betting, making it legal to bet on horses at the racetrack! His system was widely adopted and it became the popular form of betting used elsewhere. He is responsible for making the Kentucky Derby "the most exciting two minutes in sports"!

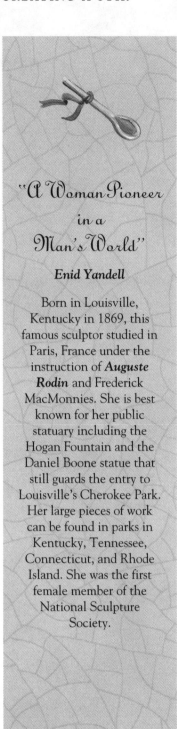

Chicken and Spinach Lasagna

You'll love this lighter version of the classic.

1 tablespoon butter
1 onion, finely chopped
3 cups sliced fresh mushrooms
1 teaspoon dried basil
1 teaspoon dried oregano
1 pound fresh spinach, stemmed and washed

2½ pounds chicken breasts, cooked and cut into thin slices
9 lasagna noodles, cooked
1 (16-ounce) container ricotta cheese
3 cups (12 ounces) shredded mozzarella cheese
2 cups freshly grated Parmesan cheese
Alfredo Sauce

- Melt butter in a skillet over medium heat; add onion, mushrooms, basil, and oregano and sauté until tender. Add spinach and cook until wilted. Stir in chicken.

- Layer 3 lasagna noodles, half each of chicken mixture and ricotta cheese, and one-third each of mozzarella and Parmesan cheese in a lightly greased 9 x 13 x 2-inch baking dish. Top with one-third of Alfredo Sauce. Repeat layers once. Top with remaining lasagna noodles, sauce, and mozzarella and Parmesan cheese.

- Bake at 350° for 1 hour or until cheese is melted and bubbly.

Alfredo Sauce

½ cup butter
1½ cups half-and-half

1½ cups grated Parmesan cheese

- Cook butter and half-and-half in a saucepan over medium heat, stirring constantly. Add Parmesan and cook, stirring constantly, until thickened.

Serves 8 to 10

Company Lasagna with Balsamella Sauce

This dish is not difficult to prepare, just a little time consuming.
The results are well worth the effort and will yield you an abundance of praise!
The Balsamella sauce makes this otherwise traditional dish exceptional!

2-3	garlic cloves, chopped	4	cups ricotta cheese
¼	cup olive oil	2	tablespoons chopped fresh parsley
1½	pounds sweet sausage, crumbled	4	large eggs
4	shallots	1	teaspoon sugar
4	pounds canned tomatoes, pureed	2	cups Balsamella Sauce
¼	cup minced fresh or 2 teaspoons dried basil	1	large package lasagna noodles, cooked
2	teaspoons salt	2	cups fontina cheese
	Freshly ground pepper to taste	¾	cup freshly grated Parmesan cheese

- Sauté garlic in hot oil in a large saucepan over medium heat until lightly browned; add sausage and cook 2 to 3 minutes.

- Add shallots to pan and sauté 1 minute; stir in tomato puree and basil. Bring to a boil; reduce heat and simmer 40 to 45 minutes. Add salt and pepper and set aside.

- Combine ricotta, parsley, eggs, sugar, and pepper to taste, stirring until smooth; set aside.

- Preheat oven to 350°.

- Spoon a small amount of Balsamella Sauce in the bottom of a 9 x 13 x 2-inch baking dish; top with lasagna noodles to cover. Layer one-third each of ricotta mixture, remaining Balsamella Sauce, and fontina cheese. Sprinkle with 1 tablespoon Parmesan cheese and top with one-fourth of tomato sauce. Cover with a layer of noodles. Repeat layers twice.

- Top with remaining tomato sauce and Parmesan cheese.

- Bake at 350° for 50 to 55 minutes. Let stand at room temperature 20 minutes before serving.

Balsamella Sauce

6	tablespoons butter	1	teaspoon salt
6	tablespoons all-purpose flour		Pinch of ground white pepper
1	cup milk		Pinch of ground nutmeg
1	cup heavy cream		

- Melt butter in a saucepan over medium heat; remove from heat and add flour, stirring well.

- Add milk and cream to saucepan and beat with a wooden spoon until smooth.

- Bring to a boil over medium heat, stirring constantly; boil, stirring constantly, until thickened. Reduce heat and simmer 2 to 3 minutes. Stir in salt, pepper, and nutmeg

Serves 10 to 12 generously!

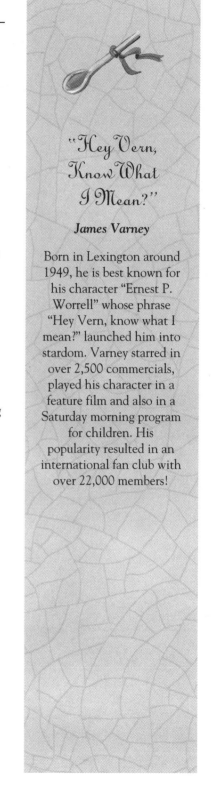

"Hey Vern, Know What I Mean?"

James Varney

Born in Lexington around 1949, he is best known for his character "Ernest P. Worrell" whose phrase "Hey Vern, know what I mean?" launched him into stardom. Varney starred in over 2,500 commercials, played his character in a feature film and also in a Saturday morning program for children. His popularity resulted in an international fan club with over 22,000 members!

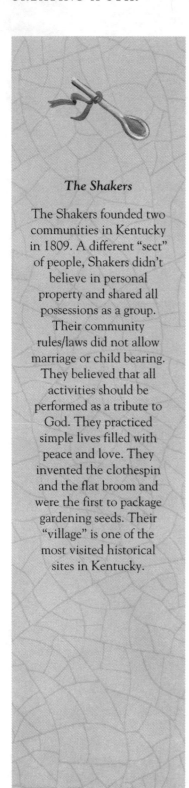

Baked Manicotti
with Spinach, Cheese, and Sausage Filling

1½	cups diced onion	1-3	teaspoons salt
1	garlic clove, crushed	1	tablespoon sugar
⅓	cup olive oil	½	teaspoon dried basil
1	(2-pound 3-ounce) can or 2½ (14.5-ounce) cans Italian tomatoes	¾	teaspoon dried oregano
		1½	cups water
			Cheese Filling
1	(6-ounce) can tomato paste	3	packages manicotti, cooked
2	tablespoons chopped fresh parsley		Freshly grated Parmesan cheese

- Sauté onion and garlic in hot oil in a 5-quart Dutch oven 5 minutes; add tomatoes, tomato paste, parsley, salt, sugar, basil, oregano, and water, mashing tomatoes with a fork. Bring to a boil; cover, reduce heat, and simmer, stirring occasionally, 1 hour.

- Spoon ¼ cup Cheese Filling into each cooked manicotti shell.

- Spoon 1½ cups tomato sauce into the bottom of each of 2 (9 x 13 x 2-inch) baking dishes. Place 8 manicotti in each dish in a single layer; top with 5 more in each dish.

- Spoon 1 cup sauce over manicotti in each dish. Sprinkle evenly with Parmesan cheese.

- Bake at 350° for 30 minutes or until bubbly.

Cheese Filling

2	pounds ricotta cheese	1	tablespoon chopped fresh parsley
2	cups (8 ounces) shredded mozzarella cheese	1	(10-ounce) package frozen chopped spinach, thawed and well drained
⅓	cup grated Parmesan cheese	2	(12-ounce) packages sausage, browned
2	large eggs		
1	teaspoon salt		

- Combine all ingredients in a large bowl, stirring well.

To freeze, line baking dishes with aluminum foil and assemble as directed. Fold foil over and fold to close. Freeze in dishes. When frozen remove foil packages from dishes. To serve, unwrap and place in baking dishes. Let stand at room temperature 1 hour. Bake, covered, at 350° for 1 hour.

Serves 12

Saucy Stuffed Shells with Four Cheeses

A fabulously hearty dish . . . sure to please a hungry crowd.

1   pound ground beef
1   pound sweet Italian sausage, with casings removed
1   teaspoon garlic salt
3   (6-ounce) cans tomato paste
3   cups water
½   teaspoon dried Italian seasoning
½   teaspoon dried basil
1   teaspoon salt
½   teaspoon pepper
1   (16-ounce) container ricotta cheese
2   large eggs, lightly beaten
1   cup grated Parmesan cheese
3   cups (12 ounces) shredded mozzarella cheese
    Jumbo pasta shells, cooked
8   (1-ounce) provolone cheese slices
    Freshly grated Parmesan cheese

- Cook ground beef, sausage, and garlic salt in a large saucepan over medium heat, stirring often with a fork, until meat is finely crumbled and browned. Drain well.

- Add tomato paste, water, Italian seasoning, basil, salt, and pepper to meat, stirring well; reduce heat and simmer 1 hour.

- Combine ricotta and eggs, stirring well; add 1 cup Parmesan and mozzarella cheese, stirring well. Spoon mixture generously into stuffed shells (shells will be overflowing with cheese mixture).

- Arrange stuffed shells in a 9 x 13 x 2-inch baking dish lightly coated with vegetable cooking spray. Place provolone slices over shells. Top with meat sauce.

- Bake, covered, at 350° for 45 minutes. Uncover and bake 15 minutes. Let stand at room temperature 10 to 15 minutes before serving.

- Serve with freshly grated Parmesan cheese.

Serves 12

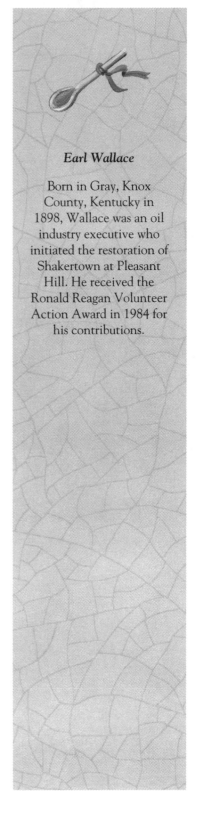

Earl Wallace

Born in Gray, Knox County, Kentucky in 1898, Wallace was an oil industry executive who initiated the restoration of Shakertown at Pleasant Hill. He received the Ronald Reagan Volunteer Action Award in 1984 for his contributions.

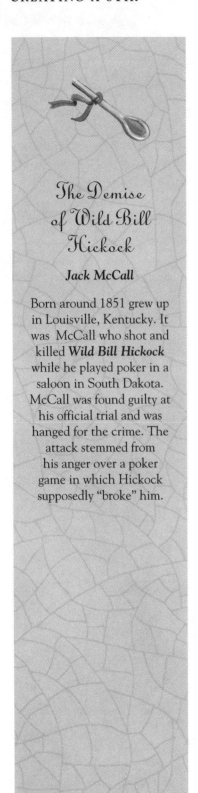

The Demise of Wild Bill Hickock

Jack McCall

Born around 1851 grew up in Louisville, Kentucky. It was McCall who shot and killed **Wild Bill Hickock** while he played poker in a saloon in South Dakota. McCall was found guilty at his official trial and was hanged for the crime. The attack stemmed from his anger over a poker game in which Hickock supposedly "broke" him.

Mott's Spaghetti and Meatballs

1	onion, chopped	1	(6-ounce) can tomato paste
1	tablespoon vegetable oil	1	bay leaf
1	tablespoon red wine vinegar	1	teaspoon salt
1	tablespoon sugar	½	teaspoon pepper
1	(14.5-ounce) can tomatoes, undrained	2	tablespoons chopped fresh parsley
1	(8-ounce) can tomato sauce		Mott's Meatballs
			Hot cooked spaghetti

- Sauté onion in hot oil in a large saucepan over medium heat until tender. Add vinegar, sugar, tomatoes, tomato sauce and paste, bay leaf, salt, pepper, and parsley; reduce heat and simmer 30 minutes.

- Add meatballs to sauce and simmer 30 minutes.

- Discard bay leaf. Serve over hot cooked spaghetti.

Mott's Meat Balls

1	white bread slice	¼	cup grated Parmesan cheese
1	pound lean ground beef	1	teaspoon salt
3	tablespoons chopped fresh parsley	½	teaspoon pepper
1	garlic clove, chopped	1	large egg, lightly beaten

- Soak bread in water; squeeze out all liquid.

- Combine bread, ground beef, parsley, garlic, Parmesan, salt, pepper, and egg; form into golf ball-size balls.

- Brown meatballs in hot oil in a skillet over medium heat; drain on paper towels.

Serves 4 to 6

Noodles with Fresh Green Cabbage and Caraway

A great change from potatoes and rice-this makes a nice vegetarian meal as well.

1	large green cabbage	1	teaspoon caraway seeds
1	teaspoon salt	¼	teaspoon pepper
5	tablespoons butter or margarine	8	ounces wide noodles, cooked
6	garlic cloves, diced		

- Cut cabbage into quarters and cut quarters into thin long shreds, discarding heart. Measure 4 cups shredded cabbage, reserving remaining cabbage for another use.

- Sprinkle salt over cabbage and let stand 30 minutes. Squeeze cabbage to drain.

- Melt butter in a large saucepan over medium heat; add cabbage, garlic, caraway seeds, and pepper. Cook, stirring often, 5 minutes or until cabbage is crisp-tender. Remove from heat.

- Add hot cooked noodles, tossing to coat. Transfer to a serving platter.

Serves 6

Company Noodles

A nice alternative to rice or potatoes!

1	(16-ounce) container sour cream, divided	1	teaspoon salt
1	cup small-curd cottage cheese	8	ounces egg noodles, cooked
1	medium onion, diced		Grated Parmesan cheese

- Combine 1 cup sour cream, cottage cheese, onion, and salt in a large bowl; add hot cooked noodles, tossing gently.

- Pour mixture into a 2-quart baking dish lightly coated with vegetable cooking spray. Spread remaining 1 cup sour cream over top. Cover generously with Parmesan cheese.

- Bake at 350° for 40 to 45 minutes or until golden.

Serves 6 to 8

Do not substitute light or nonfat sour cream.

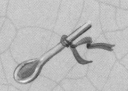

"Lets all go to the Lobby!"

Herman Ellis

Herman Ellis founded the Ellis Popcorn Company, a mail order business started in the early 1950's. If you've eaten popcorn at the movie theater, odds are you've eaten Ellis "blue ribbon" popcorn! Theaters are one of the company's biggest markets. Murray, Kentucky is home for the company, which grows its own corn. The company is still owned and operated by the Ellis family.

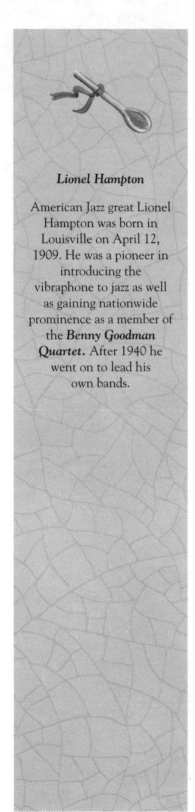

Chicken and Gruyère Stuffed Shells

Impress your guests with this savory and sophisticated pasta dish.

16 ounces jumbo shells, cooked and
    drained

Chicken Pecan Filling

3	cups finely chopped cooked chicken	2	cups ricotta cheese
1	cup coarsely chopped pecans	⅓	cup Parmesan cheese
½	cup finely chopped parsley	½	cup shredded Gruyère or Swiss cheese
2	eggs		

- Combine all ingredients together, mix well.

- Stuff cooked shells with Chicken Pecan Filling.

- Place stuffed shells in buttered casserole dish and bake at 350° for 30 minutes or until sauce is hot and bubbly.

Gruyère Sauce

¼	cup butter	½	cup dry sherry
½	cup minced shallots		Salt and white pepper to taste
6	tablespoons flour	1	cup shredded Gruyère or Swiss cheese
2½	cups chicken broth	½	cup heavy cream

- Melt butter in a saucepan, stir in shallots and cook 1 minute. Add flour and cook an additional 2 minutes.

- Gradually add chicken broth and sherry. Cook over low heat, stirring constantly until sauce thickens. Remove from heat and stir in salt, pepper, grated cheese and cream.

- Spoon sauce over prepared shells.

Serves 6 to 8

The Main Course

"We need food to sustain us, not only physically but emotionally. A home cooked meal shared with family and friends reminds us that the simple things make our lives rich. Every time my life gets too complicated, I pull myself back to the dinner table with family and close friends, and we all end up happier."

Laura Freeman
Owner and Operator, Laura's Lean Beef Company

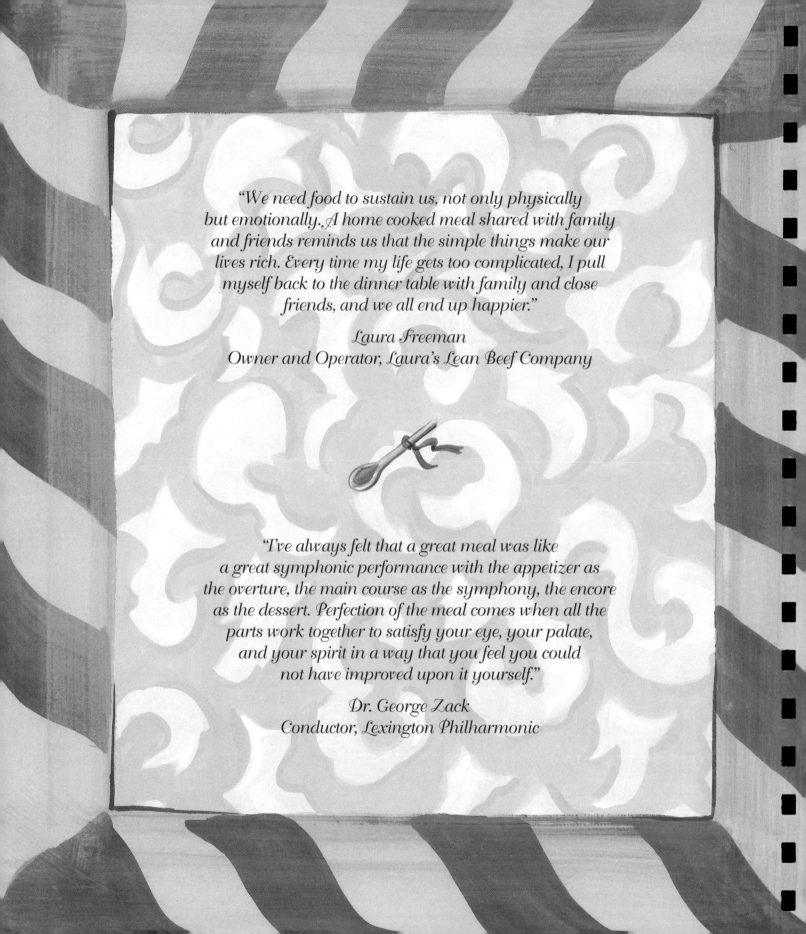

"I've always felt that a great meal was like a great symphonic performance with the appetizer as the overture, the main course as the symphony, the encore as the dessert. Perfection of the meal comes when all the parts work together to satisfy your eye, your palate, and your spirit in a way that you feel you could not have improved upon it yourself."

Dr. George Zack
Conductor, Lexington Philharmonic

Beef Tenderloin with Walnut-Feta Stuffing

An outstanding stuffing for tenderloin-you'll love the compliments!

1 (2-pound) whole beef tenderloin	2½ teaspoons dried oregano, divided
⅔ cup crumbled feta cheese	Salt and pepper to taste
2½ tablespoons chopped walnuts	⅔ cup canned beef broth
2½ tablespoons chopped fresh parsley	

- Preheat oven to 425°.

- Starting ½ inch from 1 end, cut tenderloin lengthwise to within ½ inch of opposite end, forming a long pocket.

- Combine feta, walnuts, parsley, and 1 teaspoon oregano; spoon into tenderloin pocket. Press tenderloin to enclose filling and secure with kitchen string at the center and ends.

- Rub remaining 1½ teaspoons oregano on outside of tenderloin and sprinkle with salt and pepper. Place in a 9 x 13 x 2-inch pan.

- Bake at 425° for 30 to 40 minutes or until a meat thermometer inserted into thickest portion registers 135° (medium-rare).

- Transfer tenderloin to a serving platter, reserving drippings in pan.

- Add broth to pan drippings and bring to a boil over medium-high heat, stirring to loosen browned particles. Transfer juices to a serving dish.

- Slice tenderloin and arrange on a serving platter. Serve with juices.

Serves 4 to 6

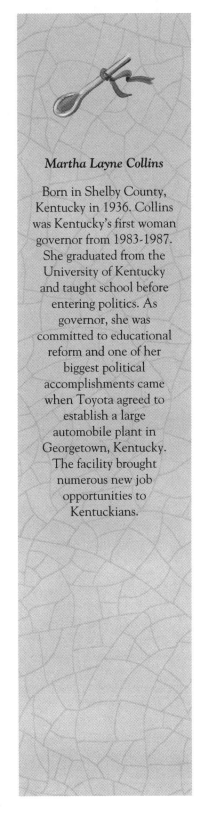

Martha Layne Collins

Born in Shelby County, Kentucky in 1936. Collins was Kentucky's first woman governor from 1983-1987. She graduated from the University of Kentucky and taught school before entering politics. As governor, she was committed to educational reform and one of her biggest political accomplishments came when Toyota agreed to establish a large automobile plant in Georgetown, Kentucky. The facility brought numerous new job opportunities to Kentuckians.

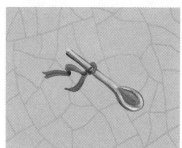

Where's The Beef?!!

Laura Freeman

Laura Freeman owns and operates Laura's Lean Beef Company, America's most successful all-natural lean beef company. It began as one woman's quest to eat healthier food and save the family farm. Started in the mid-1980's by Laura Freeman, a seventh generation Kentucky cattle farmer, Laura's Lean Beef is now sold by approximately 1600 stores in 23 states. Several hundred farmers provide beef for the company, agreeing to strict requirements regarding feed and herd management. In her first year, Freeman made $10,000. In 1998, company retail sales were close to $50 million! Laura believes the demand for her product is a real shift in lifestyle, that people truly desire a healthier, better tasting food and it isn't just a trend. Freeman didn't originally plan to become a farmer. She worked as a journalist for several years after graduating summa

Spectacular Beef Tenderloin with Port Sauce and Puff Pastry Garnish

Good recipes don't have to be complicated!
This one looks and tastes impressive but is actually very easy.

1	frozen puff pastry sheet, thawed	½	teaspoon dried crushed rosemary
1	(3- to 4-pound) beef tenderloin	1	bay leaf
2	cups beef broth	3	tablespoons butter, melted
¾	cup tawny port	3	tablespoons all-purpose flour
3	tablespoons minced shallots or onion		Fresh rosemary sprigs for garnish

- Cut puff pastry into leaf shapes using small cookie cutters or a knife. Transfer to cookie sheets.

- Bake at 400° for 10 minutes or until golden. Remove from oven and set aside.

- Place tenderloin on a rack in a shallow roasting pan, tucking long narrow ends under to form a rounded shape.

- Bake at 400° for 45 to 60 minutes. Remove from oven and cut into 8 to 10 slices.

- Bring broth, port, shallots, rosemary, and bay leaf to a boil in a saucepan over medium-high heat; boil until reduced to 1½ cups. Reduce heat and simmer 20 minutes.

- Combine butter and flour, stirring until smooth. Whisk into broth mixture; cook, stirring often, until thickened. Discard bay leaf.

- Place 1 to 2 tenderloin slices on each individual plate. Pour ¼ cup sauce over meat and top with 2 to 3 pastry leaves. Garnish with a fresh rosemary sprig.

Do not omit the puff pastry garnish. It is the combination of flavors from the meat, sauce, and pastry together that make this dish so delicious!

Serves 4 to 6

Beef Tenderloin with Rich Béarnaise

This is an excellent recipe for a cocktail buffet! The sauce is prepared the day before and chilled in the refrigerator, making it very thick and rich.

1   beef tenderloin, trimmed
    Salt and pepper to taste

½   cup butter
    Béarnaise Sauce

- Preheat oven to 450°.
- Place tenderloin on a rack in a roasting pan; season with salt and pepper.
- Bake at 450° for 30 minutes. Reduce oven temperature to 350° and bake 15 minutes.
- Remove from oven and spread ½ cup butter on top. Cover with aluminum foil and let stand at room temperature 15 minutes.
- Serve with Béarnaise Sauce and garnish with a fresh tarragon sprig.

Serves 8 for a main course and up to 12 for a cocktail buffet

Béarnaise Sauce

8   egg yolks
¼   cup lemon juice
1   teaspoon salt
2   cups melted butter (hot)
¼   cup tarragon vinegar

2   teaspoons dried tarragon
½   cup white wine
2   tablespoons chopped green onions
½   teaspoon pepper

- Process yolks, lemon juice, and salt at low speed in a blender until smooth. Heat butter to the bubbling stage but do not brown. With blender running, add 2 cups hot melted butter in a slow, steady stream.
- Bring vinegar, tarragon, wine, green onions, and pepper to a boil in a saucepan; boil until reduced to ¼ cup. Pour mixture into blender and process at high speed 15 seconds. Chill overnight.
- Bring sauce to room temperature and serve with sliced tenderloin.

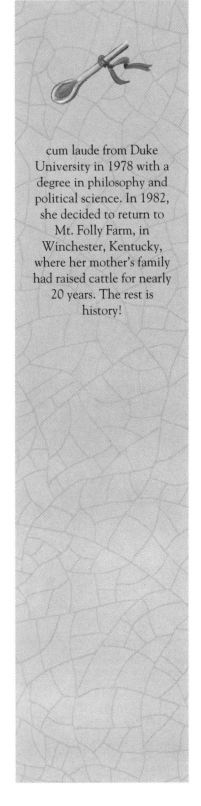

cum laude from Duke University in 1978 with a degree in philosophy and political science. In 1982, she decided to return to Mt. Folly Farm, in Winchester, Kentucky, where her mother's family had raised cattle for nearly 20 years. The rest is history!

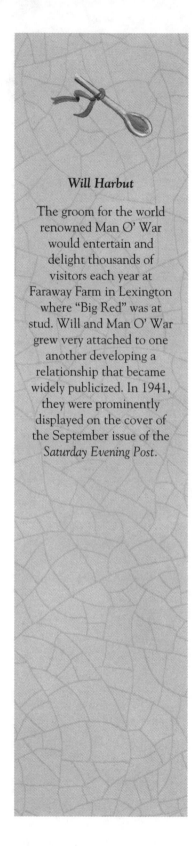

Will Harbut

The groom for the world renowned Man O' War would entertain and delight thousands of visitors each year at Faraway Farm in Lexington where "Big Red" was at stud. Will and Man O' War grew very attached to one another developing a relationship that became widely publicized. In 1941, they were prominently displayed on the cover of the September issue of the *Saturday Evening Post*.

Tenderloin of Beef with Blue Cheese and Herb Crust

A savory but simple entrée you'll make again and again!

1	(2¼-pound) beef tenderloin, cut into medallions	1	tablespoon chopped fresh parsley
½	cup soft white breadcrumbs, toasted	1	tablespoon chopped fresh chives
¼	cup blue cheese	1	pinch freshly ground white pepper
		¼	cup Madeira

- Shape medallions similarly and chill.
- Process breadcrumbs and next 4 ingredients in a food processor until a coarse paste forms.
- Sear medallions on both sides in a dry cast-iron or nonstick skillet over medium-high heat until nicely browned. Transfer to a rack in a roasting pan, reserving drippings.
- Top medallions evenly with cheese mixture and bake at 350° until desired degree of doneness.
- Add Madeira to drippings in skillet and cook over medium heat, stirring to loosen browned particles. Cook until slightly reduced.
- Serve Madeira sauce with medallions.

Serves 10

Best Beef Brisket

*A deliciously different way to prepare brisket . . .
this easy recipe is perfectly suited for a large crowd.*

1	beef brisket, trimmed	2	tablespoons Worcestershire sauce
	Lemon pepper to taste		Juice of 1 lemon
	Ground black pepper to taste	1	tablespoon beef consommé
1	(1-ounce) package dry onion soup mix	¼	cup red wine
¼	cup soy sauce	1	garlic clove, minced

- Sprinkle both sides of brisket with lemon pepper and black pepper. Place brisket in a 9 x 13 x 2-inch pan.
- Combine soup mix, soy sauce, Worcestershire sauce, lemon juice, beef consommé, wine, and garlic; pour over brisket. Cover with aluminum foil.
- Bake at 250° to 275° for 5 to 6 hours.

Serves 8 to 10

Beef with Roasted Red Pepper Sauce

*Drizzle tender, grilled steaks with this tantalizing
sauce for a superior meal worthy of company.*

4   garlic cloves
4   (½-inch-thick) rib-eyes or filet
     mignons
18   whole allspice berries
1   (1-inch) cinnamon stick
1   teaspoon black peppercorns
1   teaspoon coriander seeds
½   teaspoon whole cloves

3   tablespoons chili powder
3   tablespoons dark brown sugar
1   tablespoon dried thyme
2   teaspoons dry mustard
1½   teaspoons salt
1   teaspoon ground nutmeg
     Fresh thyme leaves for garnish
     Roasted Red Pepper Sauce

- Rub garlic on both sides of steaks; set aside.

- Cook allspice, cinnamon stick, peppercorns, coriander, and cloves in a small dry skillet over medium heat, stirring constantly, until toasted and starting to smoke. Process in a small electric spice or coffee grinder until ground.

- Combine ground spice mixture, chili powder, brown sugar, thyme, mustard, salt, and nutmeg. Reserve 2 tablespoons mixture for sauce.

- Rub remaining mixture on both sides of steaks. Cover and chill 8 hours.

- Grill steaks on a lightly greased food rack over medium heat (300° to 350°) 4 to 5 minutes on each side (rare to medium-rare) or until desired degree of doneness.

- Serve steaks on individual plates in a pool of Roasted Red Pepper Sauce. Garnish with fresh thyme leaves.

Roasted Red Pepper Sauce
1   cup sweet roasted red peppers
1   cup chicken stock
1   cup dry red wine
2   tablespoons honey

2   teaspoons Asian or favorite chili
     sauce
2   teaspoons reserved rub

- Process peppers, chicken stock, wine, honey, and chili sauce in an electric blender until smooth; stir in reserved rub and transfer to a saucepan.

- Bring sauce to a boil over high heat; boil until reduced to 1½ cups. Let cool and chill.

Serves 4

*You can also broil steaks 4 inches from heat (with electric oven door partially open)
3 minutes on each side or until desired degree of doneness.*

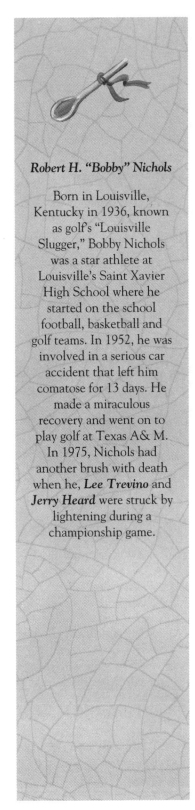

Robert H. "Bobby" Nichols

Born in Louisville, Kentucky in 1936, known as golf's "Louisville Slugger," Bobby Nichols was a star athlete at Louisville's Saint Xavier High School where he started on the school football, basketball and golf teams. In 1952, he was involved in a serious car accident that left him comatose for 13 days. He made a miraculous recovery and went on to play golf at Texas A&M. In 1975, Nichols had another brush with death when he, **Lee Trevino** and **Jerry Heard** were struck by lightening during a championship game.

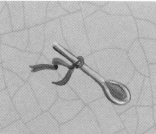

Beef Stroganoff with Crème Fraîche

3 cups Crème Fraîche
1½ tablespoons Dijon mustard
3 tablespoons tomato paste
3 tablespoons Worcestershire sauce
2 teaspoons paprika
¾ teaspoon salt
  Freshly ground pepper
1 teaspoon demi-glace

10 tablespoons butter, divided
2 (8-ounce) packages fresh mushrooms, stemmed and thinly sliced
24 medium-size white pearl onions
3 pounds beef filet tips, thinly sliced on the diagonal
  Hot cooked wide noodles, buttered
  Chopped fresh parsley

- Simmer Crème Fraîche, mustard, tomato paste, Worcestershire sauce, paprika, salt, pepper, and demi-glace in a medium saucepan 20 minutes. Remove from heat and cover.

- Melt 3 tablespoons butter in a large skillet over medium heat; add mushrooms and sauté 10 minutes or until golden. Transfer to a bowl and set aside.

- Cut an X in the root end of each onion. Bring a saucepan of water to a boil; add onions and cook 10 minutes. Drain and rinse under cold water; peel.

- Melt 2 tablespoons butter in skillet over medium heat; add onions and sauté until lightly browned. Add to mushrooms.

- Melt remaining 5 tablespoons butter in skillet over high heat; add beef tips and cook 3 to 4 minutes or until browned.

- Bring sauce to a simmer over medium heat; add mushrooms and onions and simmer 5 minutes. Add beef and simmer 2 minutes or until thoroughly heated.

- Serve beef mixture over buttered wide noodles; sprinkle with parsley.

Crème Fraîche

1½ cups heavy cream   1½ cups sour cream

- Whisk together heavy cream and sour cream in a small bowl. Cover loosely with plastic wrap and let stand in a warm spot overnight.

- Cover and chill at least 4 hours.

Serves 6

You can find demi-glace at specialty food stores.

Grits and Grillades

Wonderfully spicy and very satisfying!
(pronounced [gree-YAHDS])

4	pounds (½-inch-thick) beef round steak, trimmed	1	teaspoon dried tarragon
3	tablespoons all-purpose flour	¾	teaspoon dried thyme
½-¾	cup bacon drippings	1	cup water
½	cup all-purpose flour	1	cup red wine
2	cups chopped green onions	3	teaspoons salt
1	cup chopped onion	½	teaspoon pepper
1	cup chopped celery	2	bay leaves
1½	cups chopped green bell pepper	2	dashes hot sauce
2	garlic cloves, minced	2	tablespoons Worcestershire sauce
2	cups chopped tomato	3	tablespoons chopped fresh parsley
			Grits

- Place steak between 2 sheets of plastic wrap and flatten to ¼-inch thickness using a meat mallet or a rolling pin. Dredge steak in 3 tablespoons flour.
- Brown steak in 4 to 5 tablespoons hot bacon drippings in a large Dutch oven over medium heat. Transfer to a platter, reserving drippings; keep steak warm.
- Add 4 to 5 more tablespoons hot bacon drippings to reserved drippings in Dutch oven. Gradually add ½ cup flour and cook, stirring constantly, 30 to 40 minutes or until browned.
- Add green onions, chopped onion, celery, bell pepper, and garlic to roux and cook until onion is opaque. Add tomato, tarragon, and thyme and cook 3 minutes.
- Stir in 1 cup water and wine. Add steak, salt, pepper, bay leaves, hot sauce, and Worcestershire sauce; reduce heat and simmer at least 2 hours.
- Discard bay leaves and stir in parsley.
- Serve steak mixture over Grits.

Serves 6

Grits

6	cups water	2	cups (8-ounces) shredded cheddar or garlic cheese (optional)
1½	cups quick-cooking grits		
¾	teaspoon salt	2	tablespoons butter

- Bring 6 cups water to a boil in a saucepan over high heat; gradually add grits and salt, stirring well.
- Reduce heat to medium-low and cook, covered, 5 to 7 minutes. (Do not over thicken.)
- Add cheese, if desired, stirring until melted. Add butter, stirring well.
- If too thick when ready to serve, reheat and stir in a small amount of milk.

Serves 6

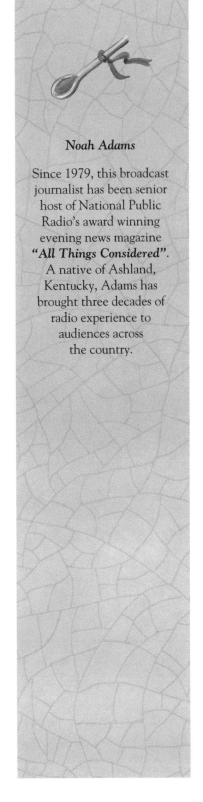

Noah Adams

Since 1979, this broadcast journalist has been senior host of National Public Radio's award winning evening news magazine *"All Things Considered"*. A native of Ashland, Kentucky, Adams has brought three decades of radio experience to audiences across the country.

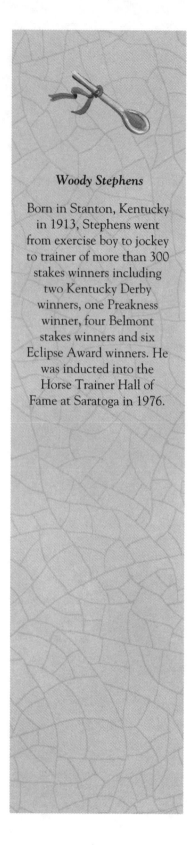

Woody Stephens

Born in Stanton, Kentucky in 1913, Stephens went from exercise boy to jockey to trainer of more than 300 stakes winners including two Kentucky Derby winners, one Preakness winner, four Belmont stakes winners and six Eclipse Award winners. He was inducted into the Horse Trainer Hall of Fame at Saratoga in 1976.

Father's Day Ribs

Saucy and delicious! These ribs should not be reserved for Father's Day alone . . . Dads love them anytime!

6 cups beer	2 teaspoons salt
2½ cups firmly packed dark brown sugar	2 teaspoons dried crushed red pepper
1½ cups apple cider vinegar	2 bay leaves
1½ tablespoons chili powder	8 pounds baby back pork ribs, cut into 4-rib sections
1½ tablespoons ground cumin	Salt to taste
1 tablespoon dry mustard	

- Bring beer, brown sugar, vinegar, chili powder, cumin, mustard, salt, red pepper, and bay leaves to a boil in a large Dutch oven; reduce heat and simmer 1 minute.

- Add half of ribs to sauce; cover and simmer 25 minutes or until ribs are tender. Transfer ribs to a baking sheet. Repeat procedure with remaining ribs.

- Bring sauce to a boil; boil 40 minutes or until reduced to 3 cups. Discard bay leaves.

- Brush ribs with sauce and season with salt. Grill over medium heat (300° to 350°) 6 minutes on each side or until browned, basting occasionally with sauce.

Honey-Ginger Marinated Flank Steak

The simple ingredients in this marinade come together to produce a spectacular flavor for mainstay flank steak.

¼ cup soy sauce	1½ teaspoons ground ginger
3 tablespoons honey	¾ cup vegetable oil
2 tablespoons vinegar	5-6 green onions, chopped
1½ teaspoons garlic powder	1 (1½- to 2-pound) flank steak

- Whisk together soy sauce, honey, vinegar, garlic powder, ginger, oil, and green onions.

- Place steak in a shallow dish; pour marinade over top. Cover and chill at least 6 hours, longer if possible.

- Drain steak, reserving marinade. Bring marinade to a boil in a saucepan; boil 2 minutes.

- Grill steak over medium heat (300° to 350°) 15 to 20 minutes. Slice steak thin on the diagonal and serve with sauce.

Serves 4 to 6

Glazed Flank Steak
with Orange and Rosemary Garnish

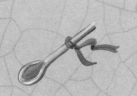

1 cup teriyaki marinade
½ cup chopped onion
⅓ cup honey
⅓ cup orange juice
1 tablespoon dark sesame oil

1 garlic clove, crushed
Pepper to taste
1 (2-pound) beef flank steak
Orange slices
Fresh rosemary sprigs

- Whisk together teriyaki marinade, onion, honey, orange juice, sesame oil, garlic, and pepper in a medium-size shallow dish. Reserve ¾ cup.
- Lightly score flank steak in a crisscross pattern. Place in marinade mixture, turning to coat. Chill 15 minutes on each side.
- Drain steak, reserving marinade.
- Grill steak over medium heat (300° to 350°) 17 to 21 minutes (medium-rare), basting occasionally with marinade. Transfer to a serving platter.
- Bring reserved ¾ cup marinade to a boil in a small saucepan.
- Spoon hot marinade over steak; slice and serve garnished with orange slices and fresh rosemary sprigs.

Serves 4 to 6

Tangy Bar-B-Q Beef Sandwiches

3 cups diced celery
1 cup diced onion
1 cup ketchup
1 cup barbecue sauce
1 cup water
2 tablespoons apple cider vinegar
2 tablespoons Worcestershire sauce

2 tablespoons brown sugar
1 teaspoon salt
1 teaspoon pepper
1 teaspoon chili powder
½ teaspoon garlic powder
1 (3- to 4-pound) chuck roast

- Combine first 12 ingredients in a slow cooker, stirring well.
- Add roast to slow cooker; cover and cook on HIGH 6 to 7 hours.
- Remove roast and let cool. Shred and return to sauce.
- Serve on buns with sliced onion, pickles, and relish.

Serves 6 to 10

"String Music"!

Orlando "Tubby" Smith-A native of Scotland, Maryland, was named Head Basketball Coach at the University of Kentucky on May 12, 1997. Tubby became the Wildcats' 5th coach since 1930 and the 20th coach in school history. He first came to UK as assistant coach for two seasons. He left to become head coach at Tulsa and then the University of Georgia, reviving distressed programs at both schools. In 6 years as head coach, he has amassed an incredible 124-62 record, coaching teams to the last 4 NCAA Tournaments including three Final 16 finishes. During his first season at UK he led his Wildcat team to a National Championship title, sending hoards of Big Blue fans into a frenzy! This explains his well deserved reputation as one of the nation's finest college basketball coaches. Coach Smith is known for his remarkable ability to lead young men and instill in them, a strong sense of sportsmanship, self-respect, reverence and determination.

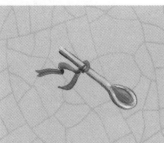

"There She Is . . ."

Phyllis George Brown

The life of Phyllis George Brown reads like a colorful patchwork quilt much like those she writes about in her latest book. In 1971 she won the Miss America title representing Texas and she is the central character in Frank DeFord's legendary book about the pageant, *There She Is*. She was a pioneer female sportscaster, the first in U.S. sports history. She made her Network Television debut in 1974 hosting "NFL Today" where she stayed for eight seasons earning an Emmy Award for her work. During her marriage to John Y. Brown, a restaurateur turned politician, she was Kentucky's first lady. Her grace and charm for which she is legendary made her popular among Kentuckians. She was also a highly successful businesswoman, marketing her own ready-to-cook chicken, "Chicken By George" and is the author of two books "Kentucky Crafts" and "Living With Quilts".

Molasses Mopped Steaks

The hearty glaze is "mopped" on for a full, rich flavor.

1	medium-size sweet onion, minced	1½	cups dark molasses
4	tablespoons olive oil, divided	2	tablespoons fresh cracked pepper
1	tablespoon grated fresh ginger	1¼	teaspoons salt
3	garlic cloves, minced	1	(1-pound) flank steak or 4 (8-ounce)
¼	cup plus 2 tablespoons dark rum		filet mignons or 2 (1½-inch-thick)
4½	cups orange juice		boneless top loin steaks

- Sauté onion in 3 tablespoons hot oil in a skillet over medium-high heat until tender. Add ginger and garlic and cook 1 minute.

- Add rum to mixture and cook 5 minutes or until liquid is evaporated.

- Add orange juice, molasses, pepper, and salt and cook 20 to 25 minutes or until mixture is reduced to 1½ cups. Remove from heat and let cool to room temperature.

- Brush steak with remaining 1 tablespoon oil and sprinkle with salt.

- Grill steak over medium heat (300° to 350°) 5 minutes; turn and begin "mopping" meat with glaze. Cook 10 to 15 minutes, turning and mopping often.

Serves 4

Eye of Round with Oriental Citrus Marinade

½	cup soy sauce	¼	teaspoon garlic powder
1¼	cups orange juice	1	(3- to 4-pound) eye of round roast
2	tablespoons wine vinegar		

- Combine soy sauce, orange juice, vinegar, and garlic powder, stirring well.

- Place roast in a shallow dish; pour marinade over top. Cover and chill overnight, turning occasionally. Transfer roast to a roasting pan, reserving marinade.

- Bake at 375° for 30 minutes. Pour reserved marinade over top. Reduce oven temperature to 350° and bake, covered, 3 hours, basting occasionally.

Serves 6 to 10

Roast can be prepared in a slow cooker. Pour marinade over meat in slow cooker and cook on LOW 6 to 8 hours or until meat is done and tender.

Grilled Beef Fajitas with Fresh Pico de Gallo

Slice flank steak on the diagonal to keep the meat tender.

¼-½ cup butter, melted
    Juice of 2 medium lemons
¼ cup Worcestershire sauce
¼ cup soy sauce
3 pounds flank or round steak

6 flour tortillas
    Toppings: guacamole, chopped tomato, Pico de Gallo, sour cream, shredded cheddar cheese

- Combine butter, lemon juice, Worcestershire sauce, and soy sauce in a large shallow dish.
- Add steak to marinade, turning to coat. Cover and chill 4 to 6 hours.
- Remove steak from marinade, discarding marinade.
- Grill over medium heat (300° to 350°) 5 to 10 minutes on each side. Slice steak on the diagonal into thin strips.
- Warm tortillas on the grill or in the oven. Divide meat evenly into 6 portions and place on tortillas. Serve with desired toppings and Pico de Gallo.

Pico de Gallo

1 medium or large sweet onion, finely diced
2-3 large tomatoes, finely diced with juice reserved

2-4 jalapeño peppers, seeded and finely diced
⅓ cup finely minced fresh cilantro
    Juice of 1 lime
1 tablespoon sugar

- Combine all ingredients, stirring well.

Serves 6

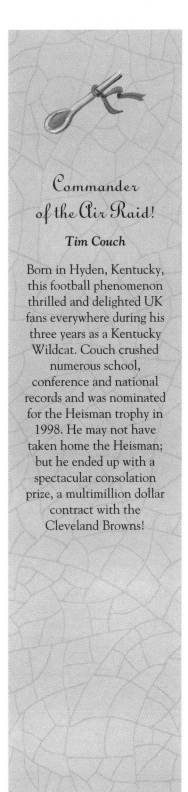

Commander of the Air Raid!

Tim Couch

Born in Hyden, Kentucky, this football phenomenon thrilled and delighted UK fans everywhere during his three years as a Kentucky Wildcat. Couch crushed numerous school, conference and national records and was nominated for the Heisman trophy in 1998. He may not have taken home the Heisman; but he ended up with a spectacular consolation prize, a multimillion dollar contract with the Cleveland Browns!

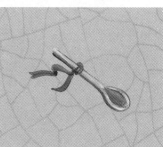

Olympic Redemption

Col. Maxine "Micki" King (USAF, Ret.)

Micki King, resident of Lexington, Kentucky, diving's Olympic gold medal winner in 1972, suffered heartbreak at the 1968 Olympic Games. Leading the springboard diving competition through eight dives, she shattered her left arm on the diving board during dive #9. King courageously finished the competition, placing fourth. She found redemption four years later in Munich, easily winning the gold medal. Other honors include NCAA diving coach of the year three times and was also the first woman to coach and teach at the then all-male U.S. Air Force Academy. Her leadership and devotion to the Olympic movement resulted in the formation of the Athlete's Advisory Council, and President Ford selected King to serve on his Olympic Sports Commission. She served as President of U.S. Diving (1990-1994) and was selected as U.S. Diving's Team Leader for the 1996 Olympic Games.

Oriental Beef and Vegetable Kabobs

Great for a cookout!

2   pounds sirloin tips, cut into 1½-inch cubes
2   onions, cut into chunks
2   green bell peppers, cut into 2-inch pieces
1   (8-ounce) package fresh mushrooms, stemmed
1   (6-ounce) jar marinated artichoke hearts
½   pint cherry tomatoes
2   yellow squash, thickly sliced

2   zucchini, thickly sliced
½   cup vegetable oil
¼   cup honey
3   tablespoons white vinegar
2   tablespoons soy sauce
1   garlic clove, minced
2   tablespoons minced fresh parsley
1   teaspoon ground ginger
1   teaspoon salt
½   teaspoon pepper

- Thread sirloin tips, onion, and bell pepper alternately on skewers. Thread mushrooms, artichokes, tomatoes, squash, and zucchini alternately on separate skewers. Place skewers in a shallow glass baking dish.

- Whisk together oil, honey, vinegar, soy sauce, garlic, parsley, ginger, salt, and pepper; pour over skewers. Cover and chill 1 to 24 hours.

- Grill skewers over medium heat (300° to 350°) 6 to 7½ minutes on each side for meat (medium-rare) and 2½ to 4 minutes on each side for vegetables. Serve kabobs with rice.

Serves 6

Spicy Rubbed Beef Brisket

This simple and tasty recipe brings the barbecue inside!

1½	teaspoons salt	1	teaspoon crushed bay leaf
1½	teaspoons pepper	1	(4- to 5-pound) beef brisket, trimmed
2	tablespoons chili powder		Barbecue Sauce

- Combine salt, pepper, chili powder, and crushed bay leaf; rub evenly on brisket. Place brisket, fat side up, in a Dutch oven. Sprinkle with remaining rub.

- Bake, covered, at 275° for 4 hours. Remove from oven and scrape off rub mixture.

- Cut brisket into thin slices and place on a serving platter. Pour Barbecue Sauce over top.

Barbecue Sauce

1	cup ketchup	1	teaspoon chili powder
⅛	teaspoon salt	2	tablespoons chopped onion
1	cup water	¼	cup Worcestershire sauce
½	cup cider vinegar	3	medium bay leaves
1	teaspoon sugar	1	garlic clove, minced
1	teaspoon paprika		Dash of pepper

- Bring all ingredients to a boil in a large saucepan. Reduce heat and simmer 15 minutes. Discard bay leaves.

Serves 8 to 10

Party Pork Tenderloin

Great for parties, picnics, and tailgating!

1	cup soy sauce	⅛	teaspoon pepper
½	cup sherry	1	medium onion, diced
½	cup firmly packed brown sugar	2	(1-pound) boneless pork
1	teaspoon salt		tenderloins

- Combine soy sauce, sherry, brown sugar, salt, pepper, and onion, stirring well.

- Place tenderloins in an aluminum foil-lined roasting pan; pour marinade over top. Cover and chill 2 hours.

- Bake at 400° for 10 minutes. Reduce oven temperature to 325° and bake 1 hour and 40 minutes or until done.

- Let cool and chill thoroughly.

- Cut tenderloins into 2½- x 1-inch slices as thin as a quarter. Arrange on a platter and serve at room temperature with hot mustard.

Serves 8 to 12

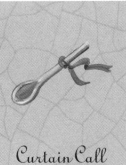

Curtain Call

Mae West, the Marx Brothers, Helen Hayes, Fannie Brice, George M. Cohan, and Lillian Russell are just a sampling of the legendary stars that have graced the historic stage of The Lexington Opera House in Lexington, Kentucky. Its history is as lavish as its velvet and gilt interior. Local performing arts groups continue to perform there. The Opera House opened in 1887 and was quickly billed as "The best one-night stand in America." In 1906 a production of "Ben Hur" included an onstage chariot race! Since its restoration in 1975 the Opera House has played home to a variety of Broadway plays and musicals as well as performances by the Lexington Ballet.

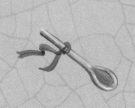

Neil and Mary Beth Van Uum

Owners and operators of **Joseph-Beth Booksellers.** Joseph-Beth, named Publisher's Weekly National Bookseller of the year, opened its first store in Lexington in November 1986. The original store has gone through two expansions from 6,500 square feet originally to over 40,000 square feet today! The opening of a second store in Cincinnati in 1993 gave the Van Uums, graduates of the University of Cincinnati, the perfect opportunity to return to their alma mater. Since then Joseph-Beth has acquired four more stores (Davis-Kidd Booksellers in Tennessee) tripling the size of the Joseph-Beth family. Although Neil had no background in the book business, he had a solid background in marketing. Mary Beth on the other hand, was from a family that "knew books". She is the sister of **Thomas and Louis Borders,** the founders and former

Mother's Roast Beef and Gravy

*The aroma of this garlic studded roast,
wafting from the kitchen, is absolutely heavenly!*

1	(4½- to 5-pound) rump roast	1-2	tablespoons vegetable oil
4	garlic cloves	¼	cup all-purpose flour
1	tablespoon salt	4-5	cups water or beef broth
1	teaspoon freshly ground pepper		

- Make 4 evenly spaced holes in roast with a sharp knife; push 1 garlic clove into each hole, making sure garlic is not exposed. Pat roast dry with paper towels and rub with salt and pepper. Let stand at room temperature 10 minutes.
- Brown roast on all sides in hot oil in a large Dutch oven over medium heat. (Roast should be mahogany colored before turning.) Cover, reduce heat, and cook 3 hours or until meat is tender and close to falling apart.
- Transfer roast to a serving platter, reserving drippings in Dutch oven.
- Combine flour and 2 cups water, stirring until smooth. Add to pan drippings and cook over low heat, stirring constantly, until smooth. Add remaining water, ½ cup at a time, until desired consistency is reached. Season to taste.
- Serve gravy over sliced roast with mashed potatoes.

Serves 8

Sesame-Ginger Pork Tenderloin

*Easy preparation and superb flavor makes this
recipe perfect for entertaining family and friends!*

1½	cups soy sauce	1	teaspoon garlic salt
¾	cup water	4	tablespoons sesame seeds
¾	cup vegetable oil	2	(1-pound) pork tenderloins
2	teaspoons ground ginger		

- Whisk together soy sauce, ¾ cup water, oil, ginger, garlic salt, and sesame seeds.
- Place tenderloins in a shallow dish; pour marinade over top. Cover and chill at least 6 hours.
- Remove tenderloins from marinade, reserving marinade.
- Grill tenderloins over high heat (400° to 500°) 10 minutes on each side, basting with marinade occasionally during the first 10 minutes.

Serves 6 to 8

Pork Tenderloin Scaloppine with Citrus Balsamic Sauce

The sauce is superb-an excitingly different dish!

1	(1-pound) pork tenderloin, cut crosswise into ½-inch-thick slices
	Salt and pepper to taste
1½	teaspoons butter
1½	teaspoons olive oil
¼	cup minced green onions or scallions
1	tablespoon honey
⅛	teaspoon ground allspice
1	cup chicken stock or rich chicken broth
1	tablespoon fresh lemon juice
¼	cup heavy cream
1	tablespoon balsamic vinegar

- Place pork slices between 2 sheets of plastic wrap and flatten to ¼-inch thickness using a meat mallet or rolling pin. Season with salt and pepper.

- Melt butter and oil in a large skillet over high heat; add pork in batches and cook 30 to 60 seconds on each side. Transfer pork to a serving platter.

- Reduce heat to medium-high; add green onions, honey, and allspice and cook, stirring often, 1 to 2 minutes or until green onions are soft.

- Increase heat to high and add chicken stock and lemon juice. Bring to a boil, stirring to loosen browned particles; boil until reduced by half.

- Add cream to skillet and boil 1 minute or until thickened. Add vinegar and season with salt and pepper; return to a boil.

- Spoon sauce over pork and serve immediately.

Serves 4

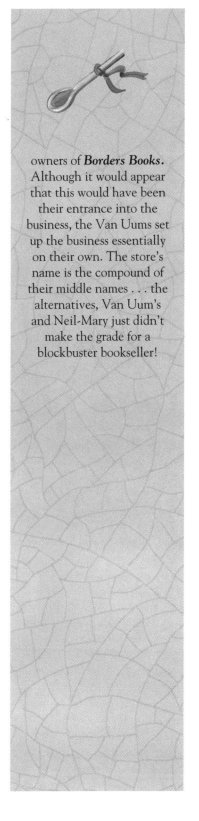

owners of **Borders Books.** Although it would appear that this would have been their entrance into the business, the Van Uums set up the business essentially on their own. The store's name is the compound of their middle names . . . the alternatives, Van Uum's and Neil-Mary just didn't make the grade for a blockbuster bookseller!

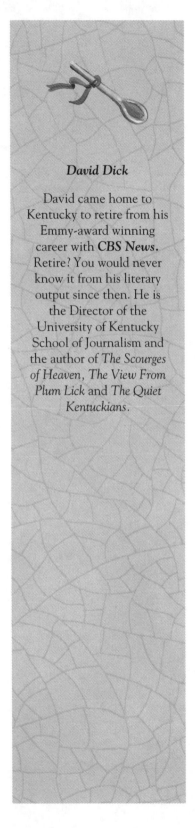

David Dick

David came home to Kentucky to retire from his Emmy-award winning career with **CBS News.** Retire? You would never know it from his literary output since then. He is the Director of the University of Kentucky School of Journalism and the author of *The Scourges of Heaven, The View From Plum Lick* and *The Quiet Kentuckians.*

Pork Tenderloin with Apples and Mustard Glaze

A multitude of flavors are fabulously blended and "stuffed" into this show stopping dish!

½	cup vegetable oil	1	small Granny Smith apple, thinly sliced
⅓	cup hoisin sauce		
½	cup cola soda	1	small onion, thinly sliced
½	cup orange juice	6	garlic cloves, halved
2	tablespoons soy sauce	1	tablespoon chopped fresh rosemary
2	(1-pound) pork tenderloins	¼	cup maple syrup
⅓	cup bourbon or apple juice	2	tablespoons brown sugar
¼	cup raisins	2	tablespoons Dijon mustard

- Combine oil, hoisin sauce, soda, orange juice, and soy sauce, stirring well.

- Place tenderloins in shallow dish; pour marinade over top. Cover and chill 6 hours or overnight.

- Combine bourbon or apple juice and raisins in a small bowl and let stand 45 minutes.

- Butterfly tenderloins lengthwise and lay open flat. Alternate apple and onion slices down the center of each. Top evenly with raisins, garlic, and rosemary. Close tenderloins over filling and place on aluminum foil.

- Combine syrup, brown sugar, and mustard; brush half of mixture over tenderloins. Fold foil closed and place in a 9 x 13 x 2-inch pan.

- Bake at 325° for 25 minutes. Pour remaining syrup mixture over tenderloins and close foil. Bake an additional 20 to 25 minutes or until a meat thermometer inserted into thickest portion registers 160°.

Serves 6

Marinated Pork and Onion Kabobs

You'll love what the marinade does for these deliciously different kabobs!

¼ cup soy sauce
2 tablespoons chili sauce
2 tablespoons honey
1 tablespoon vegetable oil
1 tablespoon minced green onion

1 teaspoon curry powder
1 (2-pound) fresh pork butt, trimmed
    and cut into 1-inch cubes
3 medium onions, quartered

- Combine soy sauce, chili sauce, honey, oil, green onion, and curry powder in a nonmetallic bowl.

- Place pork in a shallow dish; pour marinade over top, tossing to coat. Cover and chill at least 3 hours, stirring occasionally.

- Remove pork from marinade, reserving marinade.

- Thread pork and onion alternately on skewers. Grill over medium heat (300° to 350°) 20 to 25 minutes or until pork is tender, basting often with reserved marinade.

Serves 4 to 6

You can also broil skewers on a rack in a roasting pan 10 minutes on each side, basting often.

Mongolian Pork Chops

This spicy blend of ingredients works magic on ordinary pork chops.

1½ cups rice wine vinegar
¾ cup soy sauce
3 tablespoons black bean sauce or
    black bean garlic
1½ cups chopped green onions
¾ cup chopped fresh cilantro

3 teaspoons chopped fresh chives
4-5 garlic cloves, minced
1½ teaspoons ground coriander
6-8 (¾-inch-thick) boneless butterflied
    pork chops or boneless pork loin
    chops

- Combine vinegar, soy sauce, black bean sauce or garlic, green onions, cilantro, chives, minced garlic, and coriander, stirring well.

- Place pork chops in a shallow dish; pour marinade over top. Cover and chill 4 to 24 hours.

- Drain pork chops, reserving marinade.

- Grill pork chops over medium-high heat (350° to 400°) 15 minutes or until center is white but still moist, basting occasionally with marinade.

Serves 6 to 8

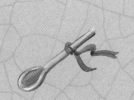

Cliff Hagan

Born in Owensboro, Kentucky in 1931, this high school All-American took his basketball skills to the University of Kentucky in 1950 where he was a two-time All-American helping the Wildcats win 86 of 91 games during his four year career there. Included in his collegiate career is a 1951 national championship under legendary coach Adolph Rupp. As a senior, Hagan helped lead UK to a perfect 25-0 record. After college he had a highly successful NBA career with the St. Louis Hawks. Following his retirement from professional basketball in 1970, he returned to Lexington where he started a restaurant chain, Cliff Hagan's Ribeye. In 1975 he replaced the late Harry Lancaster as the Athletic director for the University of Kentucky during which time he upgraded the athletic facilities that included a new football stadium, an aquatics center and an indoor tennis center. The men's basketball team also won a national championship under his reign as athletic director.

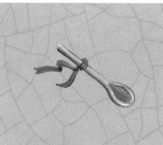

"Baron of the Bluegrass"

Adolph Rupp

Born in 1901 in Kansas, Coach Rupp is credited with bringing "big time" basketball to the South and to the University of Kentucky in 1930 where he reigned as "Baron of the Bluegrass" for 42 years. He introduced the fast break, honed offensive execution, created an excitement for the game and produced thousands of die-hard Kentucky fans that to this day "bleed blue"! Rupp didn't just win games (876 to be exact), he won championships . . . 28 SEC titles, 5 Sugar Bowl Tournament titles, 1 NIV tournament championship, 21 appearances in the NCAA Tournament, 4 NCAA championship titles and an Olympic Gold Medal in 1948. His success is unparalleled, his contribution to the sport unrivaled. He is a legend and his presence will live on forever.

Braised Pork Chops with Onions and Sticky Rice

6 (½-inch-thick) lean center-cut pork chops, trimmed
4 tablespoons soy sauce, divided
1 teaspoon sugar
1 tablespoon rice wine or pale dry sherry
2 teaspoons all-purpose flour
3 tablespoons vegetable oil
3 medium-size sweet onions, finely shredded
2 tablespoons cold water
3 cups cooked Japanese sticky rice

- Place pork chops between 2 sheets plastic wrap and flatten as thin as possible using a meat mallet or rolling pin. Transfer to a shallow dish.
- Combine 2 tablespoons soy sauce, sugar, and rice wine; pour over pork chops, turning to coat. Transfer pork chops to a sheet of wax paper.
- Lightly sprinkle flour over pork chops on both sides.
- Cook 3 pork chops in 2 tablespoons hot oil in a wok or skillet over high heat (reduce heat to medium if oil starts to smoke) 2 minutes on each side or until golden. Transfer to a plate. Repeat procedure with remaining 1 tablespoon oil and pork chops.
- Add onion to wok and stir-fry over medium heat 1 minute or until opaque. Return pork chops to wok and sprinkle with remaining 2 tablespoons soy sauce and 2 tablespoons water. Cover tightly, reduce heat, and simmer 20 minutes.
- Transfer pork chops to a large serving platter and spread onions over top. Serve with Japanese sticky rice.

Serves 6

Pan-Seared Veal Scallops with Mushrooms and Tomatoes

Elegant and impressive!

½ teaspoon salt
¼ teaspoon pepper
½ cup all-purpose flour
2 pounds (¼-inch-thick) veal scallops
5 tablespoons butter, divided
2 tablespoons olive oil
1½ pounds fresh mushrooms, sliced

2 tablespoons chopped onion
¾ cup beef broth
¾ cup dry white wine
2 large tomatoes, diced
1 teaspoon dried tarragon
½ teaspoon dry mustard
2 tablespoons chopped fresh parsley

- Combine salt, pepper, and flour in a shallow dish; dredge veal in mixture, coating lightly.

- Bring 3 tablespoons butter and oil to a boil in a large skillet over medium heat; add veal and brown on both sides, adding butter as needed. Transfer veal to a plate.

- Melt remaining 2 tablespoons butter in skillet; add mushrooms and sauté until golden. Add to veal.

- Bring onion, broth, and wine to a boil in skillet; reduce heat and simmer, whisking to loosen browned particles.

- Add tomato, tarragon, mustard, veal, and mushrooms to skillet; cover and cook over low heat, turning veal occasionally, 30 minutes.

- Serve warm and sprinkle with chopped parsley.

Serves 6

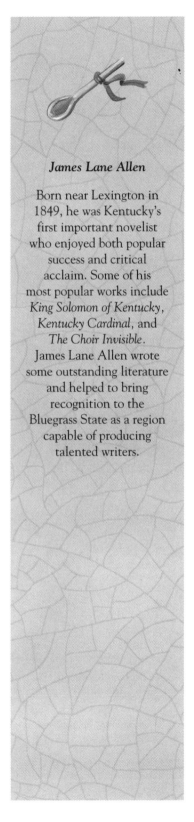

James Lane Allen

Born near Lexington in 1849, he was Kentucky's first important novelist who enjoyed both popular success and critical acclaim. Some of his most popular works include *King Solomon of Kentucky, Kentucky Cardinal,* and *The Choir Invisible.* James Lane Allen wrote some outstanding literature and helped to bring recognition to the Bluegrass State as a region capable of producing talented writers.

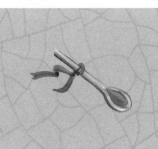

Thomas Merton

Born in Prades, France in 1915, Thomas Merton, was a Trappist monk and writer, and became one of the most famous American Roman Catholics of the 20th century. As a young man Merton traveled with his artist parents in France and studied briefly at Cambridge University, England, before coming to the United States in 1939. He earned a master's degree from Columbia University and it was during those years that he gradually changed from an agnostic to a devout Roman Catholic. After teaching English for a while and working in a Harlem settlement house, Merton decided to become a monk, choosing the Trappist order for its discipline of silence and solitude. In 1941 he entered the Abbey of Our Lady of Gethsemani south of Bardstown, Kentucky. Within the monastery he served for years as master of students and novices. Outside it, his writing,

Lamb Shanks with Garlic and Herbs

6	garlic cloves, minced	1½	cups sliced onion
2	teaspoons salt, divided	2	tablespoons chopped fresh rosemary
1	teaspoon freshly ground pepper, divided	3	tablespoons chopped fresh mint
4	lamb shanks	1	tablespoon chopped fresh thyme
2	tablespoons all-purpose flour	1	tablespoon chopped fresh parsley
2	tablespoons olive oil	1	cup white wine
		3	cups veal or chicken broth

- Preheat oven to 325°.

- Combine 1 teaspoon minced garlic, 1 teaspoon salt, and ½ teaspoon pepper; rub over lamb shanks. Dredge lamb in flour.

- Brown lamb on all sides in hot oil in a Dutch oven over medium heat. Transfer to a plate.

- Add onion and remaining garlic to Dutch oven and cook 3 to 5 minutes or until softened. Add rosemary, mint, thyme, and parsley and cook 3 to 4 minutes.

- Add wine to Dutch oven and increase temperature to high; cook until reduced by half. Stir in broth and remaining salt and pepper; bring to a simmer.

- Return lamb to Dutch oven; cover and bake at 325° for 2 hours or until meat is tender.

- Uncover and increase oven temperature to 500°. Bake 20 minutes, basting occasionally.

- Remove shanks from Dutch oven and skim off fat from drippings. Cook drippings over high heat until reduced by half.

- Serve whole shanks with gravy or remove meat from bone and return to Dutch oven; serve as stew over rice and potatoes.

Serves 8

Chef Harriet Dupree
Dupree Catering
Lexington, Kentucky

Butterflied Leg of Lamb with Sauce Champignon

1½ cups dry white wine
¼ cup lemon juice
1 tablespoon sugar
1 teaspoon salt
1 teaspoon chopped fresh rosemary
2 teaspoons chopped fresh chives
½ teaspoon pepper
1 leg of lamb, boned and butterflied
1 (10-ounce) can condensed beef broth, undiluted
3 tablespoons all-purpose flour
½ cup mushrooms

- Combine wine, lemon juice, sugar, salt, rosemary, chives, and pepper, stirring well.

- Place lamb in a shallow dish; pour marinade over top. Cover and chill several hours, turning occasionally.

- Drain lamb, reserving marinade. Place lamb on a rack in a roasting pan.

- Bake at 325° for 2 hours or until a meat thermometer inserted into thickest portion registers 170° (medium).

- Pour marinade through a wire-mesh strainer into a glass liquid measuring cup; add enough broth to measure 2 cups.

- Combine ¼ cup broth mixture and flour, stirring until smooth. Pour remaining broth mixture into a saucepan and cook over medium heat until thoroughly heated. Add flour mixture, stirring constantly.

- Add mushrooms to broth mixture and bring to a boil; boil several minutes. Reduce heat and simmer 15 minutes.

- Serve sauce over lamb.

Serves 8

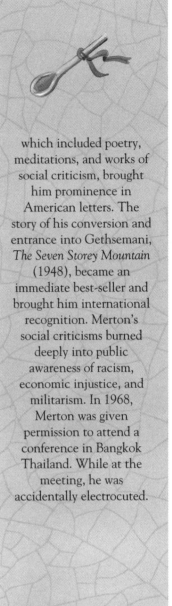

which included poetry, meditations, and works of social criticism, brought him prominence in American letters. The story of his conversion and entrance into Gethsemani, *The Seven Storey Mountain* (1948), became an immediate best-seller and brought him international recognition. Merton's social criticisms burned deeply into public awareness of racism, economic injustice, and militarism. In 1968, Merton was given permission to attend a conference in Bangkok Thailand. While at the meeting, he was accidentally electrocuted.

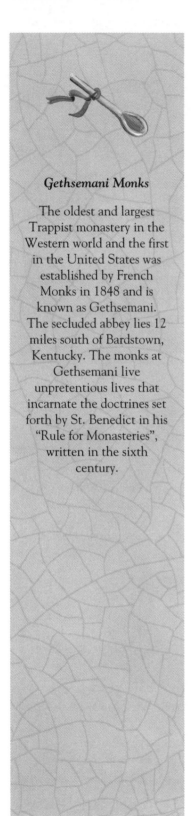

Gethsemani Monks

The oldest and largest Trappist monastery in the Western world and the first in the United States was established by French Monks in 1848 and is known as Gethsemani. The secluded abbey lies 12 miles south of Bardstown, Kentucky. The monks at Gethsemani live unpretentious lives that incarnate the doctrines set forth by St. Benedict in his "Rule for Monasteries", written in the sixth century.

Osso Buco

Try this classic Northern Italian dish for something enticingly different!

¼ cup all-purpose flour	2 garlic cloves, crushed
2 teaspoons salt	½ cup diced celery
¼ teaspoon pepper	1 (8-ounce) can tomato sauce
6 (¾- to 1-pound) veal shanks	1 cup dry white wine
3 tablespoons butter	1 teaspoon dried basil
3 tablespoons olive oil	1 teaspoon dried thyme
1 cup chopped onion	1 teaspoon grated lemon zest
1 cup thinly sliced carrot	3 fresh parsley sprigs
1 bay leaf	

- Combine flour, salt, and pepper on wax paper; rub mixture into veal shanks until well coated.

- Melt butter and oil in a Dutch oven over medium heat; add veal and cook 30 minutes or until browned on all sides. Transfer veal to a plate.

- Add onion, carrot, bay leaf, and half each of garlic and celery to Dutch oven and sauté until tender. Add tomato sauce, wine, basil, and thyme; bring to a boil.

- Reduce heat and return shanks to Dutch oven (the liquid should come halfway up the shanks). Cover and simmer 2 hours and 30 minutes.

- Combine remaining celery and garlic, lemon zest, and parsley, stirring well. Add to veal and simmer 5 to 10 minutes. Discard bay leaf.

- Serve veal with boiled new potatoes or over rice or pasta.

Serves 6

Grilled Butterflied Leg of Lamb

Simply seasoned with succulent results.

½	cup soy sauce	2	teaspoons dry mustard
2	garlic cloves, minced	1	bay leaf
1	tablespoon dried oregano	½	cup olive oil
1	tablespoon dried thyme	1	leg of lamb, butterflied and boned
1	tablespoon dried rosemary		

- Process soy sauce, garlic, oregano, thyme, rosemary, mustard, and bay leaf in a blender until smooth; with machine running, add oil in a slow, steady stream.

- Place lamb in a shallow dish; pour marinade over top. Cover and chill 24 hours.

- Drain lamb, reserving marinade

- Grill lamb over medium heat (300° to 350°) to desired degree of doneness, basting occasionally with reserved marinade.

Serves 8

Roasted Mediterranean Chicken

1	(3- to 4-pound) whole roasting hen or chicken	Garlic spray or minced garlic rub
	Extra-virgin olive oil pressed with lemons (Agrumato)	Spanex Seasoning Blend

- Wash hen both inside and out and dry thoroughly.

- Rub oil over hen and coat with garlic spray inside and out.

- Sprinkle Spanex lightly over outside of hen.

- Place hen on a vertical roaster in a pan. Bake at 350° for 1 hour and 30 minutes.

Place vertical roaster in a pan to catch the drippings.

John Kennan
The Mousetrap
Lexington, Kentucky

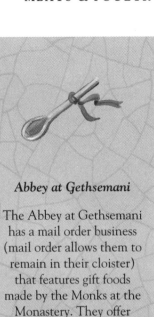

Abbey at Gethsemani

The Abbey at Gethsemani has a mail order business (mail order allows them to remain in their cloister) that features gift foods made by the Monks at the Monastery. They offer their Trappist cheese, fudge and world famous fruitcakes. Former White House Chef Henry Haller served Trappist Cheese at White House state dinners and world renowned Chef John D. Folse thinks their fruitcake is the best! It was also the cheese of choice for Pope John Paul II!

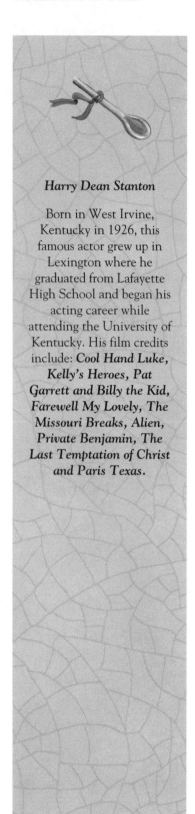

Harry Dean Stanton

Born in West Irvine, Kentucky in 1926, this famous actor grew up in Lexington where he graduated from Lafayette High School and began his acting career while attending the University of Kentucky. His film credits include: *Cool Hand Luke, Kelly's Heroes, Pat Garrett and Billy the Kid, Farewell My Lovely, The Missouri Breaks, Alien, Private Benjamin, The Last Temptation of Christ and Paris Texas.*

Lime Grilled Chicken with Black Bean Salsa

Wonderfully succulent! The salsa and chicken in this dish complement each other beautifully.

3	limes	2	garlic cloves, minced
2	tablespoons olive oil	6-8	skinned and boned chicken breasts
½	teaspoon salt		Black Bean Salsa
¼	teaspoon freshly ground pepper		

- Grate zest from 1 lime and squeeze juice from 3 limes.

- Combine lime zest, juice, oil, salt, pepper, and garlic, stirring well; pour over chicken and chill several hours.

- Grill chicken over medium-high heat (350° to 400°) 8 to 10 minutes on each side or until done.

- Serve chicken with Black Bean Salsa

Black Bean Salsa

2	(15-ounce) cans black beans, rinsed and drained	1	purple onion, chopped
1	(17-ounce) can corn, rinsed and drained	⅛	cup chopped fresh cilantro
2	large tomatoes, seeded and chopped	¼	cup lime juice
1	large avocado, chopped	2	tablespoons olive oil
		1	teaspoon salt
		½	teaspoon freshly ground pepper

- Combine all ingredients, stirring well.

Serves 6 to 8

Chicken and Artichoke Bake

*Served with a wonderful salad and crusty bread,
this dish becomes comfort food at its best!*

4-5 skinned and boned chicken breasts
2 bay leaves
1 cup cooking sherry, divided
   Salt and pepper to taste
3 tablespoons butter
1 (8-ounce) package fresh
   mushrooms, sliced
½ cup chopped green onions

1-2 garlic cloves
1 (14-ounce) can artichoke hearts,
   drained and chopped
¾ cup mayonnaise
½ cup sour cream
1½ cups freshly grated Parmesan
   cheese, divided

- Bring chicken, bay leaves, ½ cup sherry, salt and pepper, and water to cover to a boil in a Dutch oven; boil 1 hour or until chicken is done.

- Drain chicken; cut into bite-size pieces.

- Melt butter in a saucepan over medium heat; add mushrooms, green onions, and garlic and sauté until tender.

- Combine chicken and artichoke hearts in a large bowl; stir in sautéed vegetables.

- Fold mayonnaise, sour cream, ½ cup Parmesan cheese, and remaining ½ cup sherry into chicken mixture.

- Spoon mixture into a lightly greased 2-quart baking dish and sprinkle with remaining 1 cup Parmesan cheese.

- Bake at 350° for 30 to 45 minutes or until golden and bubbly.

- Serve over hot cooked rice or spinach noodles.

Serves 6 to 8

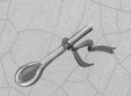

William Stamps Farish III

Born in 1939, this business mogul and lifelong horseman, established Lane's End Farm in Woodford County, Kentucky in 1978. Lane's End is one of the world's premier Thoroughbred farms. Farish is president of W. S. Farish Company, an investment firm named after his grandfather who founded Humble Oil (now part of Exxon) and was former president of Standard Oil. By 1999, Lane's End had raced over 100 stakes winners and bred more than 160 stakes winners including the 1972 Preakness winner, Summer Squall, the 1999 Kentucky Derby and Preakness winner, Charismatic and the 1999 Belmont winner Lemon Drop Kid. Farish and his wife Sarah are frequent hosts to former president and first lady *George and Barbara Bush* and *Queen Elizabeth II of England* who visits Kentucky to inspect thoroughbreds.

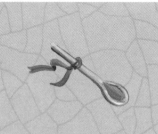

Its Finger Lickin' Good!

Colonel Harland Sanders

Creator of Kentucky Fried Chicken. It all started in 1930 in Corbin, Kentucky behind a service station in a lunchroom that seated 6 people! The business continued to grow and by 1937 Sanders' Café was opened accommodating 142 customers. His secret recipe chicken was the most popular item on the menu. After a fire destroyed the café, Sanders rebuilt the restaurant and added a motel. Business was good until the construction of Interstate 75. Sanders started selling franchises and by 1959, more than 200 outlets existed throughout the United States and Canada. Sanders' daughter Margaret developed the idea of "take-out" an innovation at the time. In 1964, Sanders sold the company to John Y. Brown, Jr. and Jack Massey for $2 million. They sold the business in 1971 to Heublein, Inc. for

Cashew Crusted Chicken with Tangerine Salsa

Spicy and hot, cool and tangy-they all come together to create an explosion of flavor and color in this spectacular dish!

1½ cups soft breadcrumbs
1½ cups cashews
1½ teaspoons dried thyme
1½ teaspoons ground coriander
1 teaspoon Chinese five spice
½ cup buttermilk
½ cup molasses

6-8 skinned and boned chicken breast halves
1½ teaspoons salt
½ teaspoon ground black pepper
¼ cup peanut oil
   Tangerine Salsa

- Process breadcrumbs, cashews, thyme, coriander, and Chinese five spice in a food processor until cashews are finely ground. Pour mixture onto wax paper.

- Combine buttermilk and molasses in a shallow dish.

- Season chicken with salt and pepper.

- Dip chicken in buttermilk mixture, letting excess drip off. Dredge in breadcrumb mixture, shaking off excess.

- Cook chicken in hot oil in a large skillet over medium heat 3 to 5 minutes on each side. Transfer to a baking dish and bake at 375° for 10 to 12 minutes or until chicken is golden brown.

- Cut chicken into thin slices and arrange on a serving plate, overlapping slices. Serve with Tangerine Salsa.

Tangerine Salsa

2 tangerines, sectioned, seeded, and cut into small pieces
1-2 plum tomatoes, seeded and diced
⅓ cup chopped purple onion
¼ cup diced poblano chile pepper
⅓ cup diced red bell pepper

1½ tablespoons lime juice
1 tablespoon vegetable oil
½ teaspoon ground coriander
½ teaspoon salt
½ teaspoon ground black pepper

- Combine all ingredients.

Serves 6 to 8

Greek Feta Chicken with Olives and Sun-Dried Tomatoes

This outstanding dish boasts the flavors of traditional Greek fare.
It is absolutely fantastic . . . you'll enjoy the compliments!

4	large skinned and boned chicken breasts	1	cup dry white wine, divided
	Salt and pepper to taste	¼	cup lemon juice
½	cup all-purpose flour	1	cup crumbled feta cheese
1	garlic clove, crushed	1	teaspoon dried oregano
1	tablespoon olive oil	½	cup chopped kalamata olives
		¼	cup chopped sun-dried tomatoes

- Season chicken with salt and pepper; dredge in flour, shaking off excess.
- Cook chicken and garlic in hot oil in a large skillet over medium heat until chicken is browned on both sides.
- Add ½ cup wine and lemon juice; cover, reduce heat, and simmer 5 minutes.
- Add remaining ½ cup wine and simmer 20 minutes.
- Sprinkle feta over chicken and cook until slightly melted.
- Sprinkle olives and chopped tomato over top. Sprinkle with oregano; cover and cook until cheese is melted.

Serves 4

Grilled Chicken with Citrus Dijon Marinade

1	cup olive oil	¼	cup chopped fresh oregano
1	cup dry white wine		Juice of 2 to 4 lemons
¼	cup coarse-grained Dijon mustard		Salt and pepper to taste
4	garlic cloves, minced	2	pounds chicken pieces

- Combine oil, wine, mustard, garlic, oregano, lemon juice, salt, and pepper, stirring well. Set aside 1 cup marinade.
- Combine remaining marinade and chicken in a zip-top plastic bag or shallow dish. Seal or cover and chill 4 hours, turning often.
- Grill chicken over medium-high heat (350° to 400°) 30 to 45 minutes, basting often with reserved 1 cup marinade.

Serves 6 to 8

$275 million and in 1978 it was sold to the R.J. Reynolds Company which in turn sold it to Pepsico, Inc. for $840 million in 1986. From Corbin, Kentucky to Hong Kong, everyone still enjoys that famous Kentucky fried chicken!!

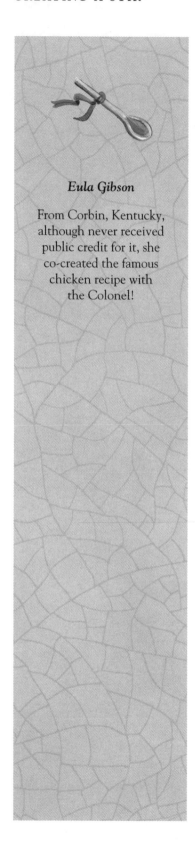

Eula Gibson

From Corbin, Kentucky, although never received public credit for it, she co-created the famous chicken recipe with the Colonel!

Tandoori Roasted Chicken

*This spicy Indian-inspired marinade makes
the chicken both delicious and extremely tender.*

2	teaspoons paprika	3	tablespoons fresh lemon juice
1½	teaspoons ground cumin	½	cup plain nonfat yogurt
¾	teaspoon ground coriander	2	garlic cloves, minced
¾	teaspoon ground ginger	½	teaspoon salt
½	teaspoon cayenne pepper	½	teaspoon ground black pepper
8	bone-in chicken breasts or mixed pieces		

- Cook paprika, cumin, coriander, ginger, and red pepper in a small heavy skillet over medium-low heat, shaking constantly, 30 seconds or until toasted. Transfer to a small bowl.

- Place chicken in a nonmetallic dish and make ½-inch-deep diagonal slices approximately 1 inch apart on each piece of chicken.

- Rub lemon juice into cuts.

- Stir yogurt, garlic, salt, and black pepper into spice mixture. Pour over chicken, tossing to coat. Cover and chill 4 hours or overnight.

- Remove chicken from marinade and let stand at room temperature 30 minutes before cooking.

- Preheat oven to 450°.

- Place chicken on a lightly greased rack in an aluminum foil-lined roasting pan.

- Bake at 450° for 40 to 50 minutes.

Serves 6 to 8

Chicken with Kiwi and Raspberry Glaze

*A ruby red glaze and bright green kiwifruit
mingle together for a dish that's pretty and tasty.*

4	bone-in chicken breast halves	1	cup raspberry preserves
1	teaspoon salt	½	cup port wine
¼	teaspoon pepper		Grated zest of 1 lemon
½	cup butter, melted	4	kiwifruit, sliced

- Place chicken in a shallow roasting pan and season with salt and pepper.

- Bake, skin side up, at 400° for 40 to 45 minutes, basting occasionally with melted butter.

- Remove chicken from oven and remove skin.

- Simmer preserves, port, and lemon zest in a medium saucepan 3 to 5 minutes or until thickened.

- Spoon raspberry glaze over chicken and top with kiwi slices.

- Bake an additional 3 minutes.

Serves 4

Fiery Cajun Rubbed Chicken with Apricot-Mustard Sauce

This fiery hot chicken gets cooled off with a sweet apricot-mustard sauce.

3½	teaspoons ground black pepper	2½	teaspoons cayenne pepper
4	teaspoons dried thyme		6-8 skinned and boned chicken breasts
3	teaspoons garlic salt		6-8 tablespoons butter
2½	teaspoons ground white pepper		Apricot-Mustard Sauce

- Combine black pepper, thyme, garlic salt, white pepper, and cayenne pepper; rub evenly on chicken breasts. Cover and chill 1 to 2 hours.

- Melt 2 tablespoons butter in a large heavy skillet over medium heat; add 2 chicken breasts and cook on both sides until golden and done. Drain chicken and transfer to a serving platter. Repeat procedure with remaining butter and chicken.

- Serve chicken with Apricot-Mustard Sauce.

Apricot-Mustard Sauce

2	cups apricot preserves	¾	cup spicy brown mustard

- Combine all ingredients, stirring well.

Serves 6 to 8

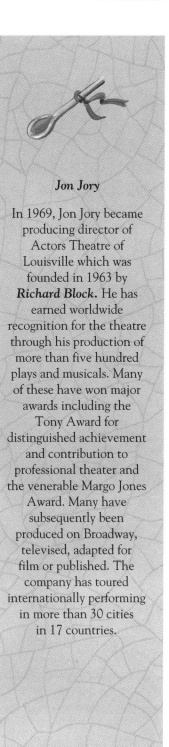

Jon Jory

In 1969, Jon Jory became producing director of Actors Theatre of Louisville which was founded in 1963 by **Richard Block.** He has earned worldwide recognition for the theatre through his production of more than five hundred plays and musicals. Many of these have won major awards including the Tony Award for distinguished achievement and contribution to professional theater and the venerable Margo Jones Award. Many have subsequently been produced on Broadway, televised, adapted for film or published. The company has toured internationally performing in more than 30 cities in 17 countries.

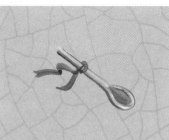

Making The Grade

Alice Lloyd

In 1915, Boston native Alice Lloyd came to Eastern Kentucky, starting her personal crusade to bring education to the mountains of central Appalachia. In 1923, she founded, along with **Jane Buchanan,** Alice Lloyd College, a private, liberal arts, interdenominational Christian institution in Pippa Passes, Kentucky, stands as the fruit of her labors. Accredited by the Commission on Colleges of the Southern Association of Colleges and Schools, Alice Lloyd now offers two bachelors degrees, with 13 majors to choose from. The college continues to be a beacon of hope to hundreds of young leaders from Kentucky, West Virginia, Virginia, Ohio and Tennessee. At Alice Lloyd College, young people discover purpose in their lives through developing their intellectual gifts, deepening their character, learning the value of work, and maintaining a strong sense of service to the Appalachian region.

Citrus Marinated Chicken with Orange and Lemon Garnish

1 medium onion, grated
4-5 garlic cloves, minced
¼ cup olive oil
½ cup orange juice
¼ cup freshly squeezed lemon juice
¼ cup chicken broth
1 teaspoon sugar
1½ teaspoons salt
½ teaspoon pepper
1½ teaspoons cider vinegar
1 (4-pound) whole chicken or 4 pounds bone-in chicken breasts

- Cook onion and garlic in hot oil in a skillet over medium heat 3 to 5 minutes.
- Add orange juice, lemon juice, chicken broth, sugar, salt, pepper, and vinegar and bring to a boil, stirring constantly.
- Remove from heat and let cool. Set aside ½ cup marinade.
- Combine chicken and remaining marinade in a shallow dish; cover and chill 6 to 8 hours or overnight.
- Remove chicken from marinade and place on a lightly greased rack in a roasting pan.
- Bake at 400° for 15 minutes.
- Reduce oven temperature to 350° and bake 1 hour to 1 hour and 30 minutes, basting often with reserved ½ cup marinade.

Serves 4

This chicken is best if it marinates overnight. You may need to cover chicken with aluminum foil after baking 45 minutes to prevent over browning.

Fusion Chicken

The melody of spices in this recipe fuses several Caribbean cuisines.

½ cup slivered almonds	⅓ cup water
3 tablespoons olive oil, divided	3 tablespoons dried currants
6 garlic cloves, minced	1½ tablespoons honey
8 skinned and boned chicken thighs	1¼ tablespoons ground cumin
2½ cups salsa	¾ teaspoon ground cinnamon

- Cook almonds in 1 tablespoon hot oil in a large skillet over medium heat 1 to 2 minutes or until golden brown. Remove from skillet.

- Sauté garlic in remaining 2 tablespoons hot oil in skillet, stirring constantly, 30 seconds.

- Add chicken to skillet and cook 2½ minutes on each side or until browned.

- Combine salsa, water, currants, honey, cumin, and cinnamon, stirring well. Pour over chicken.

- Cover chicken; reduce heat to medium and cook, stirring occasionally, 20 minutes or until tender.

- Sprinkle chicken with almonds. Serve chicken and glaze with rice or couscous.

Serves 4 to 6

Bruce's Bluegrass BBQ'd Chicken

An old Paducah, Kentucky recipe . . . this mustard-vinegar based sauce is a nice change from the typical hickory smoke types that are common in this area.

½ cup margarine	1 teaspoon chili powder
½ cup water	½ (8-ounce) jar horseradish mustard
½ cup cider vinegar	2 teaspoons salt
¼ bottle Worcestershire sauce	1-1½ whole chickens, cut into pieces

- Bring margarine, ½ cup water, vinegar, Worcestershire sauce, chili powder, mustard, and salt to a boil in a saucepan over medium heat. Remove from heat and let cool.

- Combine sauce and chicken in a shallow dish, tossing to coat. Chill up to 12 hours, if desired.

- Grill slowly over medium-low heat (300° to 325°), turning often, 1 hour or until chicken is browned and done.

This recipe can be doubled, if desired.

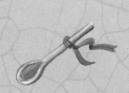

Mary Anderson

Born in 1859, this Shakespearean actress was reared in Louisville, Kentucky. She made her stage debut at the age of sixteen as Juliet in Shakespeare's *Romeo and Juliet*. Her performance launched a career that would make her the toast of the American stage. She was known for her exceptional talent and beauty not only in the United States but throughout Britain and Ireland as well. After retiring (at age 30!) at the peak of her career she sailed to England where she met her husband. She spent the remainder of her days there with her family and often entertained a wonderful array of notable friends that included: ***Henry James, Lord Tennyson, Sir James Barrie, Sir Edward Elgar, John Masefield*** and ***A.E. Housman!***

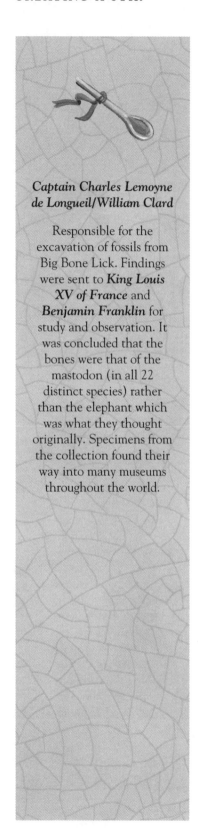

Honey-Mustard Baked Chicken

The sauce created from baking is excellent!

2	tablespoons butter		1	teaspoon ground cinnamon
¼	cup all-purpose flour		1	cup plain yogurt
½	cup honey		4	skinned and boned chicken breast halves
¼	cup prepared mustard			
1	teaspoon salt		⅓	cup white wine

- Melt butter in a large saucepan over medium heat; add flour and cook, stirring constantly, until bubbly.

- Stir honey, mustard, salt, and cinnamon into mixture; remove from heat and let cool.

- Combine honey mixture and yogurt in a shallow dish; add chicken, tossing to coat. Cover chicken and chill 2 to 3 hours.

- Transfer chicken to a baking dish, reserving marinade.

- Combine reserved marinade and wine and pour over chicken.

- Bake at 350° for 1 hour or until chicken is done.

Serves 2 to 4

Mahogany Glazed Chicken

This beautifully glazed chicken is nice served with Japanese Sticky Rice

1⅓	cups soy sauce		¼	cup dry mustard
½	cup vegetable oil		¼	cup molasses
1-2	garlic cloves, minced		6	skinned and boned chicken breast halves
4	teaspoons ground ginger			
3-4	tablespoons freshly grated gingerroot			

- Whisk together soy sauce, oil, garlic, ginger, gingerroot, mustard, and molasses.

- Combine marinade and chicken in a shallow dish and chill 6 hours or overnight.

- Drain chicken, reserving marinade.

- Grill chicken over medium-high heat (350° to 400°), basting occasionally with marinade, 15 to 20 minutes.

Serves 4 to 6

Enchiladas Monterey

This dish is a bit time-consuming but extremely tasty and
worth all of the compliments you'll get for a true Mexican taste!

1	tablespoon chopped onion	1	tablespoon chopped jalapeño
3	ounces vegetable oil	1	dozen soft corn tortillas
1	pound chopped cooked chicken		Monterey Sauce
	Salt and pepper to taste	2	cups (8 ounces) shredded Monterey
4	ounces cream cheese, softened		Jack cheese

4-6 ounces sour cream

- Sauté onion in hot oil in a skillet over medium heat until tender.

- Stir in chicken, salt, and pepper; remove from heat.

- Beat cream cheese and sour cream in a large bowl at medium speed with a hand held mixer until creamy; stir in chicken mixture and jalapeño. Season with salt and pepper.

- Cook tortillas on both sides in a lightly greased skillet over medium heat until softened.

- Spoon filling evenly into tortillas; roll up and place, seam side down, in a baking dish. Cover with Monterey Sauce and sprinkle evenly with Monterey Jack cheese.

- Bake at 350° for 20 to 30 minutes or until thoroughly heated.

Monterey Sauce

¾	cup butter	1	tablespoon chopped pimientos
¾	cup all-purpose flour	1	tablespoon chopped green chiles
1	quart warm chicken broth	1	tablespoon chopped fresh cilantro
¾	cup warm heavy cream	1	teaspoon salt
	or half-and-half	¼	teaspoon ground white pepper

- Melt butter in a saucepan over low heat; gradually add flour, stirring until well blended. (Do not let brown.)

- Remove from heat and gradually stir in chicken broth.

- Cook over low heat until smooth and thickened. Stir in cream. (Do not let boil.)

- Add pimientos, chiles, cilantro, salt, and pepper to sauce; cook, stirring often, until thoroughly heated. Keep warm.

Serves 6 to 8

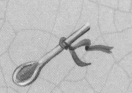

Cave Man . . .

Stephen Bishop

Born into slavery in 1821 in Glasgow, Kentucky, Bishop was one of the most celebrated guides in the history of Mammoth Cave. His wit and charm delighted tourists until his death in 1857. Visitors started requesting him and in the published travel logs of the 40's and 50's, he is the guide most often written about. On one particular cave tour, he and his guide group encountered the "bottomless pit" which heretofore had forced tour groups to turn back. With the help of a visitor, Bishop became the first person to cross the deep chasm by suspending a log pole across the "pit" and shinnying across. **Mammoth Cave** is the world's longest known cave system, with more than 340 miles of underground passages. It was Kentucky's first major tourist attraction and the second oldest in the United Sates, preceded only by **Niagara Falls.** This momentous natural and cultural site has attracted millions of visitors from around the world.

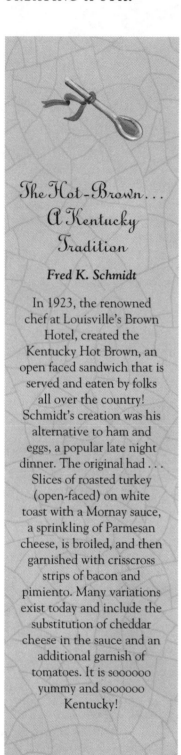

The Hot-Brown...
A Kentucky
Tradition

Fred K. Schmidt

In 1923, the renowned
chef at Louisville's Brown
Hotel, created the
Kentucky Hot Brown, an
open faced sandwich that is
served and eaten by folks
all over the country!
Schmidt's creation was his
alternative to ham and
eggs, a popular late night
dinner. The original had . . .
Slices of roasted turkey
(open-faced) on white
toast with a Mornay sauce,
a sprinkling of Parmesan
cheese, is broiled, and then
garnished with crisscross
strips of bacon and
pimiento. Many variations
exist today and include the
substitution of cheddar
cheese in the sauce and an
additional garnish of
tomatoes. It is soooooo
yummy and soooooo
Kentucky!

Kentucky Hot Brown Sandwiches

This popular Kentucky dish originated at The Brown Hotel in Louisville.

8 white bread slices, toasted with crusts removed	Sliced turkey or hen breast
	8 bacon slices, cooked

Béchamel Sauce

⅓ cup butter	1 teaspoon salt
½ medium-size onion, minced	Dash of cayenne pepper
⅓ cup all-purpose flour	Chopped fresh parsley
3 cups hot milk	Dash of ground nutmeg

- Melt butter in a saucepan over medium heat; add onion and cook 15 to 20 minutes or until lightly browned. Add flour, stirring until smooth. Add milk and next 4 ingredients and cook 25 to 30 minutes.

Mornay Sauce

2 cups Béchamel Sauce	1 tablespoon butter
2 egg yolks	¼ cup whipping cream, whipped
½ cup grated Parmesan cheese, divided	

- Cook Béchamel Sauce and yolks in a saucepan over medium heat, stirring constantly, until thoroughly heated (do not boil). Remove from heat immediately.
- Stir in ¼ cup cheese and butter; fold in whipped cream.
- Place 1 bread slice in the bottom of each of 4 ovenproof au gratin dishes. Top evenly with turkey and cheese sauce.
- Place 1 of remaining bread slices diagonally over sauce in each au gratin dish. Top evenly with bacon and sprinkle with remaining Parmesan cheese.
- Broil until lightly browned.

Sliced country ham can also be added to hen or turkey white meat.

Serves 4

Buttermilk-Cider Chicken with Apples and Pecans

A magnificent blending of flavor and texture . . .
a superb entrée that satisfies both the eye and the palate.

8 (4-ounce) skinned and boned chicken breast halves
1 cup buttermilk
½ cup margarine
1 Granny Smith apple, cut into wedges
1 Red Delicious apple, cut into wedges
1 cup apple cider
1 cup chicken broth
1 cup whipping cream
   All-purpose flour
2 tablespoons vegetable oil
2 tablespoons chopped fresh chives
¾ cup coarsely chopped pecans

- Place chicken in a 9 x 13 x 2-inch baking dish; pour buttermilk over top. Cover and chill overnight.
- Melt margarine in a large skillet over medium heat; add apple wedges and sauté until browned.
- Add cider to apple wedges and bring to a boil; boil until cider is reduced to ¼ cup.
- Add broth and cream and boil 15 minutes.
- Drain chicken; dredge in flour, coating well.
- Cook chicken in hot oil in a separate skillet over medium heat until done.
- Drain apple wedges, reserving sauce; add apple wedges to chicken and cook until thoroughly heated.
- Add reserved sauce and chives to chicken. Sprinkle with pecans and cook until thoroughly heated.

Serves 6 to 8

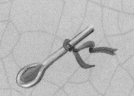

Jerome Lederer

Jerome Lederer is the founder of Jerrico, Inc., better known as the parent company of **Long John Silver's Seafood Shoppes,** the quick service seafood chain. The original company started as small six-seater hamburger stands, called The White Tavern Shoppes in Shelbyville, Kentucky. The chain grew to 13 before closing during World War II due to the shortage of meat and sugar. Following the war, Lederer opened a new chain of restaurants called **Jerry's.** He was joined by **Warren Rosenthal** in 1948. The company pioneered the theory of franchising to activate growth. Long John Silvers opened its first restaurant on Southland Drive in Lexington, Kentucky. By the late 80's there were more than 1,500 Long John Silvers in 36 states, the District of Columbia, Canada and Singapore!

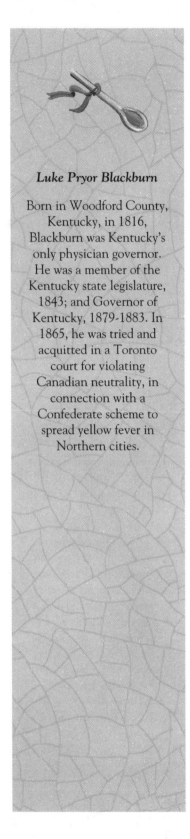

Jamaican Jerk Chicken

Sweet, hot, and very spicy! Jerk cooking refers to the Jamaican method of marinating and barbecuing chicken, pork, or beef. Try this recipe the next time you plan to barbecue!

6	green onions, diced	½	teaspoon freshly ground black pepper
1	medium-size yellow onion, diced	½	teaspoon ground ginger
3	Scotch bonnet or jalapeño peppers, seeded and minced	½	teaspoon ground cloves
¾	cup soy sauce	½	teaspoon ground nutmeg
½	cup red wine vinegar	½	teaspoon ground allspice
¼	cup vegetable oil	¼	teaspoon ground cinnamon
¼	cup firmly packed brown sugar	2-2½	pounds skinned and boned chicken breasts
2	tablespoons fresh thyme leaves		

- Puree all ingredients except chicken in a food processor 15 seconds or until smooth.
- Place chicken in a shallow dish and prick with a fork several times. Pour marinade over top. Cover and chill 6 to 12 hours, turning occasionally.
- Remove chicken from marinade, discarding marinade.
- Grill chicken over medium heat (300° to 350°) 10 to 15 minutes or until center is white.

Chicken can also be cut into strips prior to marinating. Serve Jamaican Jerk Chicken with a cool mango-papaya salsa or with San Juan Couscous Salad (see recipe index).

Sesame Crusted Chicken

1	cup finely crushed crackers	½	teaspoon pepper
1	cup grated Parmesan cheese	2	pounds skinned and boned chicken breast halves
¼	cup minced onion	½	cup butter, melted
3	tablespoons dried parsley flakes, crushed	2	tablespoons butter, softened
1	teaspoon salt	1	tablespoon sesame seeds

- Combine crackers, Parmesan cheese, onion, parsley, salt, and pepper in a shallow dish.
- Dip chicken in melted butter and dredge in Parmesan cheese mixture, coating well. Arrange chicken pieces in a shallow pan 1 inch apart.
- Dot chicken evenly with softened butter and sprinkle with sesame seeds.
- Bake at 350° for 1 hour or until done.

Serves 4

Sautéed Chicken in Lemon Cream Sauce

Rich and elegant.

6	skinned and boned chicken breast halves	¾	cup whipping cream
	Salt and pepper to taste	½	cup canned reduced-sodium chicken broth
¼	cup butter	½	cup freshly grated Parmesan cheese, divided
2	tablespoons dry vermouth		
2	teaspoons grated lemon zest		Chopped fresh parsley
2	tablespoons fresh lemon juice		Lemon wedges for garnish

- Place chicken between 2 sheets of plastic wrap and flatten to ½-inch thickness using a meat mallet or a rolling pin. Season chicken with salt and pepper.

- Melt butter in a large skillet over medium-high heat; add chicken and cook 3 minutes on each side or until done.

- Transfer chicken to a serving platter; cover with aluminum foil and keep warm.

- Pour butter from skillet; add vermouth, lemon zest, and juice to skillet. Bring to a boil; boil 1 minute, scraping to remove browned particles.

- Add cream, broth, and any juices accumulated from chicken to skillet; boil 8 minutes or until sauce consistency.

- Stir in ¼ cup Parmesan cheese. Season with salt and pepper.

- Pour sauce over chicken and sprinkle with remaining Parmesan cheese and parsley. Garnish with lemon wedges.

Serves 6

Provençal Turkey Breast

This recipe is excellent served warm with gravy made from pan drippings or chilled for sandwiches.

1	fresh or thawed turkey breast	2-3	tablespoons herbes de Provence
	Olive oil or vegetable cooking spray		Paprika to taste (add enough to create a warm color)
	Garlic salt to taste		
	Pepper to taste	1	(14-ounce) can chicken broth

- Place turkey in roasting pan, breast side up; rub with oil.

- Sprinkle turkey with garlic salt, pepper, herbes de Provence, and paprika.

- Pour broth into pan and bake according to turkey directions, basting occasionally.

For a one-pot meal, add chopped vegetables during last hour of baking.

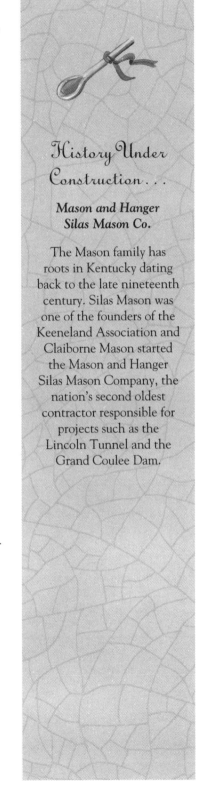

History Under Construction...

Mason and Hanger Silas Mason Co.

The Mason family has roots in Kentucky dating back to the late nineteenth century. Silas Mason was one of the founders of the Keeneland Association and Claiborne Mason started the Mason and Hanger Silas Mason Company, the nation's second oldest contractor responsible for projects such as the Lincoln Tunnel and the Grand Coulee Dam.

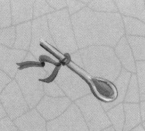

John Maxwell

Born in 1747, John Maxwell settled in Kentucky and signed the petition sent to the Virginia Assembly requesting official establishment of the town of Lexington. He was known for his generosity to the citizens of the town, allowing them free use of the natural springs on his land. He was also responsible for the annual 4th of July celebration held at Maxwell Springs. A sizeable portion of the land was often used as a park and gathering place for the city where picnics, barbecues and fairs were held. The area became so popular that Henry Clay once wrote, "No man can call himself a true Kentuckian who has not watered his horse at Maxwell Springs"!

Spicy Kung Pao Chicken

Flavor erupts from this dish! It is spicy and delicious!

2	tablespoons cornstarch
¼	teaspoon salt
½	egg white
2-3	teaspoons minced garlic
5	tablespoons black bean garlic
5	tablespoons hoisin sauce
3	tablespoons sherry
3	tablespoons red wine vinegar
1	tablespoon chile garlic sauce or chili paste
3	celery ribs, sliced
3	carrots, sliced
1	bunch green onions, chopped
3	tablespoons peanut oil
3	skinned and boned chicken breasts, cut into bite-size pieces
¼	cup peanut oil
	Hot cooked rice
½-¾	cup cashews

- Combine cornstarch, salt, and egg white, stirring well. Stir in minced garlic, black bean garlic, hoisin sauce, sherry, vinegar, and chile garlic sauce or chili paste

- Cook celery, carrot, and green onions in 3 tablespoons hot oil in a skillet over high heat, stirring constantly, 2 to 3 minutes. Transfer vegetables to a bowl.

- Cook chicken in ¼ cup hot oil in skillet over high heat, stirring constantly, 5 minutes or until done.

- Add garlic sauce and vegetables to chicken, stirring well.

- Serve over hot cooked rice and sprinkle with cashews.

Serves 4 to 6

All of these spices are readily available in the ethnic section of most grocery stores.

Pollo Cacciatore

2   medium onions, chopped
¼   cup extra-virgin olive oil
2   garlic cloves, minced
1   (3-pound) chicken, cut into 8
     pieces
1   cup dry white wine
1   (28-ounce) can peeled whole
     tomatoes, undrained and chopped

1   bay leaf
1   teaspoon minced fresh rosemary
¼   cup minced fresh flat-leaf parsley
     Salt and pepper to taste
1   cup condensed chicken broth
     Chopped fresh parsley for garnish

- Sauté onion in hot oil in a saucepan over medium-high heat 10 minutes.

- Add garlic and cook 2 minutes.

- Push onion to side of pan; add chicken and cook 4 minutes on each side or until browned.

- Add wine and cook 5 minutes or until liquid evaporates. Stir in chopped tomato with juice.

- Add bay leaf, rosemary, parsley, salt, and pepper and reduce heat. Cover partially and simmer 45 minutes, gradually adding broth as tomato juice evaporates.

- Discard bay leaf. Garnish with chopped fresh parsley. Serve with steamed potatoes, rice, or pasta.

Serves 4 to 6

Apricot Glazed Cornish Hens

1   (18-ounce) jar apricot preserves or
     orange marmalade
1   (16-ounce) bottle light or regular
     French dressing

1   (1.31-ounce) package dry onion
     soup mix (we used Lipton's)
2-3 tablespoons Worcestershire sauce
4-6 Cornish hens

- Combine orange marmalade, dressing, onion soup mix, and Worcestershire sauce, stirring well; set aside.

- Place hens in individual aluminum pans.

- Bake at 350° for 1 hour and 10 minutes.

- Add sauce evenly to hens; cover with foil and cook 20 minutes.

- Serve hens with wild rice.

Serves 4 to 6

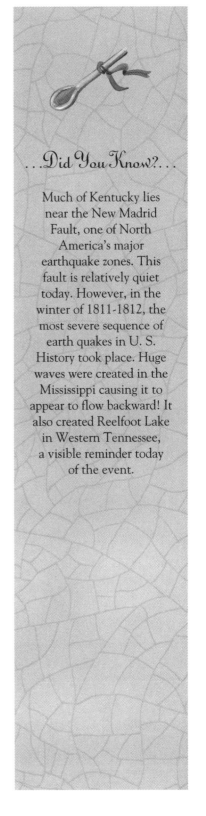

...Did You Know?...

Much of Kentucky lies near the New Madrid Fault, one of North America's major earthquake zones. This fault is relatively quiet today. However, in the winter of 1811-1812, the most severe sequence of earth quakes in U. S. History took place. Huge waves were created in the Mississippi causing it to appear to flow backward! It also created Reelfoot Lake in Western Tennessee, a visible reminder today of the event.

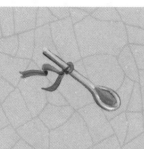

Marsha Norman

Born in Louisville in 1947, this playwright's work with mentally disturbed children and strict religious upbringing was the basis for the subject matter and dramatic and emotional content of her plays. Her first play was the award winning *Getting Out* which was published in The Best Plays of 1977-78, the first non-New York production included in the annual collection. Her production of *'night Mother* in 1982, received the Pulitzer Prize in 1983 for drama and was later made into a movie starring **Sissy Spacek** and **Anne Bancroft.**

Savory Sautéed Chicken on Fresh Greens with Tarragon-Dijon Vinaigrette

4 skinned and boned chicken breast halves	1 large head loose-leaf lettuce, torn into small pieces
1 medium onion, sliced into thin rings	¼ cup (1 ounce) shredded sharp cheddar cheese
1 yellow bell pepper, cut into thin strips	4-5 bacon slices, cooked and crumbled
1 red bell pepper, cut into thin strips	8 sun-dried tomatoes, rehydrated and sliced
1 teaspoon vegetable oil	Tarragon-Dijon Vinaigrette

- Sear chicken in a nonstick skillet over medium-high heat 4 to 5 minutes on each side or until done. Remove from skillet and set aside.

- Sauté onion and bell peppers in hot oil in skillet over medium-high heat until crisp-tender. Remove from heat.

- Arrange lettuce in a serving bowl or on individual plates. Top evenly with onion and bell peppers.

- Slice chicken and arrange over vegetables. Sprinkle with cheese, bacon, and sliced tomato.

- Serve immediately with Tarragon-Dijon Vinaigrette.

Tarragon-Dijon Vinaigrette

1 garlic clove, minced	½ teaspoon prepared horseradish
2 tablespoons tarragon vinegar	½ teaspoon salt
1 teaspoon Worcestershire sauce	¼ teaspoon pepper
1 teaspoon Dijon mustard	¼-⅓ cup olive oil

- Whisk together garlic, vinegar, Worcestershire sauce, mustard, horseradish, salt, and pepper; add oil in a slow, steady stream, whisking constantly.

Serves 4 to 6

King Ranch Chicken

1	onion, chopped	1-2	teaspoons chili powder
1	bell pepper, chopped	⅓-½	cup dry white wine (optional)
2	celery ribs, chopped	1	small package corn or flour tortillas, quartered
1	garlic clove, chopped		
	Olive oil	2	cups (8 ounces) shredded longhorn or medium cheddar cheese
2	cups chopped boiled chicken, with broth reserved		
1	(10¾-ounce) can cream of mushroom soup, undiluted	1	(10-ounce) can diced tomatoes with green chiles
1	(10¾-ounce) can cream of chicken soup, undiluted		

- Sauté onion, bell pepper, celery, and garlic in hot oil in a saucepan over medium heat until tender.
- Combine sautéed vegetables, chicken, mushroom soup, cream of chicken soup, chili powder, and, if desired, wine.
- Dip tortilla quarters into warm reserved chicken broth with a fork 1 at a time.
- Layer half each of tortilla quarters, chicken mixture, and cheese in a 9 x 13 x 2-inch baking dish. Repeat layers once. Chill overnight.
- Pour diced tomatoes over casserole.
- Bake at 350° for 45 to 50 minutes.

Serves 6 to 8

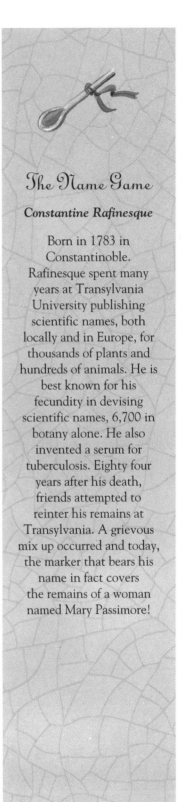

The Name Game

Constantine Rafinesque

Born in 1783 in Constantinoble. Rafinesque spent many years at Transylvania University publishing scientific names, both locally and in Europe, for thousands of plants and hundreds of animals. He is best known for his fecundity in devising scientific names, 6,700 in botany alone. He also invented a serum for tuberculosis. Eighty four years after his death, friends attempted to reinter his remains at Transylvania. A grievous mix up occurred and today, the marker that bears his name in fact covers the remains of a woman named Mary Passimore!

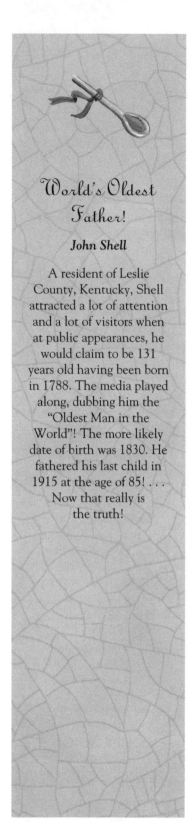

Chicken with Creamed Spinach, Gruyère, and Tomatoes

This recipe requires minimum effort for maximum enjoyment!

6	skinned and boned chicken breasts	6	tomato slices
6	egg whites, lightly beaten	6	thick Gruyère or Jarlsberg cheese
2	cups seasoned breadcrumbs		slices (large enough to cover
	Butter		chicken breast)
2	(10-ounce) packages frozen		
	creamed spinach, thawed		

- Preheat oven to 350°.

- Dip chicken in egg whites and dredge in breadcrumbs.

- Melt butter in a large skillet over medium-low heat; add chicken and cook 5 minutes on each side or until browned.

- Place creamed spinach in a 9 x 13 x 2-inch baking dish; arrange chicken over top.

- Top each chicken breast with a tomato slice and a cheese slice. Chill, if desired.

- Bake, covered, at 350° for 20 minutes. Uncover and bake until cheese is melted and chicken is done.

Serves 6

Citrus-Brown Sugar Grilled Chicken

Simple but very satisfying!

¼	cup Dijon mustard	½	cup olive oil
½	cup firmly packed brown sugar	2	teaspoons salt
	Juice of 1 lime	1	teaspoon pepper
¼	cup vinegar	2-3	crushed garlic cloves
	Juice of 1 lemon	4	skinned and boned chicken breasts

- Combine mustard, brown sugar, lime juice, vinegar, lemon juice, oil, salt, pepper, and garlic, stirring well.

- Place chicken in a shallow dish; pour marinade over top. Chill 4 hours.

- Remove chicken from marinade, discarding marinade.

- Grill chicken over medium-high heat (350° to 400°) 5 to 7 minutes on each side or until done.

Serves 4

Mushroom, Garlic, and Cilantro Stuffed Chicken

*An interesting combination of ingredients
creates a delightfully different stuffing for this main dish.*

½ cup chopped onion
3 tablespoons olive oil
12 ounces fresh mushrooms, chopped
7 garlic cloves, crushed
¾ teaspoon salt
¼ teaspoon freshly ground pepper
3 tablespoons chopped fresh cilantro

6 skinned and boned chicken breasts, butterflied and flattened slightly
6 white bread slices, finely crumbled
3 tablespoons olive oil
¼ cup chopped fresh cilantro
¾ teaspoon salt
¾ teaspoon freshly ground pepper
½ cup milk

- Sauté onion in hot oil in a skillet over medium-high heat 2 minutes.

- Stir in mushrooms, garlic, salt, and pepper; cover and cook 3 minutes. Uncover and cook, stirring occasionally, until liquid is evaporated.

- Stir in cilantro. Transfer mixture to a plate and let cool.

- Place one-sixth of filling in the center of each chicken breast; fold edges to center to completely cover filling.

- Combine breadcrumbs, oil, cilantro, salt, and pepper. Dip chicken in milk and dredge in breadcrumb mixture, coating well. Place, folded side down, on a baking sheet.

- Bake at 400° for 20 to 25 minutes or until done.

Serves 6

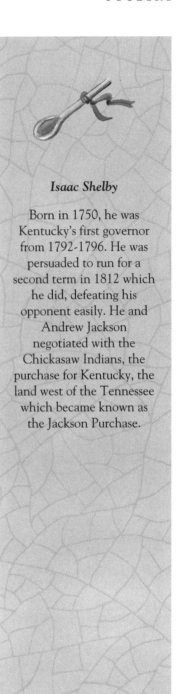

Isaac Shelby

Born in 1750, he was Kentucky's first governor from 1792-1796. He was persuaded to run for a second term in 1812 which he did, defeating his opponent easily. He and Andrew Jackson negotiated with the Chickasaw Indians, the purchase for Kentucky, the land west of the Tennessee which became known as the Jackson Purchase.

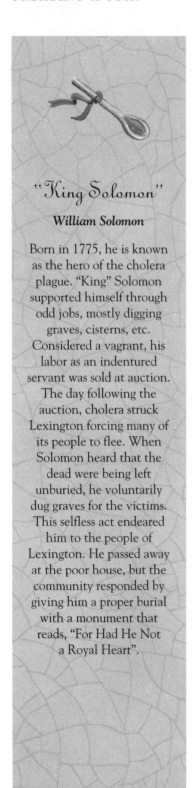

"King Solomon"

William Solomon

Born in 1775, he is known as the hero of the cholera plague. "King" Solomon supported himself through odd jobs, mostly digging graves, cisterns, etc. Considered a vagrant, his labor as an indentured servant was sold at auction. The day following the auction, cholera struck Lexington forcing many of its people to flee. When Solomon heard that the dead were being left unburied, he voluntarily dug graves for the victims. This selfless act endeared him to the people of Lexington. He passed away at the poor house, but the community responded by giving him a proper burial with a monument that reads, "For Had He Not a Royal Heart".

Grilled Dove

A great dish for a fall buffet!

15	small fresh jalapeño peppers, seeded and sliced in half	1	cup red wine	
30	dove breasts, rinsed	¾	cup olive oil	
15-30	maple cured bacon slices (depending on length of bacon and size of dove breasts)	½	cup vinegar	
			Cracked black pepper to taste	
		1	teaspoon garlic salt	
½	cup Worcestershire sauce	½	teaspoon onion powder	

- Place a jalapeño half in the cavity of each dove breast; wrap with bacon and secure with a wooden pick. Place dove in a nonmetallic container.
- Combine Worcestershire sauce, red wine, oil, vinegar, pepper, garlic salt, and onion powder; pour over dove.
- Chill dove, turning occasionally, 12 to 24 hours. Remove from marinade, reserving marinade.
- Grill dove over medium heat (300° to 350°), turning and basting occasionally with marinade, until dove is done. Serve on a bed of hot cooked wild rice.

Serves 8

Some people prefer to pre-marinate dove in buttermilk to decrease the "gamey" flavor. To do so, simply rinse dove breasts and place in a nonmetallic container. Cover with buttermilk and chill 12 to 24 hours. Drain, rinse, and drain again before proceeding with recipe.

Dove and Oyster Pie

In Central Kentucky, dove season is open during the months of September and October. Many of the farms in the Bluegrass painstakingly grow sunflowers, wheat, and millet for the doves to feed on. The doves fly in to feed around 3 to 5 o'clock in the early evening. There is a limit for each shooter, so unless you hunt everyday, these little dove breasts become valuable jewels to the dove hunter and his family and friends. In some families this is a generational experience, with young shooters starting at ages 8 to 9 to shoot with fathers!

15-16 dressed doves	1½ pints select oysters
1 cup chopped celery	Hot sauce
1 cup chopped onion	4-5 tablespoons Worcestershire sauce
Salt and pepper to taste	12 bacon slices, cooked and
2 tablespoons all-purpose flour	crumbled
Butter	½ cup chopped fresh parsley
1½ cups fresh mushrooms, sliced	Pastry

- Simmer doves, celery, onion, salt, pepper, and water to cover in a large Dutch oven until doves are tender. Drain doves, reserving broth in Dutch oven; let cool.

- Pick dove meat from bones; set aside.

- Combine flour and ¼ cup dove broth, stirring until smooth. Add to remaining broth and cook over low heat until thickened. Remove from heat.

- Melt butter in a skillet over medium heat; add mushrooms and sauté until tender.

- Add mushrooms, oysters, hot sauce, and Worcestershire sauce to broth.

- Line a 3-quart oblong baking dish with your favorite pastry.

- Bake at 350° for 10 minutes. Remove from oven and let cool.

- Place half of dove meat in prepared crust and top with half of oyster mixture; top with remaining dove meat and oyster mixture.

- Fit pastry over top and bake at 350° for 20 minutes or until browned and bubbly. Remove from oven and sprinkle with bacon and parsley. Serve with a green salad.

Serves 6

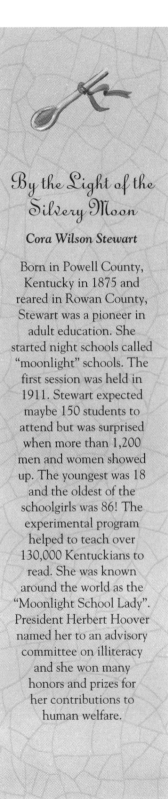

By the Light of the Silvery Moon

Cora Wilson Stewart

Born in Powell County, Kentucky in 1875 and reared in Rowan County, Stewart was a pioneer in adult education. She started night schools called "moonlight" schools. The first session was held in 1911. Stewart expected maybe 150 students to attend but was surprised when more than 1,200 men and women showed up. The youngest was 18 and the oldest of the schoolgirls was 86! The experimental program helped to teach over 130,000 Kentuckians to read. She was known around the world as the "Moonlight School Lady". President Herbert Hoover named her to an advisory committee on illiteracy and she won many honors and prizes for her contributions to human welfare.

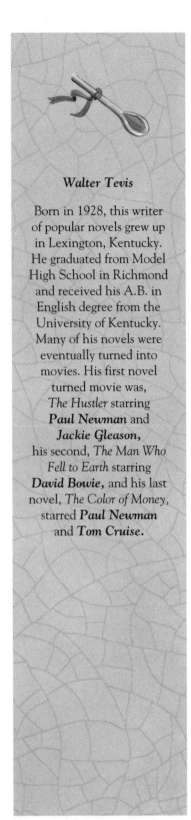

Quail with Shallot Sauce

If you don't have a hunter to supply you with quail, you should be able to purchase them at many better grocery stores. They are domestically raised rather than shot in the wild, but they are still tasty. This dish is wonderful for an elegant brunch served with grits!

4-6 dressed quail	½ cup butter, melted
Vegetable oil	1 tablespoon Worcestershire sauce
Salt and freshly ground pepper to taste	Juice from half a lemon
	Toasted bread slices
4-6 bacon slices	Shallot Sauce (see recipe)

- Rub quail with oil and season with salt and pepper; chill 1 hour.
- Wrap 1 bacon slice around each quail and secure with a wooden pick.
- Combine melted butter, Worcestershire sauce, and lemon juice; brush on quail.
- Preheat oven to 400°.
- Place quail on a rack in a roasting pan and bake at 400° for 15 minutes, basting occasionally with pan juices.
- Increase oven temperature to 450° and bake 10 minutes.
- Serve quail on toast with Shallot Sauce.

Serves 2 to 3

Shallot Sauce

This sauce is a marvelous accompaniment for grilled or roasted game (doves, pheasant, quail, chucker).

3-4 shallots, diced	1½ cups chicken broth
¾ cup dry white wine	Salt and freshly ground pepper to taste
¼ cup butter	
2 tablespoons all-purpose flour	

- Simmer shallots and wine in a saucepan until wine is reduced and shallots are plump.
- Melt butter in a heavy skillet over medium heat; gradually add flour, stirring constantly. Cook, stirring constantly, until browned and thickened.
- Gradually stir in broth; cook, stirring constantly, until thickened. Season with salt and pepper and stir in shallots.

Makes about 1½ cups

Wild Goose with Currant Sauce

1   cooking apple, cut into wedges
1   large orange, unpeeled and cut into
      wedges
6   pitted dried prunes, chopped
2   (2½-pound) wild geese, dressed
2   (1.31-ounce) envelopes dry onion
      soup mix
2   cups dry red wine
2   cups water
      Currant Sauce

- Combine apple, orange, and prunes, stirring well; spoon half of mixture into each goose cavity.

- Place each goose, breast side up, in an oven cooking bag.

- Combine soup mix, wine, and 2 cups water; pour half of mixture into each bag.

- Seal bags and cut 6 small slits in the top of each bag to allow steam to escape. Place bags in a large shallow roasting pan.

- Bake at 350° for 3 to 3½ hours.

- Serve goose with Currant Sauce.

Serves 4

Currant Sauce
¼   cup red currant jelly
¼   cup ketchup
¼   cup port wine
¼   cup Worcestershire sauce
2   tablespoons butter

- Cook all ingredients in a saucepan over low heat until thoroughly heated.

Makes 1 cup

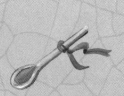

The U.S. Bullion Depository

The U.S. Bullion Depository, also known as the gold vault is located at Fort Knox. It houses pure refined gold in the form of bars and is a major part of the United States depository system. An even more interesting fact about the Depository, it has stored other famous items such as a copy of the *British Magna Carta of 1215,* a copy of the *Gutenberg Bible,* the original *U.S. Declaration of Independence,* the original *Articles of Confederation,* the original and signed copy of the *Constitution of the United States of America,* the original autographed copy of *Lincoln's Gettysburg Address* and the original autographed copy of *Lincoln's second inaugural address!*

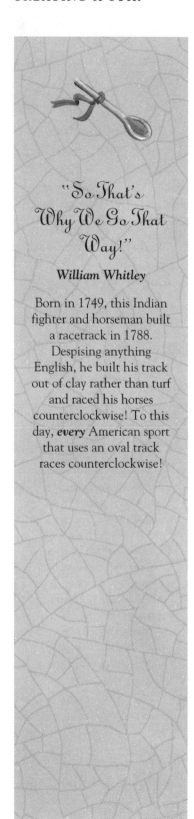

"So That's Why We Go That Way!"

William Whitley

Born in 1749, this Indian fighter and horseman built a racetrack in 1788. Despising anything English, he built his track out of clay rather than turf and raced his horses counterclockwise! To this day, *every* American sport that uses an oval track races counterclockwise!

Wild Duck à la Suan-Song Sauce Orangerie

2 dressed wild ducks
1 teaspoon salt, divided
½ cup chopped onion
½ cup chopped celery
½ cup chopped carrot
Freshly ground pepper to taste
Melted butter
Red wine (Burgundy)
White wine (Chablis)
Chopped fresh parsley
Suan-Song Sauce Orangerie

- Preheat oven to 450°.
- Rub duck cavities evenly with ½ teaspoon salt.
- Combine remaining ½ teaspoon salt, onion, celery, carrot, and pepper; spoon evenly into duck cavities.
- Place ducks, on their side, on a rack in a roasting pan. Brush all over with melted butter.
- Bake at 450° for 15 minutes. Turn ducks to other side and bake 15 more minutes.
- Turn ducks on their backs and bake 1 hour to 1 hour and 30 minutes, basting occasionally with juices and red and white wine.
- Sprinkle ducks with chopped parsley and serve with Suan-Song Sauce Orangerie.

Suan-Song Sauce Orangerie

2 tablespoons butter
1 tablespoon all-purpose flour
1 cup reserved duck juices
½ cup red wine
Zest of 1 orange, cut into thin strips
2 tablespoons brown sugar
2 tablespoons red wine
Salt to taste

- Melt butter in a skillet over low heat; gradually add flour, stirring constantly. Cook, stirring constantly, until thickened and browned.
- Gradually add 1 cup duck juices and ½ cup red wine; cook, stirring constantly, until thickened.
- Boil orange zest strips and water to cover in a small saucepan 3 minutes. Drain, reserving water.
- Cook brown sugar and reserved orange water in a small saucepan over medium heat. Add duck sauce, 2 tablespoons red wine, and salt to taste. Cook until thoroughly heated.

Serves 4

Salmon with Goat Cheese and Fresh Herbs

An exotically delicious dish with Mediterranean flair!

½-1	onion, chopped	⅛	teaspoon dried crushed red pepper flakes
2-3	garlic cloves, minced		
¼	cup olive oil, divided	½	cup canned crushed tomatoes
½	cup red wine	20	pitted ripe olives
¼	cup capers	4	(6-ounce) boned salmon fillets
¼	cup chopped fresh oregano or		Salt and pepper to taste
	1 tablespoon dried oregano	½	cup crumbled goat cheese
1	tablespoon chopped fresh rosemary	2	tablespoons anisette liqueur
	or ½ teaspoon dried rosemary	¼	cup chopped fresh cilantro

- Sauté onion and garlic in 2 tablespoons hot oil in a saucepan; add wine, capers, oregano, rosemary, red pepper flakes, tomatoes, and olives and simmer 5 minutes.

- Arrange salmon, skin side down, in an oiled baking dish; sprinkle with salt and pepper.

- Pour tomato mixture around salmon. Brush top of salmon with remaining oil and sprinkle with cheese.

- Bake at 475° for 5 to 6 minutes.

- Sprinkle with liqueur and broil 5 minutes.

- Sprinkle salmon with cilantro and serve immediately.

Serves 4

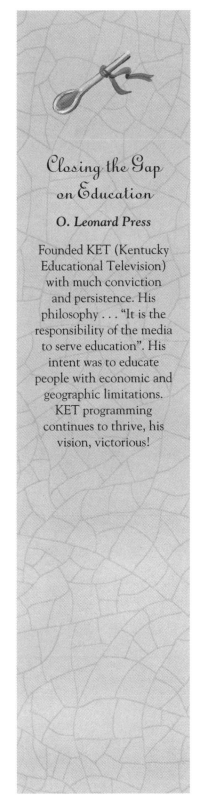

Closing the Gap on Education

O. Leonard Press

Founded KET (Kentucky Educational Television) with much conviction and persistence. His philosophy . . . "It is the responsibility of the media to serve education". His intent was to educate people with economic and geographic limitations. KET programming continues to thrive, his vision, victorious!

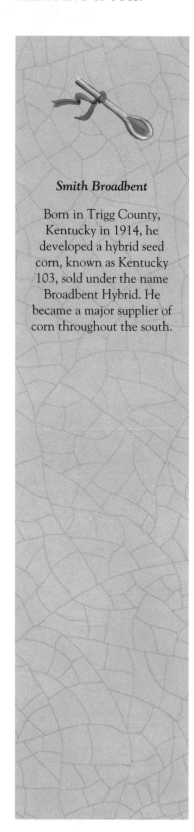

Warm Salmon Salad

This salad can be done ahead and assembled at the last minute.

3	cups cubed red potato		2	teaspoons vegetable oil
4	cups diagonally sliced 1-inch asparagus pieces		8	cups gourmet salad greens
¼	teaspoon salt		¼	cup sliced green onions
¼	teaspoon pepper		8	cherry tomatoes, quartered
1½	pounds salmon fillets (of approximately equal thickness)		2-3	tablespoons balsamic vinegar
			2-3	tablespoons pesto basil sauce (Pesto Sanrema)

• Place potatoes in a large saucepan; cover with water and bring to a boil. Reduce heat and simmer 12 minutes.

• Add asparagus to pan and cook 3 minutes or until potato is tender. Drain.

• Sprinkle salt and pepper over salmon.

• Cook salmon in hot oil in a skillet over medium-high heat 4 minutes on each side or until fish flakes with a fork.

• Flake salmon into chunks, discarding skin.

• Combine salmon, potato mixture, salad greens, green onions, and tomato quarters in a large bowl.

• Combine vinegar and pesto and drizzle over salad, tossing gently.

Serves 4

Asian Gingered Shrimp

Serve these spicy shrimp over cheese grits for a satisfying meal!

½	cup sherry		½	teaspoon garlic powder
⅓	cup sesame oil		¼	teaspoon ground ginger
½	cup soy sauce		2	pounds large fresh shrimp, peeled and deveined
½	teaspoon sugar			

• Combine sherry, oil, soy sauce, sugar, garlic powder, and ginger in a large shallow dish, stirring well. Add shrimp, tossing gently. Cover and chill 3 to 4 hours.

• Drain shrimp, reserving marinade.

• Thread shrimp onto skewers.

• Grill over medium heat (300° to 350°) 5 minutes on each side, basting often with reserved marinade.

Serves 4

Shrimp with Feta

Outstanding!

¼ cup lemon juice
1 pound medium-size fresh shrimp, peeled and deveined
1 cup minced green onions
2 garlic cloves, minced
2 tablespoons minced fresh parsley
¼ cup olive oil
1½ cups canned Italian plum tomatoes, diced

¼ cup clam juice (optional)
3 tablespoons butter
1 tomato, peeled and chopped
½ teaspoon dried oregano
1 teaspoon dried basil
¼ cup dry white wine
⅔ cup crumbled feta cheese

- Drizzle lemon juice over shrimp; set aside.

- Sauté green onions, garlic, and parsley in hot oil in a skillet until soft; add canned tomatoes and bring to a boil. Reduce heat to medium-low; cover and simmer 20 to 30 minutes.

- Add clam juice to tomato mixture, if desired, and simmer 5 minutes.

- Preheat oven to 400°.

- Melt butter in a separate skillet over medium heat; add shrimp and sauté 4 to 5 minutes or until shrimp turn pink.

- Pour tomato mixture into a 2-quart shallow baking dish; put chopped tomato in center and surround with shrimp. Sprinkle oregano and basil over shrimp.

- Pour wine over top and sprinkle with feta. Bake at 350° for 15 to 20 minutes. Serve over hot cooked angel hair pasta.

Serves 2

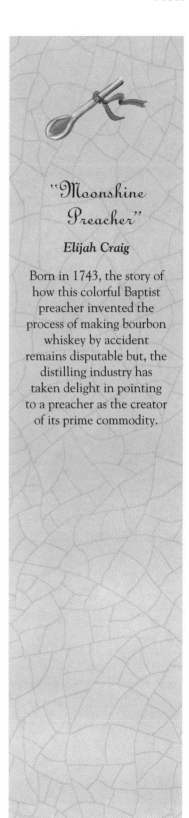

"Moonshine Preacher"

Elijah Craig

Born in 1743, the story of how this colorful Baptist preacher invented the process of making bourbon whiskey by accident remains disputable but, the distilling industry has taken delight in pointing to a preacher as the creator of its prime commodity.

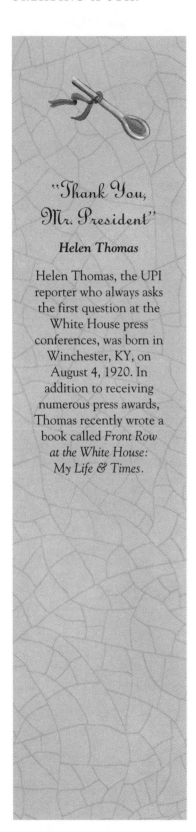

Shrimp Florentine

Great for a buffet dinner.

2	packages crab boil	½	cup butter
2	lemons	½	cup all-purpose flour
3-4	celery ribs, coarsely chopped	1	bunch green onions, chopped
2	onions, coarsely chopped	3	cups milk
	Salt to taste	1½	teaspoons salt
	Cayenne pepper to taste	1	teaspoon ground white pepper
4	pounds unpeeled, medium or large or 5 pounds unpeeled, small fresh shrimp	1	teaspoon accent
		1	cup sherry
		1½	teaspoons paprika
4	(10-ounce) packages frozen chopped spinach, thawed and well drained	4	cups (1-pound) shredded sharp cheddar cheese

- Bring crab boil, lemons, celery, onion, salt, and cayenne pepper to a boil in a large Dutch oven; add shrimp and boil 10 to 15 minutes. Remove from heat and let cool. Peel shrimp and devein.

- Press thawed and well drained spinach onto bottom and sides of a buttered 9 x 13 x 2-inch baking dish; top with shrimp.

- Melt butter in a saucepan over medium heat; gradually add flour, stirring until smooth.

- Add green onions and milk and cook, stirring constantly, until thickened.

- Add salt, white pepper, accent, and enough paprika to make mixture rose colored. Add sherry, stirring well. Pour sauce over shrimp.

- Let shrimp mixture cool. Top evenly with cheese.

- Bake at 350° for 30 to 35 minutes.

Freezes well.

Serves 8 to 10

Shrimp Creole

Don't let the lengthy ingredient list discourage you from trying this. Most are good herbs and spices! Preparation is actually very easy and the results are worth the effort.

⅔	cup vegetable oil
1¾	cups thinly sliced shallots
⅓	cup chopped celery
1	cup chopped green bell pepper
4	teaspoons minced garlic
½	cup all-purpose flour
1	pound canned whole peeled tomatoes
3	tablespoons minced fresh parsley
1	tablespoon minced fresh chives
¼	cup dry red wine
4	bay leaves, crushed
6	whole allspice
2	whole cloves
2	teaspoons salt
½	teaspoon dried thyme
¾	teaspoon ground black pepper
½	teaspoon cayenne pepper
¼	teaspoon chili powder
¼	teaspoon ground mace
¼	teaspoon dried basil
4	teaspoons lemon juice
2	cups water
1½-5	pounds medium-size fresh shrimp, peeled and deveined

- Heat oil in a large Dutch oven over medium heat. Sauté shallots, celery, bell pepper, and garlic until tender. Make a roux by gradually adding flour, stirring constantly, until browned and thickened.

- Add tomatoes and remaining ingredients, stirring well. Reduce heat and simmer 45 minutes.

- Add shrimp and simmer 15 to 20 minutes. Serve immediately with rice.

Serves 6 to 8

Bubba's Outer Banks Crab Cakes

¼	cup soft breadcrumbs
2	tablespoons milk
1	large egg
1	pound backfin crabmeat, rinsed
2	tablespoons Old Bay seasoning
2	tablespoons mayonnaise
1	tablespoon Worcestershire sauce
	Salt to taste
	Vegetable oil

- Combine breadcrumbs, milk, and egg; mix well. Add crabmeat, Old Bay seasoning, mayonnaise, Worcestershire sauce, and salt. Form into small patties.

- Fry crab cakes in hot oil in a skillet until browned on both sides. Serve with your favorite seafood sauce.

Serves 4 to 6

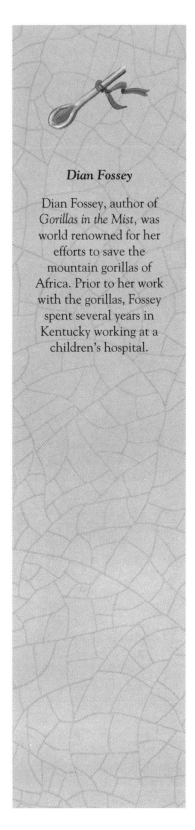

Dian Fossey

Dian Fossey, author of *Gorillas in the Mist*, was world renowned for her efforts to save the mountain gorillas of Africa. Prior to her work with the gorillas, Fossey spent several years in Kentucky working at a children's hospital.

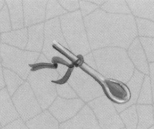

Macadamia Crusted Yellowtail with Mango-Papaya Salsa

This enticing dish is attractive and delicious!
You'll dazzle your guests with its presentation!

2	large bell peppers, cut into ¼-inch pieces	1	teaspoon finely chopped garlic
1	mango, cut into ¼-inch pieces	¼	teaspoon cayenne pepper
1	papaya, cut into ¼-inch pieces		Salt and pepper to taste
1	cup finely chopped fresh cilantro	½	cup all-purpose flour
½	small purple onion, diced	2	large eggs
2	tablespoons fresh lime juice	3	cups macadamia nuts, finely ground
1	tablespoon olive oil	6	(6-ounce) yellowtail or red snapper fillets
1	tablespoon rice vinegar	¼	cup olive oil

- Combine bell pepper, mango, papaya, cilantro, onion, lime juice, oil, vinegar, garlic, and cayenne pepper in a large bowl; add salt and pepper to taste. Cover and set aside.

- Preheat oven to 350°.

- Place flour in a shallow dish. Whisk eggs in a shallow bowl. Place ground nuts in a separate shallow dish.

- Dredge fillets in flour; dip in egg and dredge in ground nuts, coating well.

- Cook 3 fillets in 2 tablespoons hot oil in a large heavy skillet over medium heat 2 minutes on each side or until golden brown. Repeat with remaining 3 fillets.

- Transfer fillets to a baking sheet and bake at 350° for 7 minutes or until opaque in center.

- Serve fillets on individual plates with salsa mixture.

Serves 6

Stuffed Crabs

½ cup butter
8 celery ribs, finely chopped
1 bunch green onions, finely chopped
6 cups backfin or lump crabmeat, rinsed
 Several dashes of hot sauce
1 tablespoon Worcestershire sauce
1 teaspoon pepper
1 teaspoon salt
1 teaspoon accent

2 large eggs, lightly beaten
1 (8-ounce) container sour cream
2 cups soft French breadcrumbs, divided
24 crab shells or 10 to 12 small ramekins
1 tablespoon butter
 Slices of butter
 Paprika to taste

- Melt ½ cup butter in a skillet over medium heat; add celery and green onions and sauté until soft. Let cool.
- Combine crabmeat, hot sauce, Worcestershire sauce, pepper, salt, and accent in a large bowl. Add egg, sour cream, and 1 cup breadcrumbs.
- Add sautéed vegetables to crab mixture, tossing gently to not break up clumps of crab. Spoon mixture evenly into crab shells or ramekins.
- Melt 1 tablespoon butter in a skillet over medium heat; add remaining 1 cup breadcrumbs and cook until browned. Sprinkle evenly over crab mixture.
- Sprinkle crab with paprika and top each with a slice of butter.
- Bake at 350° for 20 to 25 minutes.

Yields: 10 to 12

Grilled Grouper with Toasted Almonds

4 grouper fillets
½ cup butter, melted
 Juice of 2 large lemons

1 teaspoon lemon pepper
1 cup toasted slivered almonds

- Arrange fillets in a single layer in a glass dish.; pour butter over top. Squeeze lemon juice over fillets and sprinkle with lemon pepper. Cover and chill 1 hour.
- Drain fish, reserving marinade.
- Grill fillets over medium heat (300° to 350°) 6 to 8 minutes on each side or until done, basting with marinade after turning.
- Sprinkle with almonds and serve immediately.

Serves 4

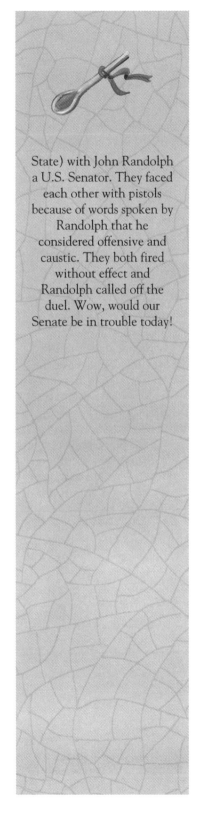

State) with John Randolph a U.S. Senator. They faced each other with pistols because of words spoken by Randolph that he considered offensive and caustic. They both fired without effect and Randolph called off the duel. Wow, would our Senate be in trouble today!

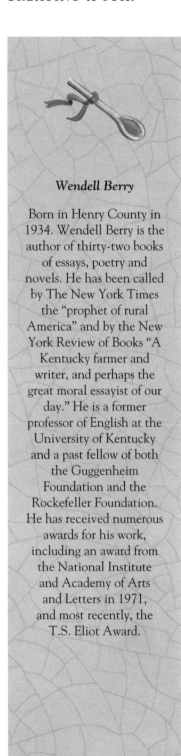

Scallop Shells

Simple and elegant.

½	cup butter	2	teaspoons lemon juice
1	cup crushed round buttery crackers or soft breadcrumbs		Salt and pepper to taste
⅛	teaspoon paprika	2	teaspoons dry vermouth (optional)
1	pint fresh or frozen scallops, thawed and cut into bite-size pieces		Fresh parsley sprigs for garnish

- Melt butter in a skillet over medium heat; add crushed crackers. Stir in paprika and cook until lightly browned. Remove from heat.
- Add scallops to cracker mixture, stirring to coat. Divide among 4 scallop baking shells.
- Sprinkle scallops with lemon juice, salt, pepper, and, if desired, vermouth. Let cool. Cover and chill.
- Bake at 350° for 20 minutes. Garnish, if desired.

Serves 4

Creole Crab Cakes with Rémoulade Sauce

Crab cakes with a hot and spicy twist!

2	celery ribs, diced	2	tablespoons dry mustard
½	red bell pepper, diced	1	teaspoon cayenne pepper
½	green bell pepper, diced	1	tablespoon garlic powder
1	large onion, diced	1	tablespoon onion powder
	Olive oil	3	egg whites
1	pound backfin or lump crabmeat, rinsed	½	cup mayonnaise
4	cups ¼-inch French bread cubes	2	cups fine, dry breadcrumbs, divided

- Sauté celery, bell peppers, and onion in hot oil in a skillet until tender. Let cool.
- Combine crab, bread cubes, mustard, cayenne pepper, garlic powder, onion powder, egg whites, mayonnaise, and 1 cup fine, dry breadcrumbs; shape into patties.
- Dredge patties in remaining 1 cup fine, dry breadcrumbs.
- Sauté crab cakes in hot oil 2 to 3 minutes on each side or until browned.

Serves 4 to 6

Rémoulade Sauce

4 tablespoons lemon juice
4 tablespoons vinegar, preferably
   tarragon
4 tablespoons prepared mustard
2 teaspoons salt
½ teaspoon black pepper

2 teaspoons paprika
   Dash of cayenne pepper
2 tablespoons ketchup
1 cup vegetable oil
½ cup finely chopped celery
½ cup minced green onions

- Combine lemon juice, vinegar, mustard, salt, pepper, paprika, cayenne, and ketchup. Gradually whisk in oil, blending well.

- Whisk in celery and onion.

Makes 2 cups

Catfish Acadiene

2 large eggs
1 cup milk
2 cups all-purpose flour
1¼ teaspoons salt, divided
2 teaspoons cayenne pepper, divided
4 catfish fillets (1½ pounds)
   Vegetable oil
12 unpeeled, large fresh shrimp

1 tablespoon butter
2 teaspoons minced garlic
¼ cup vermouth
2 cups whipping cream
¼ cup chopped green onions, divided
2 teaspoons lemon juice
3 very thin ham slices, cut into thin strips
   Lemon wedges for garnish

- Combine eggs and milk, stirring well.

- Combine flour, 1 teaspoon salt, and ½ teaspoon cayenne pepper in a shallow dish.

- Dredge fillets in flour mixture; dip in milk mixture and dredge in flour mixture again.

- Pour oil to a depth of 3 inches in a Dutch oven; heat to 360°. Fry fillets 6 to 8 minutes or until golden brown on both sides. Drain on paper towels; keep warm.

- Peel shrimp and devein, if desired.

- Melt butter in a large skillet over medium heat; add shrimp and garlic and cook, stirring often, until shrimp turn pink.

- Remove shrimp; set aside. Bring butter mixture to a boil and cook 1 minute.

- Add vermouth, whipping cream, 2 tablespoons green onions, lemon juice, remaining ¼ teaspoon salt, and remaining 1½ teaspoons cayenne pepper; cook, stirring often, 12 to 15 minutes or until sauce is thickened.

- Place catfish on a serving plate and drizzle with sauce. Top with shrimp and ham. Sprinkle with remaining green onions. Garnish with fresh lemon wedges.

Serves 4

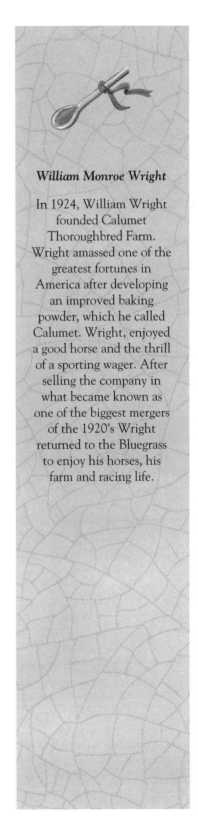

William Monroe Wright

In 1924, William Wright founded Calumet Thoroughbred Farm. Wright amassed one of the greatest fortunes in America after developing an improved baking powder, which he called Calumet. Wright, enjoyed a good horse and the thrill of a sporting wager. After selling the company in what became known as one of the biggest mergers of the 1920's Wright returned to the Bluegrass to enjoy his horses, his farm and racing life.

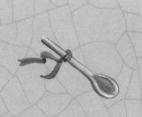

And The Story Goes...

Lucille Parker Markey

Lucille Parker Markey was born into a hard and rough life in the small town of Tollesboro in 1888. Her father was a livery stable operator and her mother who, though wheelchair bound, raised seven children. Mrs. Markey would later change this information, claiming that her ancestors were the prominent Parker family from Maysville. After marrying Warren Wright, heir to Calumet Farm, the two worked to establish Calumet as a giant in the Thoroughbred industry. Wright plucked Parker from her working-class existence, then deposited her into the fairy-tale life of multimillionaires and Kentucky socialites. But as Lucille P. Wright, she was never invited into the winner's circle with her husband when Calumet's horses won. She stayed strictly in the background. Her only publicized role at

Catfish Cakes with Sweet Red Pepper Sauce

For those who are landlocked, fresh crab can be pricey!
Try this affordable and tasty alternative!

1½ pounds catfish fillets
1 large peeled potato, boiled and mashed
2 large eggs, lightly beaten
1 large onion, finely chopped
1-2 tablespoons chopped fresh parsley
2-3 drops hot sauce
1 garlic clove, minced
1 teaspoon salt
½ teaspoon pepper
½ teaspoon dried basil
2 cups finely crushed round buttery crackers
Vegetable oil
Sweet Red Pepper Sauce or rémoulade
Lime wedges for garnish

- Poach or bake fish and drain. Cover and chill thoroughly.
- Flake fish into a large bowl; add mashed potato, eggs, onion, parsley, hot sauce, garlic, salt, pepper, and basil, stirring well. Shape into 8 patties.
- Dredge patties in cracker crumbs, coating well.
- Cook fish cakes in hot oil in a large skillet over medium heat until browned and done.
- Pour Sweet Red Pepper Sauce onto 8 serving plates; place 1 fish cake in sauce on each plate and garnish, if desired.

Sweet Red Pepper Sauce

4 red bell peppers, roasted and sliced, or 2 (7-ounce) jars roasted sweet red peppers, drained
6 tablespoons lime juice
5 tablespoons chopped fresh thyme
¼ teaspoon salt
⅛ teaspoon pepper
6 tablespoons water
4 tablespoons butter

- Process red peppers, lime juice, thyme, salt, pepper, and 6 tablespoons water in a food processor until smooth. Transfer mixture to a small saucepan.
- Cook sauce over medium heat until warmed; add butter, stirring until melted.

Serves 8

Chef Jerry Hester
Something Special Catering
Lexington, Kentucky

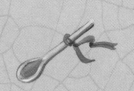

Grilled Salmon Glazed with Kentucky Bourbon Marinade

The bourbon adds a wonderful flavor to the marinade and produces a beautifully glazed fish.

½ cup vegetable oil
½ cup Kentucky bourbon
2 garlic cloves, minced
6 tablespoons soy sauce

2 tablespoons brown sugar
Salt and pepper to taste
2 pounds unskinned salmon fillets

- Combine oil, bourbon, garlic, soy sauce, brown sugar, salt, and pepper, stirring well.
- Place salmon in a shallow pan; pour marinade over top. Cover and chill 6 hours.
- Remove salmon from marinade, discarding marinade.
- Grill salmon, skin side down, over high heat (400° to 500°) 4 to 5 minutes. Turn salmon and grill 7 minutes.
- Discard skin and transfer salmon to a serving platter.

Serves 4 to 6

Swordfish with Lemon-Basil-Dijon Marinade

This marinade is excellent!

1 cup olive oil
1 cup vegetable oil
½ cup Dijon mustard
½ cup fresh lemon juice
8 garlic cloves, minced
½ teaspoon pepper

2⅔ cups chopped fresh basil
6-8 (1-inch-thick) swordfish steaks
   (8 ounces each)
Lemon slices and fresh basil sprigs
   for garnish

- Whisk together olive oil, vegetable oil, mustard, lemon juice, garlic, and pepper; stir in basil. Set aside half of marinade.
- Arrange swordfish in a single layer in a glass dish; pour remaining half of marinade over top. Cover and chill 3 to 4 hours.
- Remove fish from marinade, discarding marinade.
- Grill over medium-high heat (350° to 400°) 4 to 5 minutes on each side.
- Serve with reserved sauce and garnish with lemon slices and fresh basil sprigs.

Serves 6 to 8

Calumet was in naming the horses. She also remained in his shadow socially, and they rarely entertained in Lexington during the 1930's, although they were invited to the best of the legendary bluegrass bashes. Following Wright's death, she fled to Europe and upon her return, a new Lucille emerged. She assumed control of the farm and saw her efforts rewarded as Calumet continued at the apex of American breeding and racing. She married Gene Markey in 1952 who was thrice divorced from Joan Bennett, Hedy Lamarr, and Myrna Loy. During her association with the farm, Calumet amassed racing and breeding statistics that are unlikely to ever be challenged.

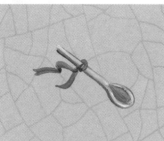

Fly Me to the Moon...!!!

Story Musgrave

Story Musgrave (M.D.), NASA Astronaut considers Lexington, Kentucky, where he received a master of science in physiology and biophysics from the University of Kentucky in 1966, to be his hometown. While living in Fayette County, he learned to fly and eventually logged over 120 types of aircraft, both civilian and military. Dr. Musgrave was selected as a scientist-astronaut by NASA in August 1967. He completed astronaut academic training and then worked on the design and development of the Skylab Program. He participated in the design and development of all Space Shuttle extravehicular activity equipment including spacesuits, and life support. His many honors include NASA Space Flight Medals (1983, 1985, 1989, 1991, 1993, 1996) and the NASA Distinguished

Grilled Tuna with Fresh Salsa

Fresh Salsa is a nice accompaniment to the grilled fish.

4	(1-inch-thick) tuna steaks	1	jalapeño pepper, seeded and minced	
¼	cup olive oil	1	garlic clove, minced	
2	large tomatoes, cored and chopped	⅓	cup chopped fresh cilantro	
1	purple onion, chopped		Salt and pepper to taste	
½	cup lime juice			

- Brush tuna with olive oil.
- Combine tomatoes, onion, lime juice, jalapeño pepper, garlic, cilantro, salt, and pepper; let stand at room temperature 1 hour.
- Grill tuna over medium heat (300° to 350°) 5 minutes on each side.
- Serve tuna immediately with salsa mixture.

Serves 4

Seared Tuna with Green Onion-Wasabi Sauce

½	cup water	1½	teaspoons minced fresh ginger	
3	tablespoons wasabi powder (horseradish powder)	4	green onions, thinly sliced	
3	tablespoons peanut oil, divided	4	(6-ounce) tuna steaks	
⅓	cup reduced-sodium soy sauce		Salt and pepper to taste	
1	tablespoon dry sherry	1	cucumber, peeled, seeded, and cut into matchstick-size pieces	
1½	teaspoons sesame oil	½	cup radish sprouts	

- Whisk together ½ cup water and wasabi powder to form a smooth paste. Whisk in 2 tablespoons peanut oil, soy sauce, sherry, sesame oil, and ginger. Stir in green onions and set aside.
- Season tuna with salt and pepper.
- Sear tuna in remaining 1 tablespoon hot peanut oil in a large heavy skillet over high heat 4 minutes on each side or until opaque in center.
- Arrange cucumber evenly on 4 serving plates; top with tuna. Spoon sauce around tuna and garnish with radish sprouts.

Serves 4

Wasabi powder can be found at Japanese food stores and some supermarkets and health food stores.

Seafood Lasagna

1 tablespoon margarine
1 cup chopped onion
1 (8-ounce) package cream cheese, softened
1½ cups cream-style cottage cheese
1 large egg, lightly beaten
2 teaspoons dried basil, crushed
12 lasagna noodles, cooked

1 (10¾-ounce) can cream of mushroom soup, undiluted
⅓ cup white wine
1 pound medium-size fresh shrimp, cooked and peeled
1 (6½-ounce) can crabmeat
1 cup grated Parmesan cheese
½ cup (2 ounces) shredded cheddar cheese

- Melt margarine in a saucepan over medium heat; add onion and sauté until tender. Add cream cheese, cottage cheese, egg, and basil.

- Cover the bottom of a greased 9 x 13 x 2-inch baking dish with 4 lasagna noodles. Spread one-third of cream cheese mixture over noodles.

- Combine soup, wine, shrimp, and crabmeat; spread one-third over cream cheese mixture. Repeat layers twice using remaining noodles, cream cheese mixture, and shrimp mixture.

- Sprinkle lasagna with Parmesan cheese and bake at 350° for 45 minutes.

- Sprinkle with cheddar cheese and bake 2 more minutes. Let stand at room temperature 10 to 15 minutes before serving.

Marinated and Grilled Halibut Steaks with Lemon Garnish

2 tablespoons fresh lemon juice
2 tablespoons fresh lime juice
½ cup soy sauce
½ cup vegetable oil
1 teaspoon grated lemon zest
2 garlic cloves, minced

3 teaspoons Dijon mustard
6 hailbut or swordfish steaks
3-4 green bell peppers, cut into thick rings
Lemon wedges and fresh parsley sprigs for garnish

- Combine lemon juice, lime juice, soy sauce, oil, lemon zest, garlic, and mustard; add swordfish and bell pepper halves, tossing to coat. Chill 2 hours.

- Drain swordfish and bell pepper halves, discarding marinade.

- Grill swordfish and bell pepper rings in a grill basket over medium heat (300° to 350°) 6 minutes on each side or until done.

- Serve on individual plates; garnish with lemon wedges and parsley sprigs.

Serves 6

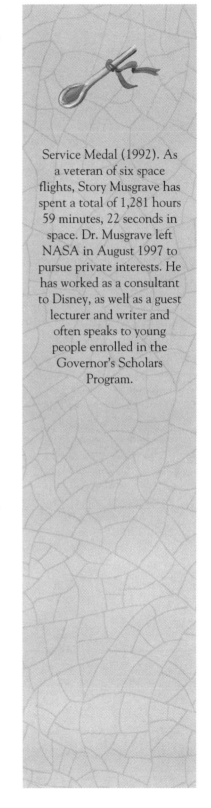

Service Medal (1992). As a veteran of six space flights, Story Musgrave has spent a total of 1,281 hours 59 minutes, 22 seconds in space. Dr. Musgrave left NASA in August 1997 to pursue private interests. He has worked as a consultant to Disney, as well as a guest lecturer and writer and often speaks to young people enrolled in the Governor's Scholars Program.

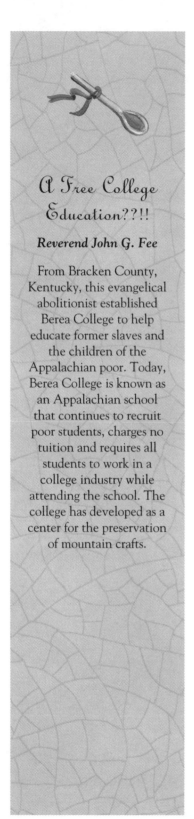

Cajun Grilled Swordfish

Cajun Spices
2 tablespoons cayenne pepper
2 tablespoons paprika
2 tablespoons garlic powder
1 tablespoon onion powder
1 tablespoon dried oregano
1 tablespoon dried thyme
1 tablespoon salt
½ teaspoon ground black pepper
½ teaspoon ground white pepper
1 tablespoon olive oil
1 tablespoon lemon juice
4-6 swordfish steaks (approximately 1 inch thick or ½ pound each)
Cucumber Salsa

- Combine all Cajun Spices, blending well.

- Combine oil and lemon juice; brush over swordfish and rub 1 teaspoon blended Cajun Spices into each fish (½ teaspoon per side).

- Grill steaks over medium-high heat (350° to 400°) 6 to 8 minutes on each side, turning when bottom of fish begins to brown nicely and becomes opaque in the center.

- Serve spicy fish with cool Cucumber Salsa

Makes 4 to 6

Cucumber Salsa
1 cup peeled, seeded, and chopped cucumber
2 tablespoons white wine vinegar
¼ cup sliced green onions
4 teaspoons chopped fresh marjoram
1 teaspoon chopped fresh thyme
2 teaspoons olive oil
Salt and freshly ground pepper to taste

- Combine all ingredients, mixing well; chill until needed.

Sweets

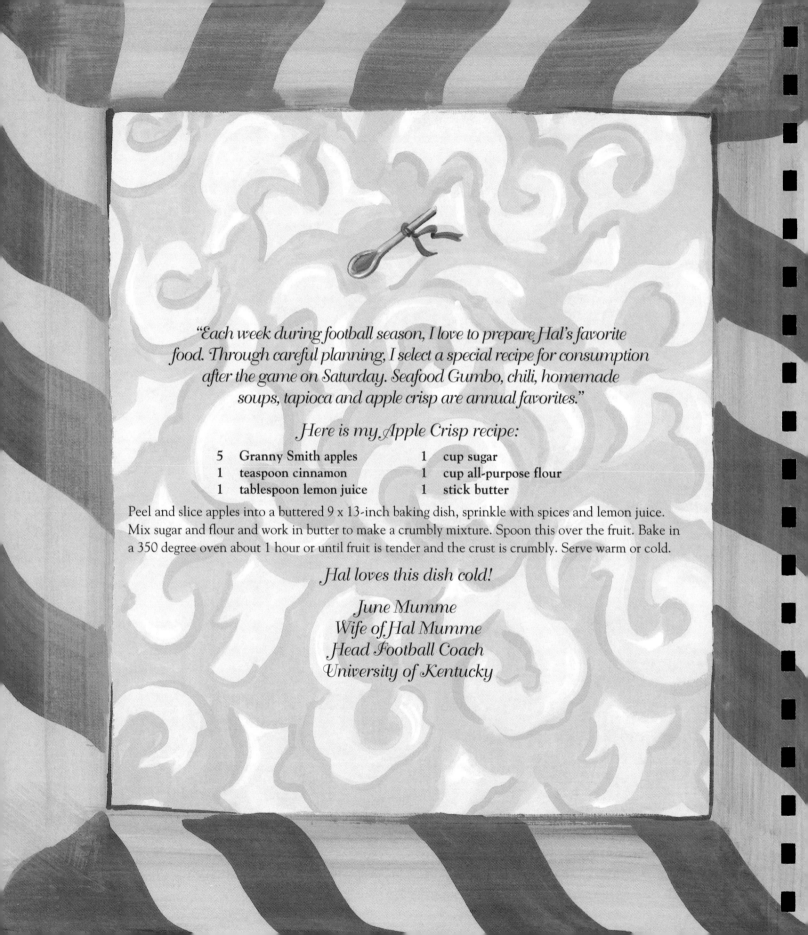

"Each week during football season, I love to prepare Hal's favorite food. Through careful planning, I select a special recipe for consumption after the game on Saturday. Seafood Gumbo, chili, homemade soups, tapioca and apple crisp are annual favorites."

Here is my Apple Crisp recipe:

5	Granny Smith apples	1	cup sugar
1	teaspoon cinnamon	1	cup all-purpose flour
1	tablespoon lemon juice	1	stick butter

Peel and slice apples into a buttered 9 x 13-inch baking dish, sprinkle with spices and lemon juice. Mix sugar and flour and work in butter to make a crumbly mixture. Spoon this over the fruit. Bake in a 350 degree oven about 1 hour or until fruit is tender and the crust is crumbly. Serve warm or cold.

Hal loves this dish cold!

June Mumme
Wife of Hal Mumme
Head Football Coach
University of Kentucky

Refreshing Lemon Cheesecake

A scrumptious marriage of tart and Sweet!

2 cups cinnamon graham cracker crumbs	3 large eggs
½ cup finely chopped pecans	2½ teaspoons grated lemon zest
6 tablespoons butter, melted	¼ cup fresh lemon juice
1 cup sugar, divided	1 tablespoon vanilla extract, divided
3 (8-ounce) packages cream cheese, softened	2 cups sour cream
	Lemon Glaze
	Mint leaves, violets for garnish

- Combine graham cracker crumbs, pecans, butter, and 2 tablespoons sugar; press onto bottom and sides of a buttered 9-inch springform pan.

- Bake at 350° for 5 minutes.

- Beat cream cheese and ¾ cup sugar at medium speed with an electric mixer until creamy; add eggs, 1 at a time, beating well after each addition.

- Add lemon zest, juice, and vanilla, beating well. Pour into cooled crust.

- Bake at 350° for 45 to 50 minutes or until set. Let cool on a wire rack 30 minutes.

- Combine sour cream, remaining 2 tablespoons sugar, and 2 teaspoons vanilla; spread over top of cake. Increase oven temperature to 500° and bake 5 minutes. Let cool slightly.

- Spread Lemon Glaze over top. Cover and chill 8 hours or until set.

- Remove sides of pan to serve. Garnish with mint leaves or violets.

Lemon Glaze

½ cup sugar	⅓ cup fresh lemon juice
4 teaspoons cornstarch	1 egg yolk, lightly beaten
Pinch of salt	1 tablespoon butter
¾ cup water	1 teaspoon grated lemon zest

- Combine sugar, cornstarch, and salt in a 1-quart heavy saucepan.

- Combine ¾ cup water, lemon juice, and egg yolk; add to sugar mixture and cook over low heat, stirring occasionally, until thickened.

- Stir in butter and lemon zest. Let cool slightly.

Serves 12

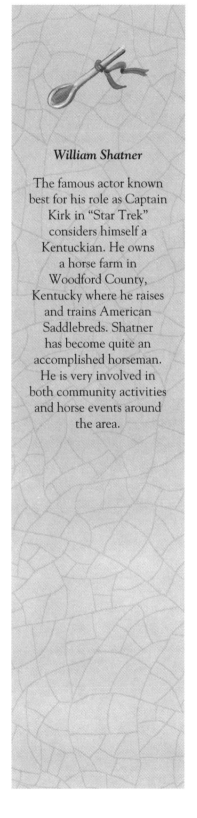

William Shatner

The famous actor known best for his role as Captain Kirk in "Star Trek" considers himself a Kentuckian. He owns a horse farm in Woodford County, Kentucky where he raises and trains American Saddlebreds. Shatner has become quite an accomplished horseman. He is very involved in both community activities and horse events around the area.

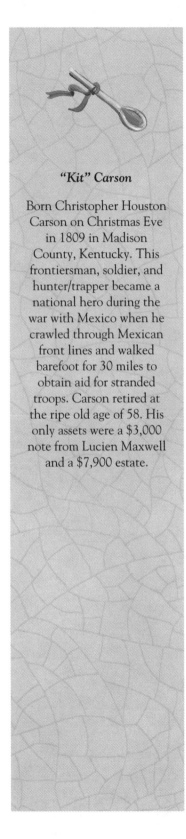

"Kit" Carson

Born Christopher Houston Carson on Christmas Eve in 1809 in Madison County, Kentucky. This frontiersman, soldier, and hunter/trapper became a national hero during the war with Mexico when he crawled through Mexican front lines and walked barefoot for 30 miles to obtain aid for stranded troops. Carson retired at the ripe old age of 58. His only assets were a $3,000 note from Lucien Maxwell and a $7,900 estate.

Key West Key Lime Cheesecake

Always a hit! This yummy combination of Key lime pie and cheesecake was developed by Tom Wiesel and his boss, Susan Taylor-Mitchel, at a restaurant in Key West, Florida

Crust

1	cup finely crushed graham cracker crumbs	⅓	cup butter, melted
½	cup walnut pieces, coarsely chopped		Key Lime Filling
¼	cup sugar		Glaze

- Preheat oven to 350°.
- Combine graham cracker crumbs, walnuts, sugar, and melted butter; press onto the bottom and sides of a 9-inch springform pan.
- Bake at 350° for 10 minutes. Let cool.
- Prepare Key Lime Filling and pour into cooled crust.
- Bake at 350° for 1 hour. Let cool on a wire rack 30 minutes.
- Prepare glaze; pour over cake. Bake an additional 10 minutes.

Key Lime Filling

3	(8-ounce) packages plus 1 (3-ounce) package cream cheese, softened	⅛	teaspoon salt
1½	cups sugar	1	teaspoon vanilla extract
4	large eggs	½	cup Key lime juice

- Beat cream cheese at medium speed with an electric mixer; gradually add sugar, beating until smooth. Add eggs, 1 at a time, beating well after each addition.
- Add salt, vanilla, and Key lime juice to cream cheese mixture, beating well.

Glaze

1	(16-ounce) container sour cream	2	teaspoons vanilla extract
¼	cup sugar		

- To prepare glaze combine sour cream, sugar, and vanilla, stirring well.

Serves 12 to 16

Portions should be small because it is so rich. May decorate with a twist of lime or other fruit.

Crème Brûlée Cheesecake

Crust
1½ cups graham cracker crumbs
2 tablespoons granulated sugar

¼ cup butter or margarine, melted

Filling
2 (8-ounce) packages cream cheese, softened
½ cup granulated sugar

1 teaspoon vanilla extract
2 large eggs
1 egg yolk

Crème Brûlée Glaze
½ cup firmly packed brown sugar

1-4 teaspoons water

- Combine graham cracker crumbs, sugar, and melted margarine; press evenly onto the bottom and sides of a 9-inch pie pan. Chill.

- Beat cream cheese, ½ cup granulated sugar, and vanilla at medium speed with an electric mixer until blended. Add eggs and egg yolk, beating well. Pour into prepared crust.

- Bake at 350° for 40 minutes or until center is set. Chill 3 hours or overnight.

- Combine brown sugar and water, 1 teaspoon at a time, until thin. Pour over cheesecake.

- Broil 4 to 6 inches from heat 1 to 1½ minutes or until bubbly (watch carefully to prevent burning).

Serves 8

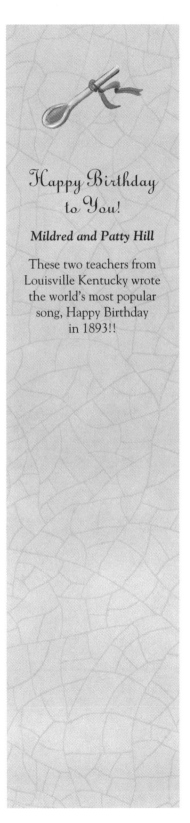

Happy Birthday to You!

Mildred and Patty Hill

These two teachers from Louisville Kentucky wrote the world's most popular song, Happy Birthday in 1893!!

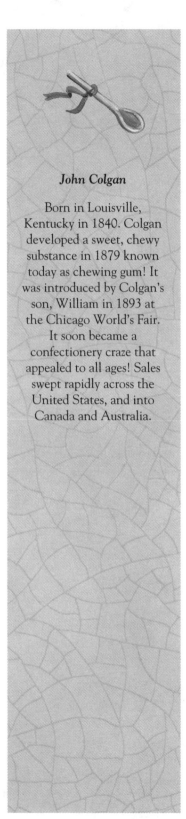

John Colgan

Born in Louisville, Kentucky in 1840. Colgan developed a sweet, chewy substance in 1879 known today as chewing gum! It was introduced by Colgan's son, William in 1893 at the Chicago World's Fair. It soon became a confectionery craze that appealed to all ages! Sales swept rapidly across the United States, and into Canada and Australia.

Decadent Peanut Butter Cup Cheesecake

Gloriously rich!

3	cups chocolate wafer crumbs	4	large eggs
3	tablespoons sugar	¾	cup creamy peanut butter
¼	cup butter, melted	10	miniature peanut butter cups,
1½	pounds cream cheese, softened		frozen and quartered
1	cup sugar		Shaved chocolate (optional)

- Combine chocolate wafer crumbs, sugar, and melted butter; press onto the bottom of a 9-inch springform pan. Chill.

- Beat cream cheese and 1 cup sugar at medium speed with an electric mixer until creamy; add eggs, 1 at a time, beating well after each addition. Add peanut butter, beating well. Fold in quartered peanut butter cups. Spoon mixture into prepared crust.

- Bake at 350° for 1 hour to 1 hour and 10 minutes or until center is set. Turn off oven and let cake cool in oven 30 minutes with door partially open. Transfer to a wire rack and let cool completely.

- Top pie with shaved chocolate, if desired.

Serves 8 to 10

Cheesecake

*This is a recipe for the cheesecake purist! The crust is a nice change from
the typical graham cracker types and the garnishing options are endless.*

Crust

1 cup sifted all-purpose flour	1 egg yolk
¼ cup sugar	¼ teaspoon vanilla extract
1 teaspoon grated lemon zest	Cheesecake Filling
½ cup butter, cut up	

- Combine flour, sugar, and lemon zest; cut in butter with a pastry blender until mixture is crumbly. Add yolk and vanilla, stirring well.
- Press one-third of mixture onto the bottom of a 9-inch springform pan with sides removed.
- Bake at 400° for 6 minutes. Let cool.
- Attach buttered sides of pan to bottom; press remaining dough evenly up 2 inches on sides. Pour Cheesecake Filling in crust.
- Bake at 500° for 5 to 8 minutes. Reduce oven temperature to 200° and bake 1 to 3 hours; or bake at 550° for 12 to 15 minutes, then reduce oven temperature to 200° and bake 1 to 2 hours..

Cheesecake Filling

5 (8-ounce) packages cream cheese, softened	3 tablespoons all-purpose flour
	Dash of salt
¼ teaspoon vanilla extract	5 large eggs
1½ teaspoons grated lemon zest	2 egg yolks
1 tablespoon fresh lemon juice	¼ cup heavy cream
1¾ cups sugar	

- Beat cream cheese at medium speed with an electric mixer until fluffy; add vanilla, lemon zest, and juice, beating well.
- Combine sugar, flour, and salt; gradually add to cream cheese mixture, beating well. Add eggs and yolks, 1 at a time, beating well after each addition. Add heavy cream, beating well.

Serves 12

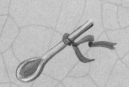

Calumet Farm

Warren Wright

Business mogul and developer of Calumet Farm in Lexington, Kentucky. Wright worked as a stock boy for the *Calumet Baking Powder Company* which was founded by his father in 1888. In 1899 he became president of the company and in 1928 engineered one of the biggest mergers of the 1920's, the $40 million buyout of the company by Postum. It was also one of the major deals that led to the birth of General Foods Corp. Wright inherited Calumet Farm as part of his father's $30 million estate turning it into one of the leading thoroughbred breeding and racing firms in the country. It produced eight Kentucky Derby winners, seven Preakness winners, two Belmont winners and two Triple Crown Winners in Whirlaway (1941) and Citation (1948).

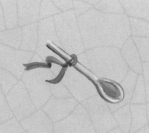

Duncan Hines

Born in Bowling Green Kentucky in 1880, Duncan Hines is one of the most recognized names in the world! He was an intelligent and funny but quiet and unassuming man. His success started, not with the food products his name is associated with today, but with the food and restaurant guides he wrote in the 30's and 40's. As he traveled, he began to chronicle his experiences at restaurants, making notes on the food, service and cleanliness of those he patronized. His publications expanded to include hotel guides, cookbooks and vacation guides. His name and approval was synonymous with quality and trust. A poll taken in the late 30's revealed that he was the most trusted name in the industry. This led to a joint business venture with Roy Park thus the creation of Hines-Park Foods. This is what most people associate his name with today. They created over 250 products under this name. Today, the brand includes approximately 60 mixes for cakes, brownies, frostings, muffins, and dessert bars.

Frosted Italian Cream Cake

A delicious cake that requires a small amount of effort for a wonderful result-extremely rich and moist

½ cup butter, softened
½ cup shortening
2 cups sugar
5 large eggs, separated
2 cups sifted all-purpose flour
1 teaspoon baking soda
1 cup buttermilk
1 teaspoon vanilla extract
1 (3.5-ounce) can flaked coconut
1 cup chopped pecans, divided
Cream Cheese Frosting

- Beat butter and shortening at medium speed with an electric mixer until creamy; add sugar, beating until smooth. Add egg yolks, beating well.
- Sift together flour and baking soda. Add flour mixture to butter mixture alternately with buttermilk, beginning and ending with flour mixture and beating well after each addition.
- Beat egg whites in a separate bowl with clean beaters at medium speed until stiff peaks form.
- Stir vanilla, coconut, and ½ cup pecans into batter. Fold in egg whites.
- Pour batter into 3 (8-inch) or 2 (9-inch) greased and floured round cake pans.
- Bake at 350° for 25 minutes. Remove from oven and let cool in pans on wire racks 10 minutes. Turn out cake layers onto wire racks and let cool completely.
- Spread Cream Cheese Frosting between layers and on top and sides of cake. Sprinkle with remaining ½ cup pecans.

Cream Cheese Frosting
1 (8-ounce) package cream cheese, softened
¼ cup butter, softened
1 (16-ounce) package powdered sugar
1 teaspoon vanilla extract

- Beat cream cheese and butter at medium speed with an electric mixer until smooth; add powdered sugar, beating well.
- Add vanilla and beat until smooth.

Serves 12

Banana-Nut Cake with Cream Cheese-Pecan Icing

Irresistible!

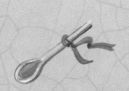

1⅔ cups sugar	1¼ teaspoons baking powder
⅔ cup shortening	1 teaspoon baking soda
2 large eggs	1 teaspoon salt
1¼ cups mashed banana	⅔ cup buttermilk
1 teaspoon vanilla extract	1 cup chopped pecans
2 cups plus 2 tablespoons all-purpose flour	Cream Cheese-Pecan Icing
	Pecan halves or chopped pecans

- Beat sugar, shortening, and eggs at medium speed with an electric mixer until light and pale; add banana and vanilla, beating well.

- Combine flour, baking powder, baking soda, and salt. Add flour mixture to sugar mixture alternately with buttermilk, beginning and ending with flour mixture and beating well after each addition. Stir in 1 cup chopped pecans.

- Pour batter into 3 greased and floured 9-inch round cake pans.

- Bake at 325° for 25 to 30 minutes. Remove from oven and let cool on wire racks 10 minutes. Turn out cake layers onto wire racks and let cool completely.

- Spread Cream Cheese-Pecan Icing between layers and on top and sides of cake. Place pecan halves around top edge or sprinkle top with chopped pecans. Chill until icing is set.

Cream Cheese-Pecan Icing

2 (8-ounce) packages cream cheese, softened	1½ (16-ounce) packages powdered sugar
1 cup margarine, softened	2 teaspoons vanilla extract
	2 cups chopped pecans

- Beat cream cheese and margarine at medium speed with an electric mixer until creamy; add sugar and vanilla, beating well. Stir in pecans.

Serves 12 to 15

"Bookmobiles"

Mrs. C.P. Barnes of Louisville, along with her Monday Afternoon Club, started a traveling book project sending books in crates to rural areas where there were no libraries. After the books were read, they were packed up and returned. At one time during the depression, women would deliver the books to remote areas on horseback. **Mary Belknap Gray** was one of the original organizers who raised enough funds to purchase vehicles to transport the books. The original bookmobiles consisted of an ambulance, a hearse and a jeep! The bookmobile project was a landmark in the expansion of the public library system.

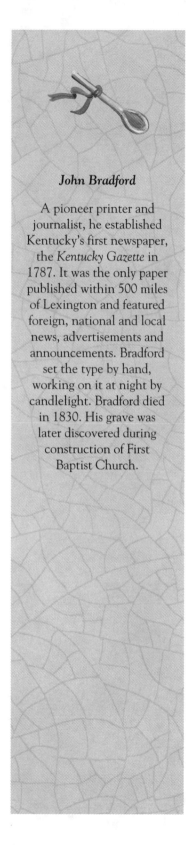

John Bradford

A pioneer printer and journalist, he established Kentucky's first newspaper, the *Kentucky Gazette* in 1787. It was the only paper published within 500 miles of Lexington and featured foreign, national and local news, advertisements and announcements. Bradford set the type by hand, working on it at night by candlelight. Bradford died in 1830. His grave was later discovered during construction of First Baptist Church.

Red Astoria Cake

This is the original recipe for Red Velvet Cake from New York's world famous Waldorf-Astoria Hotel! Following a spat with the hotel management, the head chef agreed to share the secret recipe with my family. After returning home, a sizeable bill from the hotel was mailed (C.O.D.!) requesting payment for it. The bill was paid and since then, we have wildly and widely disseminated the recipe! Enjoy!

½	cup shortening	2¼	cups all-purpose flour
1½	cups sugar	1	scant teaspoon salt
2	large eggs	1	cup buttermilk
1	ounce liquid red food coloring	1	tablespoon vinegar
2	tablespoons cocoa	1	teaspoon baking soda
1	teaspoon vanilla extract		Butter Frosting

- Beat shortening and sugar at medium speed with an electric mixer until creamy; add eggs, beating well.

- Combine food coloring and cocoa, stirring well; add to sugar mixture, beating well. Beat in vanilla.

- Add flour and salt to sugar mixture alternately with buttermilk, beginning and ending with flour and beating well after each addition.

- Combine vinegar and baking soda; stir into batter.

- Pour batter into 2 greased and floured 8-inch round cake pans.

- Bake at 350° for 30 minutes. Remove from oven and let cool on wire racks 10 minutes. Turn out cake layers onto wire racks and let cool completely. Cut cake layers in half horizontally.

- Spread Butter Frosting between layers and on top and sides of cake.

Butter Frosting

1	cup milk	1	cup butter, softened
3	tablespoons all-purpose flour	1	cup sugar
	Pinch of salt	1	teaspoon vanilla extract

- Cook milk, flour, and salt in a saucepan over medium heat, stirring constantly, until thickened. Remove from heat and let cool completely.

- Beat butter and sugar at medium speed with an electric mixer 7 minutes; gradually add flour mixture, beating until fluffy. Stir in vanilla.

For a lighter cake add ¼ teaspoon baking soda to flour.

Serves 12 to 16

Autumn Apple-Walnut Cake with Brown Sugar-Applejack Glaze

Thinking about a slice of this cake is very evocative! Cool crisp autumns, back to school, ball games, and warm hearty meals with family and friends! Indulge yourself!

1½ cups vegetable oil	1¼ teaspoons ground cinnamon
2 cups sugar	¼ teaspoon ground mace
3 large eggs	1¼ cups walnuts, coarsely chopped
2 cups all-purpose flour, sifted	3¼ cups coarsely chopped peeled apple
1 cup whole wheat flour, sifted	(we used Rome Beauty apples)
1 teaspoon baking soda	3 tablespoons applejack or Calvados
¾ teaspoon salt	Warm Brown Sugar-Applejack
⅛ teaspoon ground cloves	Glaze

- Beat oil and sugar at medium speed with an electric mixer until thickened. Add eggs, 1 at a time, beating well after each addition.

- Sift together all-purpose flour, wheat flour, baking soda, salt, cloves, cinnamon, and mace; add to oil mixture, beating well. Stir walnuts, apple, and applejack into batter.

- Pour batter into a greased Bundt pan.

- Bake at 325° for 1 hour and 15 minutes. Remove from oven and let cool on a wire rack 10 minutes. Unmold cake and pour Warm Brown Sugar-Applejack Glaze over top.

Serves 12 to 16

Warm Brown Sugar-Applejack Glaze

¼ cup butter	¼ cup sweet cider
2 tablespoons brown sugar	2 tablespoons fresh orange juice
6 tablespoons granulated sugar	2 tablespoons heavy cream
3 tablespoons applejack or Calvados	

- Melt butter in a saucepan over medium heat; add sugars, stirring to dissolve.

- Stir applejack, cider, orange juice, and heavy cream into butter mixture and bring to a boil. Reduce heat slightly and cook 4 minutes. Remove from heat and let cool slightly.

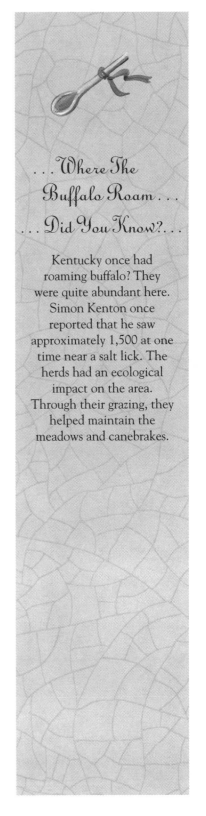

...Where The Buffalo Roam... ...Did You Know?...

Kentucky once had roaming buffalo? They were quite abundant here. Simon Kenton once reported that he saw approximately 1,500 at one time near a salt lick. The herds had an ecological impact on the area. Through their grazing, they helped maintain the meadows and canebrakes.

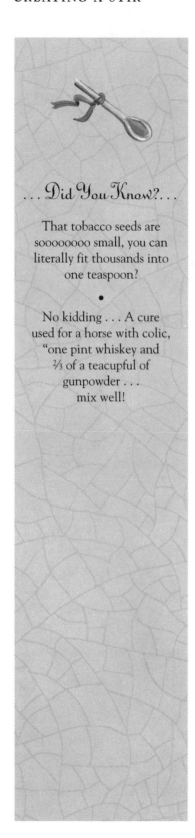

Lazy Daisy Oatmeal Cake

Delightfully different!

1	cup firmly packed brown sugar	1	teaspoon baking soda
1	cup granulated sugar	½	teaspoon salt
½	cup butter, softened	½	teaspoon ground cinnamon
2	large eggs	1	cup uncooked regular oats
1	teaspoon vanilla extract	1-1¼	cups boiling water
1⅓	cups all-purpose flour		Coconut-Walnut Frosting

• Beat sugars and butter at medium speed with an electric mixer until creamy; add eggs and vanilla, beating well.

• Combine flour, baking soda, salt, cinnamon, and oats; add to butter mixture, beating well. Add 1 cup boiling water, beating well. Gradually beat in remaining ¼ cup boiling water until a batter consistency.

• Pour batter into a greased and floured 9 x 13 x 2-inch pan.

• Bake at 350° for 45 minutes or until a wooden pick inserted in center comes out clean.

• Spread Coconut-Walnut Frosting over top of hot cake; broil 4 inches from heat (with electric oven door partially open) 1 to 2 minutes watching carefully to prevent burning.

Coconut-Walnut Frosting

1	cup firmly packed brown sugar	1	teaspoon vanilla extract
¼	cup evaporated milk	1	cup chopped walnuts
6	tablespoons butter, softened	1	cup flaked coconut

• Combine all ingredients in a bowl, stirring well.

Serves 12 to 15

Genie's Cream Cheese Pound Cake

*For something different, try toasting the slices! Eat it plain,
with fresh fruit, or topped with ice cream and your choice of sauce.*

1 (8-ounce) package cream cheese, softened	3½ cups cake flour
1½ cups margarine, softened	3 cups sugar
6 large eggs	2 teaspoons vanilla extract

- Beat cream cheese and margarine at medium speed with an electric mixer until creamy; add eggs, 1 at a time, beating well after each addition.

- Add flour, sugar, and vanilla, beating at low speed. Pour batter into a 9-inch greased and floured tube pan.

- Bake at 300° for 2-2½ hours. Test for doneness before removing. Cake is done when wooden pick inserted in center comes out clean; the top should be a nice golden color. Remove from oven and let cool completely.

Serves 12 to 18

That Pound Cake

½ cup butter, softened	¼ teaspoon almond extract
3 cups sugar	3 cups all-purpose flour
6 large eggs	½ teaspoon baking soda
1 teaspoon vanilla extract	1 (8-ounce) container sour cream
½ teaspoon lemon extract	

- Beat butter and sugar at medium speed with an electric mixer until creamy; add eggs, 1 at a time, beating well after each addition. Add extracts, beating well.

- Sift together flour and baking soda. Add flour mixture to butter mixture alternately with sour cream, beginning and ending with flour mixture and beating well after each addition.

- Pour batter into a greased and floured 10-inch tube pan.

- Bake at 350° for 1 hour and 10 minutes.

Serves 14

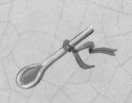

Henry Clay Morrison

A young Methodist minister, helped generate a religious revival in Wilmore, Kentucky with his preaching at the end of the 19th century. This and the collection of funds by the *Reverend John Wesley Hughes* helped to establish *Asbury College* in Wilmore, Kentucky in 1890. Asbury College was named for *Francis Asbury,* the first general superintendent or bishop of American Methodism and a pioneer in education. Francis Asbury's influence and leadership spawned the expansion of the Methodist Church as one of the most important Protestant denominations in the United States.

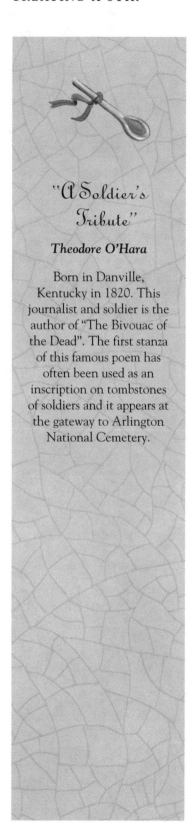

"A Soldier's Tribute"

Theodore O'Hara

Born in Danville, Kentucky in 1820. This journalist and soldier is the author of "The Bivouac of the Dead". The first stanza of this famous poem has often been used as an inscription on tombstones of soldiers and it appears at the gateway to Arlington National Cemetery.

Texas Sized Chocolate Sheet Cake

Great for large crowds, potlucks, and picnics!

2	cups all-purpose flour	¼	cup cocoa
1	teaspoon baking soda	2	large eggs
½	teaspoon salt	½	cup buttermilk
2	cups sugar	1	teaspoon vanilla extract
1	cup butter or margarine		Chocolate Buttermilk Icing
1	cup water		

- Sift together flour, baking soda, salt, and sugar in a large bowl.
- Melt butter in a saucepan over medium heat; add 1 cup water and cocoa and bring to a boil.
- Beat eggs at medium speed with an electric mixer until frothy; add buttermilk and vanilla, beating well.
- Add egg mixture to flour mixture, beating well. Add cocoa mixture, beating well.
- Pour batter into a greased and floured 10 x 15-inch jelly-roll pan.
- Bake at 350° for 15 to 20 minutes. Pour Chocolate Buttermilk Icing over warm cake. Let cool.

Chocolate Buttermilk Icing

½	cup butter or margarine	1	(16-ounce) package powdered sugar
¼	cup cocoa	1	teaspoon vanilla extract
6	tablespoons buttermilk	1	cup chopped nuts

- Bring butter, cocoa, and buttermilk to a boil in a saucepan over medium heat; add powdered sugar, vanilla, and nuts, stirring until creamy.

Iced Apple Cake

This cake is perfectly spiced . . . a simple but satisfying ending to any great fall menu!

3	large eggs	¼	teaspoon salt
1	cup vegetable oil	2	teaspoons ground cinnamon
2	cups sugar	4	apples, chopped
1	teaspoon vanilla extract	1	cup chopped nuts
2	cups all-purpose flour	1	cup raisins (optional)
1	teaspoon baking soda		Cream Cheese Icing

- Beat eggs, oil, sugar, and vanilla at medium speed with an electric mixer until fluffy.

- Combine flour, baking soda, and salt; add to sugar mixture, beating well. Stir in cinnamon, apple, nuts, and, if desired, raisins.

- Pour batter into a greased and floured 9 x 13 x 2-inch pan.

- Bake at 350° for 40 to 45 minutes. Remove from oven and let cool completely on a wire rack.

- Spread cooled cake with Cream Cheese Icing.

Serves 12 to 16

Cream Cheese Icing

1	(3-ounce) package cream cheese, softened	¼	cup butter
½	teaspoon vanilla extract	½	(16-ounce) package powdered sugar

- Beat all ingredients at medium speed with an electric mixer until creamy.

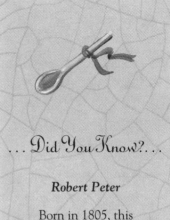

... Did You Know? ...

Robert Peter

Born in 1805, this Lexington resident physician and geologist was the first to observe that the phosphates so abundant in the Limestone of the Bluegrass plateau, contribute to the production of stronger, faster more superior thoroughbreds.

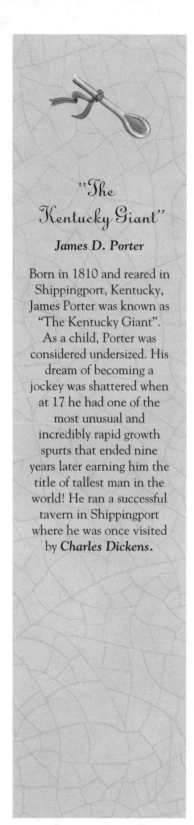

Luscious Strawberry Cake with Strawberry Buttercream Icing

The ultimate reward! This cake is just superb . . . well worth the extra effort to prepare.

½ cup butter, softened
½ cup shortening
2 cups sugar
⅔ cup water
⅔ cup milk
3 cups sifted cake flour
1 tablespoon plus 1 teaspoon baking powder

1 teaspoon salt
2 teaspoons vanilla extract
1 teaspoon almond extract
6 egg whites, at room temperature
Strawberry Puree
Strawberry Buttercream
Fresh strawberries for garnish

- Beat butter and shortening at medium speed with an electric mixer until creamy; gradually add sugar, beating well.

- Combine ⅔ cups water and milk.

- Combine flour, baking powder, and salt. Add flour mixture to butter mixture alternately with milk mixture, beginning and ending with flour mixture and beating well after each addition. Stir in flavorings.

- Beat egg whites in a separate bowl with clean beaters at medium speed until stiff peaks form; gently fold into batter.

- Pour batter into 3 greased and parchment paper-lined 8-inch round cake pans.

- Bake at 350° for 20 minutes or until a wooden pick inserted in center comes out clean. Remove from oven and let cool on wire racks 10 minutes. Turn out cake layers on wire racks and let cool completely; discard parchment paper.

- Spread 2 tablespoons Strawberry Puree on top of 1 cake layer; spread with Strawberry Buttercream and top with a second cake layer. Repeat procedure with remaining cake layers. Spread top and sides of cake with Strawberry Buttercream. Garnish with fresh strawberries.

Strawberry Buttercream

1 cup sugar
¾ cup water
6 egg yolks
1 cup unsalted butter, softened

1 teaspoon vanilla extract
¼ cup Strawberry Puree
2 tablespoons crème de cassis

- Cook sugar and ¾ cup water in a saucepan over medium heat, stirring and washing crystals from sides of pan with a pastry brush dipped in cold water, until sugar dissolves and a candy thermometer registers 234° (soft ball stage).

Luscious Strawberry Cake with Strawberry Buttercream Icing continued

- Place egg yolks in the top of a double boiler; bring water to a simmer. Beat egg yolks with a hand held mixer until frothy. Add hot syrup in a slow, steady stream, beating until smooth.

- Remove top of double boiler from bottom pan and beat frosting until thickened and completely cool.

- Add butter, 1 tablespoon at a time, beating until smooth after each addition. Stir in vanilla.

- Cover frosting and chill until firm but still spreadable. Stir in Strawberry Puree and liqueur.

Strawberry Puree

1	pound strawberries, sliced	1	teaspoon lemon juice
½	cup superfine sugar	1	tablespoon framboise

- Process strawberries in a food processor until pureed; transfer to a bowl.

- Stir sugar, lemon juice, and framboise into pureed strawberries; cover and chill 2 hours.

Serves 12 to 18

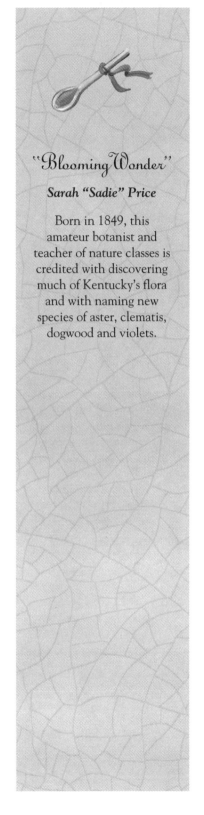

"Blooming Wonder"

Sarah "Sadie" Price

Born in 1849, this amateur botanist and teacher of nature classes is credited with discovering much of Kentucky's flora and with naming new species of aster, clematis, dogwood and violets.

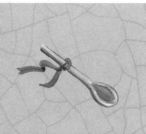

**Julia Ann
Hieronymous Tevis**

Founded The Science Hill
Academy in Shelbyville,
Kentucky in 1825. The
school was renowned,
drawing students from
around the country, from
nearly every state. It
became one of the
foremost college
preparatory schools for
women. The school taught
young women through
moral training to become
good mothers and wives
but also went beyond the
typical training and offered
math, writing, grammar,
rhetoric, astronomy,
French, music and
painting. Julia Tevis
remained active in the
school and for nearly 60
years was indeed its driving
force. The school was sold
after closing in 1939 to
Mark Scearce who opened
Wakefield Scearce
Antique Gallery on the
premises in 1940.

Decadent Fudge Cake with Double Chocolate Drizzle

This cake makes a lovely presentation and is sure to satisfy any chocolate lover's fancy!

1 cup butter	⅓ cup chocolate syrup
1½ cups sugar	2 teaspoons vanilla extract
4 large eggs	4 (1-ounce) white chocolate squares, chopped
½ teaspoon baking soda	2 tablespoons plus 2 teaspoons shortening, divided
1 cup buttermilk	Garnishes: chocolate and white chocolate leaves
2½ cups all-purpose flour	
1½ cups semisweet chocolate mini-morsels, divided	
8 (1-ounce) sweet baking chocolate squares, melted and cooled	

- Preheat oven to 300°.

- Beat butter and sugar at medium speed with an electric mixer until creamy; add eggs, 1 at a time, beating well after each addition.

- Combine baking soda and buttermilk, stirring until dissolved. Add buttermilk mixture to butter mixture alternately with flour, beginning and ending with flour and beating well after each addition.

- Add 1 cup mini-morsels, melted chocolate, chocolate syrup and vanilla extract to batter, beating just until blended (do not overbeat).

- Spoon batter into a heavily greased and floured 10-inch Bundt pan.

- Bake at 300° for 1 hour and 25 minutes to 1 hour and 35 minutes or until cake springs back when touched.

- Turn out cake immediately onto a serving plate and let cool completely.

- Combine white chocolate and 2 tablespoons shortening in the top of a double boiler; bring water to a boil and cook, stirring constantly with a wooden spoon, until melted. Drizzle over cooled cake.

- Cook remaining ½ cup mini-morsels and 2 teaspoons shortening in a small saucepan over low heat, stirring constantly. Let cool slightly and drizzle over white chocolate.

Spicy Carrot Cake

The best you'll ever have!

3	cups all-purpose flour	1½	cups vegetable oil
1	tablespoon baking soda	1	tablespoon vanilla extract
2	teaspoons salt	1½	pounds carrots, grated
3	cups sugar		Buttery Cream Cheese Frosting
1	tablespoon ground cinnamon	1	cup pecans (optional)
4	large eggs		

- Combine flour, baking soda, salt, sugar, and cinnamon in a large bowl; add eggs, oil, and vanilla, stirring until blended. Fold in grated carrot.

- Pour batter into 3 greased and parchment paper-lined 8-inch round cake pans.

- Bake at 350° for 45 minutes or until a wooden pick inserted in center comes out clean. Remove from oven and let cool on wire racks 10 minutes. Turn out cake layers onto wire racks and let cool completely; discard parchment paper.

- Spread Buttery Cream Cheese Frosting between layers and on top and sides of cake.

Buttery Cream Cheese Frosting

2	(8-ounce) packages cream cheese, softened	16	ounces powdered sugar
6	tablespoons butter, softened	2	teaspoons lemon juice
		1	teaspoon vanilla extract

- Beat cream cheese and butter at medium speed with an electric mixer until light and fluffy; add one-third of powdered sugar at a time, beating well after each addition.

- Add lemon juice and vanilla, beating until smooth.

Serves 8 to 12

Secretariat

Secretariat's world record set at the Belmont still stands! He also achieved the fastest Derby time finishing the race in under 2 minutes.

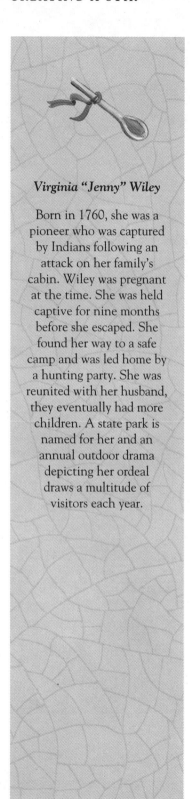

Perfect Pumpkin Cake

This easy and versatile recipe can also be used for cupcakes.

4	large eggs	2	teaspoons ground cinnamon
2	cups sugar	1	cup vegetable oil
2	cups sifted all-purpose flour	1	(16-ounce) can pumpkin
2	teaspoons baking soda		Perfect Cream Cheese Frosting
½	teaspoon salt		

- Beat eggs and sugar at medium speed with an electric mixer until light and pale.

- Sift together flour, baking soda, salt, and cinnamon. Add flour mixture to egg mixture alternately with oil, beginning and ending with flour mixture and beating well after each addition. Stir in pumpkin.

- Pour batter into a greased and floured 9 x 13 x 2-inch pan.

- Bake at 300° for 50 to 60 minutes. Remove from oven and let cool completely on a wire rack.

- Spread cake with Perfect Cream Cheese Frosting.

Serves 15

Perfect Cream Cheese Frosting

1	(16-ounce) package powdered sugar	1	(8-ounce) package cream cheese, softened
¼	cup butter, softened	1	teaspoon vanilla extract

- Beat all ingredients at medium speed with an electric mixer until creamy.

You can also bake batter in greased muffin pan cups at 350° for 15 to 20 minutes for 32 cupcakes.

Old-Fashioned Gingerbread with Lemon Curd Sauce

This spicy cake is easily and quickly prepared and the aroma is heavenly!

¼	cup butter, softened	½	teaspoon salt
¼	cup shortening	1	teaspoon ground cinnamon
½	cup sugar	1	teaspoon ground ginger
1	large egg	½	teaspoon ground cloves
1	cup dark molasses	1	cup hot water
2½	cups all-purpose flour		Whipped Cream
1½	teaspoons baking soda		Lemon Curd Sauce

- Beat butter, shortening, and sugar at medium speed with an electric mixer until creamy; add egg and molasses, beating well.

- Sift together flour, baking soda, salt, cinnamon, ginger, and cloves; add to butter mixture, beating well. Add 1 cup hot water, beating until smooth (batter will be thin).

- Pour batter into a greased 9 x 13 x 2-inch pan.

- Bake at 325° for 30 to 35 minutes.

- Serve gingerbread with a dollop of whipped cream and Lemon Curd Sauce.

Lemon Curd Sauce

1	cup sugar	⅔	cup water
3	tablespoons all-purpose flour	2	teaspoons butter
1	large egg	1	cup whipped cream
⅓	cup lemon juice		

- Sift together sugar and flour.

- Combine sugar mixture, egg, lemon juice, ⅔ cup water, and butter in the top of a double boiler; bring water to a boil and cook, stirring constantly, until thickened.

- Remove from heat and let cool. Fold in whipped cream.

Serves 15 to 20

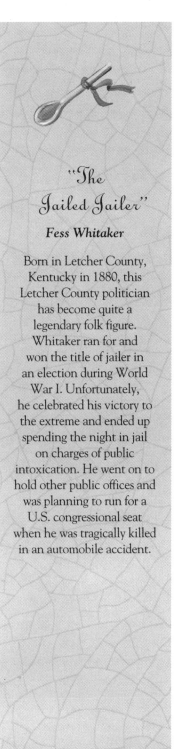

"The Jailed Jailer"

Fess Whitaker

Born in Letcher County, Kentucky in 1880, this Letcher County politician has become quite a legendary folk figure. Whitaker ran for and won the title of jailer in an election during World War I. Unfortunately, he celebrated his victory to the extreme and ended up spending the night in jail on charges of public intoxication. He went on to hold other public offices and was planning to run for a U.S. congressional seat when he was tragically killed in an automobile accident.

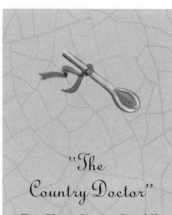

Chocolate Strawberry Shortcake

A delectable twist on a summertime favorite!

2	cups all-purpose flour	½	cup buttermilk
1	tablespoon baking powder	½	cup milk
½	teaspoon baking soda		Sugar
¼	teaspoon salt	1	quart strawberries, sliced
½	cup sugar		Whipped Cream Filling
⅓	cup cocoa		Hot Fudge Sauce
½	cup unsalted butter, chilled and cut into pieces		Chocolate Dipped Strawberries

- Preheat oven to 400°.

- Combine flour, baking powder, baking soda, salt, sugar, and cocoa in a large bowl; cut in butter with a fork or pastry blender until mixture is crumbly. Stir in buttermilk and milk until flour mixture is moist (dough will be sticky).

- Spoon batter into 2 greased 8- or 9-inch round cake pans.

- Bake at 400° for 12 to 15 minutes or until a wooden pick inserted in center comes out clean. Remove from oven and let cool on wire racks 5 minutes. Turn out layers onto wire racks and let cool completely.

- Sprinkle sugar over sliced strawberries in a medium bowl; let stand at room temperature 30 minutes, stirring occasionally.

- Place 1 shortcake layer on a serving plate; pipe two-thirds of Whipped Cream Filling through a pastry bag fitted with a star tip to within ½ inch of cake edges. Spoon sliced strawberries over filling; place remaining cake layer on top.

- Spoon remaining filling on top of cake in large swirls; drizzle with Hot Fudge Sauce. Chill until ready to serve.

- Garnish slices with Chocolate Dipped Strawberries and Hot Fudge Sauce.

Whipped Cream Filling

1	teaspoon unflavored gelatin	1	teaspoon vanilla extract
1½	tablespoons cold water	¼	cup powdered sugar
1½	cups whipping cream, divided		

- Sprinkle gelatin over 1½ tablespoons cold water in a glass liquid measuring cup; let stand at room temperature 1 minute.

- Place cup in a small saucepan and cook in a 1-inch water bath over low heat, stirring constantly, until dissolved.

- Remove cup from water and stir in 2 tablespoons cream.

Chocolate Strawberry Shortcake continued

- Beat remaining whipping cream and vanilla at medium speed with an electric mixer until slightly thickened; add gelatin, beating well. Gradually add powdered sugar, beating until stiff peaks form.

Hot Fudge Sauce

½ cup plus 2 tablespoons unsalted butter	1½ cups sugar
½ cup cocoa (we used Dutch process)	1⅓ cups evaporated milk
4 (1-ounce) unsweetened chocolate squares	¼ teaspoon salt
	2 teaspoons vanilla extract

- Melt butter in a saucepan over medium heat; add cocoa, stirring until smooth. Add chocolate squares, sugar, and milk and bring to a boil, stirring constantly.

- Remove from heat; stir in salt and let cool slightly. Stir in vanilla.

Chocolate Dipped Strawberries

½ (1-ounce) semisweet chocolate square	Whole strawberries, washed and patted dry with paper towels

- Microwave chocolate in a small bowl at HIGH, stirring often, until melted.

- Dip tips of berries in melted chocolate and place on wax paper. Chill 10 minutes or until firm.

Serves 12

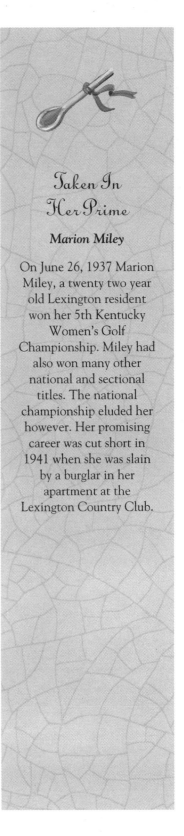

Taken In Her Prime

Marion Miley

On June 26, 1937 Marion Miley, a twenty two year old Lexington resident won her 5th Kentucky Women's Golf Championship. Miley had also won many other national and sectional titles. The national championship eluded her however. Her promising career was cut short in 1941 when she was slain by a burglar in her apartment at the Lexington Country Club.

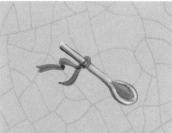

"The Book Lady"

Harriet Drury Van Meter

This Lexington resident, sometimes known as the "Book Lady", founded The International Book Project in 1966. The Project sends close to 130,000 books to 100 countries every year. It was on a State Department – sponsored trip to India and Brazil in the 60's, that she became aware of the international need for books and journals. By 1984, there were 8 million people who had access to book project books and when she retired in 1987 as its director, the project had 17,000 volunteers across the world. In the Filipino town of Baguio City, everyone knows about Lexington, Kentucky because of Harriet Van Meter. The Project has sent enough books to this city to start a library. The Harriet Van Meter Library is a visual reminder of her work there . . . Mrs. Van Meter has received a multitude of distinguished honors

Chocolate Turtle Tart

Intensely rich! This recipe is easy but has the appearance and taste of gourmet, making it suitable for a variety of gatherings.

1¾ cups pecans, toasted
⅓ cup sugar
¼ cup unsalted butter, melted and cooled

Chocolate Filling
½ cup finely chopped pecans
Warm Caramel Sauce

- Preheat oven to 350°.

- Process pecans and sugar in a food processor until finely ground; add butter and process well.

- Press mixture firmly in the bottom and up the sides of a 9-inch tart pan with removable bottom.

- Bake at 350° for 25 minutes or until golden brown. Remove from oven and let cool completely.

- Pour Chocolate Filling into prepared crust; chill for 30 minutes. Remove and sprinkle pecans around edges. Return to refrigerator and chill 3 hours or until firm.

- Loosen tart pan sides and remove; cut tart into wedges and transfer to serving plates. Spoon Warm Caramel Sauce over each serving.

Chocolate Filling

1½ cups whipping cream

12 (1-ounce) semisweet chocolate squares, chopped

- Bring cream to a simmer in a heavy medium saucepan; reduce heat to low and whisk in chocolate until melted and smooth. Remove from heat and let cool to lukewarm.

Warm Caramel Sauce

½ cup unsalted butter
1 cup sugar

1 cup whipping cream

- Melt butter in a saucepan over medium heat; add sugar and cook, stirring occasionally, 12 minutes or until deep golden brown.

- Whisk in cream until smooth. Remove from heat and let cool to lukewarm.

Serves 8

This tart can be prepared up to 3 days ahead. Cover and chill until ready to serve. Warm Caramel Sauce can be prepared up to 2 days ahead; store in refrigerator and reheat before serving.

Chocolate Chip-Pecan Tarts

½	cup butter		½	cup all-purpose flour
1	cup (6 ounces) chocolate morsels		1	cup chopped pecans or walnuts
1	teaspoon vanilla extract		12	frozen tart shells
2	large eggs, lightly beaten			Whipped cream (optional)
1	cup sugar			

- Melt butter in a saucepan over medium heat; add chocolate and vanilla and cook, stirring constantly, until melted.

- Add eggs, sugar, and flour, stirring well. Remove from heat and stir in nuts.

- Spoon filling evenly into tart shells and place on a baking sheet.

- Bake at 325° for 25 to 30 minutes. Serve warm with whipped cream, if desired.

Makes 12 tarts

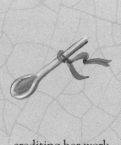

crediting her work including a Nobel Peace Prize nomination in 1986, and a Kiwanis International World Service Medal. A Harriet Van Meter Humanitarian Award is given annually to recognize volunteer efforts in the Bluegrass. Mrs. Van Meter was a member of the Fayette County Medical Auxiliary.

Upside-Down Apple Pie

*Try this fun new version of apple pie! It makes
a beautiful presentation and is absolutely delicious!*

¼	cup margarine		½	cup granulated sugar
1	(15-ounce) package refrigerated pie crusts, at room temperature		1	teaspoon ground cinnamon
			1	tablespoon lemon juice
2	packages pecan halves		1	tablespoon all-purpose flour
½	cup firmly packed brown sugar		2	teaspoons margarine, cut into pieces
6	large Granny Smith apples, peeled and thinly sliced			

- Rub ¼ cup margarine over bottom and sides of a 10-inch baking dish with sides; place pecans in bottom, flat side up. Press brown sugar over nuts.

- Unfold 1 pie crust, pressing out fold lines. Stretch crust to 10 inches and place over brown sugar and nuts.

- Combine apple slices, sugar, cinnamon, lemon juice, and flour, tossing to coat; spoon in the center of crust and dot with 2 teaspoons margarine. Place remaining crust on top, pressing edges to seal and flute.

- Bake at 400° for 1 hour. Remove from heat and let cool on a wire rack exactly 5 minutes. Place a plate over top and invert pie so pecans are on top.

Serves 8

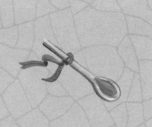

Sugar Crusted Fruit Pizza with Orange Sauce

A lovely summer dessert

1 cup butter, softened	2½ teaspoons cream of tartar
1 cup powdered sugar	Cream Cheese Filling
⅓ cup granulated sugar	Fresh sliced fruit (peaches,
1 large egg	strawberries, kiwi, bananas,
½ teaspoon vanilla extract	grapes, blueberries, or mandarin
¼ teaspoon almond extract	oranges)
2½ cups all-purpose flour	Orange Sauce
2½ teaspoons baking soda	

- Beat butter and sugars at medium speed with an electric mixer until light and fluffy; add egg, vanilla, and almond extracts, beating well.

- Combine flour, baking soda, and cream of tartar; add to butter mixture, beating well.

- Divide dough into 2 portions and pat each portion into a lightly greased pizza pan using your lightly floured hands.

- Bake at 325° for 12 to 15 minutes. Remove from oven and let cool.

- Spread Cream Cheese Filling over cooled crust; decorate with fruit slices, covering crust.

- Glaze pizzas evenly with Orange Sauce.

Cream Cheese Filling

2 (8-ounce) packages cream cheese, softened	1 cup powdered sugar
	1 teaspoon vanilla extract

- Beat all ingredients at medium speed with an electric mixer until creamy.

Orange Sauce

½ cup sugar	4 teaspoons cornstarch
1 cup fresh orange juice	¼ teaspoon grated orange zest
¼ cup fresh lemon juice	¼ teaspoon grated lemon zest

- Cook sugar, orange juice, lemon juice, and cornstarch in a small saucepan over medium heat, stirring occasionally, until thickened. Stir in orange and lemon zest and let cool.

Makes 2 pizzas

Almond Crusted Key Lime Pie

1¼ cups sugar, divided
1½ cups graham cracker crumbs
¼ cup finely chopped almonds

¼ cup butter, melted
Key Lime Filling

- Combine ¼ cup sugar, graham cracker crumbs, almonds, and melted butter; press into the bottom and 1-inch up the sides of a 10-inch pie plate or springform pan.

- Bake at 375° for 5 minutes. Remove from oven and let cool.

- Pour Key Lime Filling into cooled crust.

- Reduce oven temperature to 350° and bake 15 minutes. Remove from oven and let cool.

Key Lime Filling

6 egg yolks
1 (14-ounce) can sweetened condensed milk

2 teaspoons grated lime zest
¾ cup fresh regular or Key lime juice

- Beat egg yolks at medium speed with an electric mixer until thick and pale; add milk, beating well.

- Add lime zest and juice, beating well.

Meringue

6 egg whites

½ teaspoon tartar

- Beat egg whites at medium speed with an electric mixer until frothy; gradually add remaining 1 cup sugar and cream of tartar, beating until stiff peaks form.

- Spoon meringue over pie filling.

- Bake 5 to 6 more minutes or until golden brown.

Serves 8

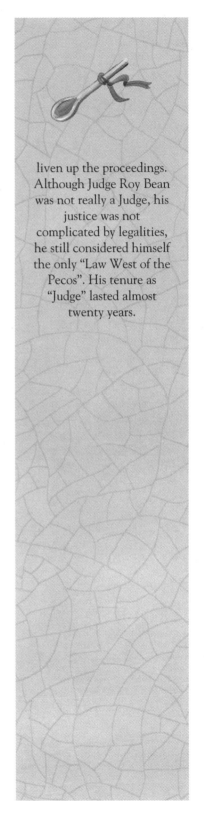

liven up the proceedings. Although Judge Roy Bean was not really a Judge, his justice was not complicated by legalities, he still considered himself the only "Law West of the Pecos". His tenure as "Judge" lasted almost twenty years.

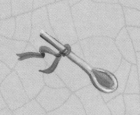

Pansy Yount

Few people in Kentucky have enjoyed cooking and tantalizing recipes as much as the lady of Spindletop Oil Fortune, Pansy Yount. And few have done more for Kentucky's children during depression times than this legend of Lexington's famed Spindletop Hall, now the Faculty/Alumni Club of the University of Kentucky. Pansy Yount came from abject poverty to become one of the world's wealthiest women when she and her husband, Meles Frank Yount, brought in the world's greatest oil gusher. Spindletop, in Beaumont, Texas in 1925. With the world to choose from, she chose Lexington, Kentucky to build her palatial Spindletop Hall, making it into one of "the" showplaces of the times. She revolutionized the American Saddlebred industry and gave us such legendary horses as Beau Peavine, Roxie Highland, and Chief of Spindletop. Unable to have children

Caramel-Apple Pie

Just like eating an old-fashioned caramel apple!

6 cups thinly sliced apple	2 tablespoons margarine, cut into
2 tablespoons lime juice	pieces
¼ cup all-purpose flour	¼ cup butter
¾ cup granulated sugar	½ cup firmly packed brown sugar
½ teaspoon ground cinnamon	2 tablespoons heavy cream
¼ teaspoon salt	½ cup chopped pecans
1 (15-ounce) package refrigerated pie crusts	

- Toss together apple slices and lime juice.

- Combine flour, sugar, cinnamon, and salt; add to apple mixture, tossing lightly.

- Unfold 1 pie crust, pressing out fold lines. Fit into a 9-inch pie plate according to package directions. Spoon apple mixture into crust.

- Dot apple mixture with margarine and top with remaining pie crust. Prick top with a fork to vent.

- Bake at 400° for 40 to 45 minutes.

- Melt butter in a saucepan over medium heat; add brown sugar and cream and bring to a boil, stirring constantly.

- Remove butter mixture from heat and stir in pecans. Pour over top of pie.

- Bake pie 3 to 4 more minutes or until bubbly. Serve warm.

Serves 8

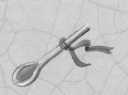

Chocolate Fudge and Walnut Pie

An easy dessert that everyone will love-serve warm with vanilla ice cream.

¾	cup margarine	½	teaspoon vanilla extract
⅓	cup cocoa	3	large eggs
⅓	cup all-purpose flour	1	cup chopped walnuts
1½	cups sugar	1	unbaked 9-inch deep-dish pie crust

- Melt margarine in a saucepan over medium heat. Remove from heat and whisk in cocoa, flour, sugar, vanilla, and eggs until smooth.

- Stir in nuts and pour filling into pie crust.

- Bake at 350° for 30 minutes or until center is set.

Serves 8

Summer Fresh Peach Pie

The perfect union of flaky crust and summer ripened fruit!

2	Pastry Crusts	6	large peaches, blanched, skinned, and sliced
¾	cup sugar		
2-3	tablespoons all-purpose flour		Cinnamon sugar
	Ground cinnamon to taste		

- Fit 1 Pastry Crust into a 9-inch pie plate.

- Combine sugar, all-purpose flour, and cinnamon; sprinkle one-third of mixture into prepared crust. Top with one-third of peaches. Repeat flour mixture and peach layers twice.

- Place remaining Pastry Crust on top, pressing edges to seal and flute. Sprinkle top with cinnamon sugar. Make slits in top to vent and place on a baking sheet.

- Bake at 425° for 20 minutes. Reduce oven temperature to 375° and bake 30 minutes.

Pastry Crust

1	cup all-purpose flour	⅓	cup plus 1 tablespoon butter
½	teaspoon salt	2-3	tablespoons water

- Beat flour, salt, and butter at medium speed with an electric mixer until blended; add water, 1 tablespoon at a time, beating until a dough forms.

- Roll pastry out flat between 2 sheets of wax paper.

Serves 8

herself, Mrs. Yount adopted her one and only child, Mildred. Pansy Yount was a benefactress to children's causes throughout her life. Through her generosity she made sure that every child that needed milk in Lexington during depression times got it. When she died, she bequeathed her jewelry—worth a small fortune—to the Shriners Hospital for Children in Lexington. Yet, despite her generosity to the Bluegrass, she was routinely snubbed by Kentucky polite society. The tragic and almost supernatural life of this lady of Spindletop is detailed in the bestselling book *Passions and Prejudice: The Secrets of Spindletop* by Linda Light—as are a few of her favorite recipes!

Spindletop Productions Lexington, Kentucky

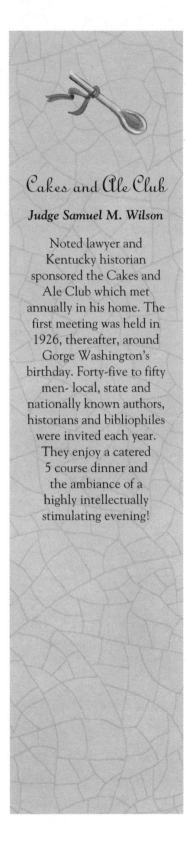

Pumpkin Pie

One of John Michael Montgomery's favorite recipes

2 cups fresh pumpkin	2 tablespoons dark cooking molasses
1 cup firmly packed light brown sugar	1½ teaspoons pumpkin pie spice or
2 large eggs, well beaten	¼ teaspoon ground nutmeg and
½ teaspoon salt	¼ teaspoon ground ginger
¼ cup evaporated milk	1 teaspoon ground cinnamon
2 tablespoons melted margarine	1 9-inch unbaked pastry shell

- Preheat oven to 450°.

- Combine all ingredients except pastry shell, stirring well.

- Pour mixture into pastry shell.

- Bake at 450° for 10 minutes. Reduce oven temperature to 350° and bake 30 minutes with oven door partially open. Pie is done when a knife inserted in center comes out clean.

Old-Fashioned Rhubarb Crunch

Grandmothers are special and their recipes are coveted. This "handed down" old-fashioned favorite received high marks from our test panel! Serve warm with ice cream or homemade whipped cream for a memorable dessert.

½ cup butter or margarine, melted	1 cup granulated sugar
1 cup sifted all-purpose flour	1 tablespoon cornstarch
¾ cup uncooked regular oats	1 cup water
1 cup firmly packed brown sugar	1 teaspoon vanilla extract
1 teaspoon ground cinnamon	Grated orange zest for garnish
4 cups diced rhubarb	

- Combine butter, flour, oats, brown sugar, and cinnamon, stirring until crumbly. Press half of mixture into a greased 9-inch square baking dish. Cover with rhubarb.

- Cook granulated sugar, cornstarch, 1 cup water, and vanilla in a saucepan over medium heat, stirring often, until thickened. Pour over rhubarb and top with remaining oat mixture.

- Bake at 350° for 1 hour. Serve warm with vanilla ice cream and garnish, if desired.

Serves 8

Zabaglione

An Italian dessert that produces a luxuriously rich,
puffy cream. Seasonal berries are the perfect compliment!

6	egg yolks	1	cup Marsala
2	large eggs	2	cups heavy cream
½	cup powdered sugar		Fresh seasonal berries for garnish

- Beat egg yolks, eggs, and powdered sugar at medium speed with an electric mixer until frothy; stir in Marsala and transfer to the top of a double boiler.

- Bring water to a boil and beat egg mixture with a hand held mixture at medium speed until thickened. Transfer top of double boiler to a bowl of ice water and beat mixture at medium speed until lukewarm.

- Beat cream in a separate bowl at medium speed until soft peaks form; fold into egg mixture.

- Pour mixture into glass serving dishes and garnish with fresh seasonal berries.

Serves 4

Barbara Bush's Apple Crisp with Orange Juice

A dessert enjoyed by the former president and his family

4	cups peeled and sliced tart apple	½	teaspoon ground cinnamon
¼	cup orange juice	¼	teaspoon ground nutmeg
1	cup sugar		Dash of salt
¾	cup all-purpose flour, sifted	⅓	cup butter, cut into pieces

- Place apple slices in the bottom of a buttered pie plate; pour orange juice over top.

- Combine sugar, flour, cinnamon, nutmeg, and salt in a bowl; cut in butter with a fork or pastry blender until crumbly. Sprinkle over apple.

- Bake at 375° for 45 minutes or until apple is tender and topping is crisp. Serve warm with whipped cream.

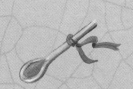

Football Frenzy!!

Hal Clay Mumme

Born in 1952 in San Antonio, Texas, Hal Mumme was named head football coach for the University of Kentucky Wildcats in 1997. Coach Mumme's combination of passing wizardry, risky but exciting fourth-down gambles, a bold and daring defense, energetic recruiting and winning games produced an unprecedented level of football frenzy in the Bluegrass. Record crowds attended games during his first season including four of the top five in school history. Mumme gave fans the excitement they had been waiting for. In 1998, he coached the Wildcats in what will be remembered as one of the best games in the history of college football when UK beat the University of Alabama for the first time in 75 years, 40-34 in overtime! That same year, he returned the Cats to post-season play when they participated in their first New Year's Day bowl game since 1952. More than 40,000 Kentucky fans attended, giving the Outback Bowl its first ever sellout!

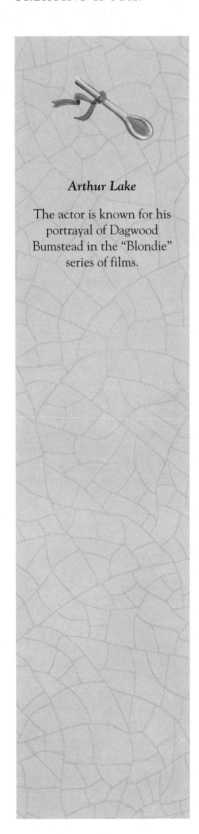

Arthur Lake

The actor is known for his portrayal of Dagwood Bumstead in the "Blondie" series of films.

Blueberry Betty
with Homemade Vanilla Bean Ice Cream

Tastes like cobbler without the crust. Just as delicious with fresh blackberries.

1	quart fresh blueberries	1	cup sugar
1	tablespoon lemon juice	½	cup butter, chilled and cut into
¼	teaspoon ground cinnamon		pieces
1	cup all-purpose flour		Homemade Vanilla Bean Ice Cream

- Preheat oven to 375°.

- Place berries in a 1½-quart baking dish; sprinkle with lemon juice and cinnamon.

- Sift together flour and sugar; cut in butter with a fork or pastry blender until crumbly. Sprinkle over berries.

- Bake at 375° for 45 minutes. Serve warm with ice cream.

Serves 6

Homemade Vanilla Bean Ice Cream

2½	cups half-and-half	1	(6-inch) vanilla bean
¾	cup sugar	1¼	cups heavy whipping cream

- Combine half-and-half, sugar, and vanilla bean in a saucepan. Heat just until mixture starts to simmer. Remove from heat and let cool.

- Slice the vanilla bean lengthwise and remove seeds, scraping them into the milk mixture. Add cream, stirring well.

- Chill mixture 6 hours. Pour mixture in freezer container of an electric freezer. Freeze according to manufacturer's instructions.

Makes 1 to 2 quarts

Lemon Soufflé with Warm Caramel Sauce

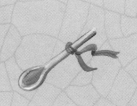

1¼ cups sugar
Pinch of cream of tartar
¾ cup water
6 tablespoons fresh lemon juice
1¾ cups milk
Grated zest of 2 lemons
5 egg yolks

3 tablespoons cornstarch
3 tablespoons sugar
7 egg whites
¼ cup sugar
⅛ teaspoon cream of tartar
Warm Caramel Sauce

- Cook 1¼ cups sugar, cream of tartar, and ¾ cup water in a saucepan over high heat until golden brown; pour into a mold and turn to coat entire surface. Let cool (sugar may crack).

- Pour lemon juice into a large bowl.

- Cook milk in a separate saucepan over medium heat. Combine lemon zest, egg yolks, cornstarch, and 3 tablespoons sugar and gradually add to milk, stirring constantly.

- Bring milk mixture to a boil, stirring constantly, until clumps disappear. Boil, stirring constantly, 1½ minutes. Add to lemon juice, stirring well.

- Beat egg whites, ¼ cup sugar, and ⅛ teaspoon cream of tartar at medium speed with an electric mixer until soft peaks form; fold into lemon mixture. Pour into prepared mold, smoothing top.

- Place mold in a warm water bath and bake at 375° for 1 hour and 15 minutes or until golden. Chill overnight.

- Unmold and serve with Warm Caramel Sauce.

Warm Caramel Sauce

6 tablespoons butter
2¼ cups sugar

2 cups heavy cream

- Melt butter in a saucepan over medium heat; add sugar and cook, stirring constantly, until golden. Add cream, stirring until smooth.

Serves 8

Edwin Carlisle Litsey

Born in Washington County, Kentucky in 1874, this novelist and poet was a lifelong employee of the Marion National Bank in Lebanon, Kentucky. He started at 17 emptying waste baskets, worked his way up to a teller and was eventually offered the bank's presidency which he declined. At 24, he made his writing debut with *The Princess of Gramfalon*. In 1954, he was appointed joint poet laureate with Jesse Stewart.

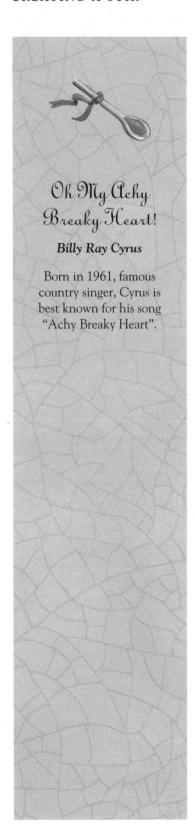

Bread Pudding Soufflé with Kentucky Whiskey Sauce

6 egg yolks	½ cup powdered sugar
½ cup granulated sugar	Unsalted butter
2½ cups French Bread Pudding	Granulated sugar
6 egg whites	Whiskey Sauce

- Preheat oven to 375°.

- Combine egg yolks and ½ cup granulated sugar in the top of a double boiler; bring water to a simmer and cook, whisking constantly, until frothy.

- Combine yolk mixture and 2½ cups French Bread Pudding in a bowl, stirring until smooth.

- Beat egg whites at medium speed with an electric mixer until frothy; gradually add powdered sugar, beating until stiff peaks form; fold into bread pudding mixture.

- Spoon pudding mixture into a buttered and lightly sugared 1½-quart soufflé dish, filling three-fourths full and wiping dish lip clean.

- Bake at 375° for 35 to 40 minutes.

- Serve soufflé immediately with Whiskey Sauce in a bowl on the side.

French Bread Pudding

1 cup sugar	1 tablespoon vanilla extract
½ cup butter, softened	¼ cup raisins
5 large eggs, lightly beaten	12 (1-inch-thick) fresh or stale French
1 pint heavy cream	bread slices
Dash of ground cinnamon	

- Preheat oven to 350°.

- Beat sugar and butter at medium speed with an electric mixer until creamy; add eggs, heavy cream, cinnamon, vanilla, and raisins, beating well. Pour mixture into a 9-inch square pan.

- Arrange bread slices flat in mixture and let stand at room temperature 5 minutes. Turn slices and let stand 5 more minutes. Press bread down until it is covered in egg mixture.

- Place dish in a ½-inch water bath and cover with aluminum foil. Bake at 350° for 35 to 40 minutes. Uncover and bake 10 more minutes.

Bread Pudding Soufflé with Kentucky Whiskey Sauce continued

Whiskey Sauce

1	cup sugar	1	tablespoon unsalted butter
1	cup heavy cream	½	teaspoon cornstarch
1	cinnamon stick or a dash of ground cinnamon	¼	cup water
		1	tablespoon bourbon

- Bring sugar, cream, cinnamon, and butter to a boil in a saucepan.

- Combine cornstarch and ¼ cup water, stirring until smooth; add to cream mixture and cook, stirring constantly, until clear.

- Remove sauce from heat and stir in bourbon.

Serves 6 to 8

Almond Crusted Chocolate Torte

½	cup chopped slivered almonds	1	cup chilled whipping cream
½	cup butter	1	quart chocolate ice cream
1	cup all-purpose flour	¼	cup golden rum or 1 tablespoon rum extract
½	cup sugar		

- Place almonds on an ungreased baking sheet. Bake at 350°, stirring occasionally, 5 minutes or until toasted (do not burn).

- Melt butter in a large skillet over medium heat; add almonds, flour, and sugar and cook, stirring constantly, 6 to 8 minutes or until golden and crumbly. Reserve ¾ cup mixture.

- Press remaining mixture in a buttered 9-inch springform pan. Freeze 3 hours.

- Beat whipping cream at medium speed with an electric mixer until soft peaks form.

- Place ice cream in a chilled large bowl and let stand at room temperature until slightly softened; fold rum and whipped cream gently into ice cream. Spoon into prepared crust. Freeze 1 hour or until partially set.

- Sprinkle with reserved ¾ cup crumb mixture. Freeze 2 hours or until firm.

Serves 8 to 12

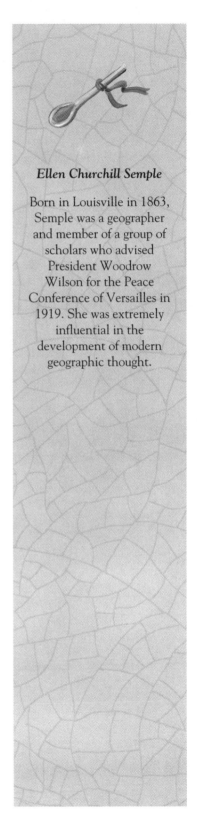

Ellen Churchill Semple

Born in Louisville in 1863, Semple was a geographer and member of a group of scholars who advised President Woodrow Wilson for the Peace Conference of Versailles in 1919. She was extremely influential in the development of modern geographic thought.

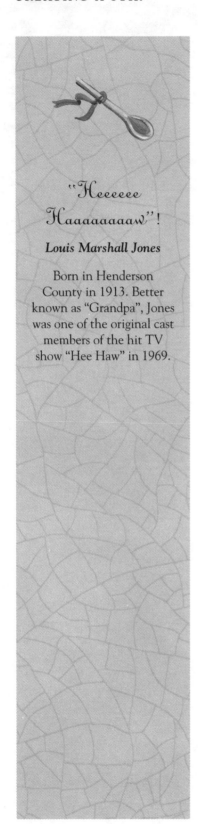

Pecan Passion

Whoaaaa! These tasty little squares are rich!

2	cups toasted pecan halves	1½	cups firmly packed light brown sugar
1	tablespoon dark rum or cognac	¼	teaspoon salt
⅓	cup whipping cream	¼	cup dark corn syrup
6	tablespoons unsalted butter		Chocolate Crust

- Place pecans on an ungreased baking sheet. Bake at 375°, stirring occasionally, 10 minutes or until toasted.

- Combine rum and cream in a bowl, stirring well.

- Melt butter in a heavy 3-quart saucepan over medium heat; add sugar, salt, and corn syrup and bring to a boil, stirring constantly. Boil 2 minutes or until a candy thermometer registers 250° (hard ball stage). (Do not overcook.)

- Remove from heat and stir in cream mixture. Stir in toasted pecans and pour over Chocolate Crust.

- Bake at 375° for 25 minutes. Remove from oven and let cool to room temperature. Chill thoroughly.

- Remove from pan and cut into pieces on a cutting board. Store in refrigerator of freezer.

Makes 24 small squares

Chocolate Crust

6	tablespoons unsalted butter, melted	1	large egg
½	cup firmly packed light brown sugar	¼	cup cocoa
⅛	teaspoon salt	¼	cup sifted all-purpose flour
½	teaspoon vanilla extract		

- Beat butter, brown sugar, salt, vanilla, and egg at medium speed with an electric mixer until smooth; add cocoa and flour, beating well.

- Pour mixture into a greased aluminum foil-lined 9-inch square pan.

- Bake at 375° for 15 minutes (layer will be thin).

Banana-Pineapple Ice Cream

4 large eggs	3 bananas, mashed
1½ cups sugar	1 (7-ounce) can crushed pineapple with juice
1 (14-ounce) can sweetened condensed milk	Rock salt
1 teaspoon vanilla extract	2 bags crushed ice
1 gallon milk	

• Combine eggs, sugar, sweetened condensed milk, vanilla, milk, bananas, and pineapple in freezer container of an electric freezer. Freeze according to manufacturer's instructions.

• Pack freezer with additional ice and rock salt and let stand 1 hour before serving.

• Serve in frosted glass bowls with petite wafer cookies.

Serves 8 to 12

Three-of-a-Kind

This "ice" is a traditional Southern treat handed down through many generations of the Showalter family in Central Kentucky and is very refreshing on hot, humid days.

Juice of 3 lemons	2 tablespoons cold water
Juice of 3 oranges	2 cups boiling water
3 ripe bananas, mashed	¾ cup sugar
1 package unflavored gelatin	

• Process lemon juice, orange juice, and banana in a blender until smooth.

• Combine gelatin and 2 tablespoons cold water in a bowl; let stand 5 minutes. Add 2 cups boiling water, stirring until dissolved.

• Add juice mixture to gelatin mixture, stirring well. Add sugar, stirring until dissolved. Transfer to a freezer-safe storage container.

• Freeze mixture, stirring occasionally. Serve with fun cookies!

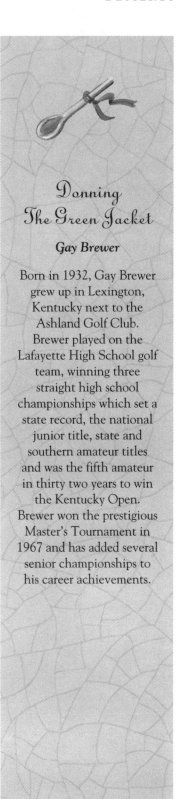

Donning The Green Jacket

Gay Brewer

Born in 1932, Gay Brewer grew up in Lexington, Kentucky next to the Ashland Golf Club. Brewer played on the Lafayette High School golf team, winning three straight high school championships which set a state record, the national junior title, state and southern amateur titles and was the fifth amateur in thirty two years to win the Kentucky Open. Brewer won the prestigious Master's Tournament in 1967 and has added several senior championships to his career achievements.

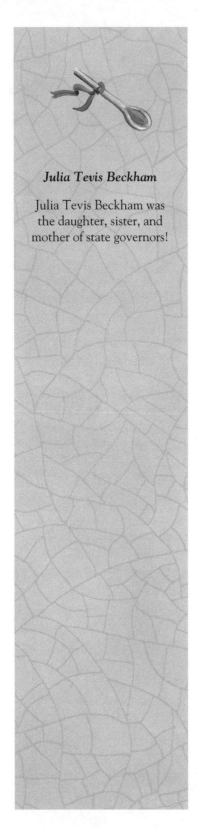

Julia Tevis Beckham

Julia Tevis Beckham was the daughter, sister, and mother of state governors!

Fresh Peach Ice Cream

1	quart plus 1 cup milk	1½	tablespoons vanilla extract
1½	cups sugar	¼	teaspoon almond extract
¼	cup all-purpose flour	1	quart plus 1 cup mashed sweetened
6	large eggs		peaches
2	cups whipping cream		

- Cook milk in a saucepan over low heat until warmed.

- Combine sugar and flour in a bowl.

- Beat eggs at medium speed with an electric mixer until frothy; add sugar mixture, beating well. Gradually add 2 to 3 cups warm milk.

- Remove remaining milk from heat; gradually add egg mixture, stirring well. Cook over low heat, stirring constantly, until thickened and mixture lightly coats the back of a spoon (do not overcook). Remove from heat and let cool.

- Add whipping cream and extracts to mixture, stirring well. Chill.

- Add cream mixture to freezer container, filling half full. Add peaches to fill. Freeze according to manufacturer's instructions.

- Pack freezer with additional ice and rock salt and let stand 1 hour before serving.

When adding sugar to sweeten the peaches, make them sweeter than you like because the taste is less sweet when it freezes.

Tortoni Squares

A make-ahead dessert that is great for summer picnics or special gatherings.

⅓	cup chopped toasted almonds	1	half-gallon vanilla ice cream,
3	tablespoons butter, melted		softened
1⅓	cups finely crushed vanilla wafers	1	(12-ounce) jar apricot preserves
1	teaspoon almond extract		

- Combine almonds, butter, vanilla wafer crumbs, and almond extract; press one-third of mixture into a buttered 5 x 9 x 3-inch loaf pan.

- Place half of ice cream over crumb layer. Repeat layers once and top with preserves. Press remaining crumb mixture on top.

- Freeze until ready to serve. Slice to serve.

Serves 9

Glazed Cheesecake Bars

A sophisticated miniature version of the classic . . . lusciously rich!

1	cup all-purpose flour	1	cup sugar
1	cup chopped pecans	3	large eggs
¼	cup firmly packed brown sugar	2	cups sour cream
½	cup butter, melted	6	tablespoons sugar
2	teaspoons vanilla extract, divided		Fresh berries and mint leaves for garnish
2	(8-ounce) packages cream cheese, softened		

- Combine flour, pecans, brown sugar, and butter; press into the bottom of an ungreased 9 x 13 x 2-inch baking dish.

- Bake at 350° for 10 to 15 minutes or until golden.

- Beat 1 teaspoon vanilla, cream cheese, sugar, and eggs at medium speed with an electric mixer until creamy; pour over prepared crust. Bake 20 minutes.

- Combine remaining 1 teaspoon vanilla, sour cream, and 6 tablespoons sugar; pour over filling. Bake 3 to 5 minutes. Remove from oven and let cool on a wire rack.

- Chill thoroughly. Cut into bars and garnish with fresh berries and mint leaves.

Makes 18 to 24 squares

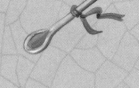

Henry Green

Henry Green, from Owensboro opened one of Kentucky's first commercial BBQ stands. We all know it as Moonlight BBQ and today, the Moonlight Inn in Owensboro remains famous for its pit-cooked barbecue.

Norwegian Almond Squares

1¾	cups all-purpose flour	1	teaspoon ground cinnamon
1	cup sugar	½	teaspoon salt
¼	cup ground almonds	1	egg white
1	cup butter, softened	¾	cup sliced almonds
1	large egg		

- Preheat oven to 350°.

- Beat flour, sugar, ground almonds, butter, egg, cinnamon, and salt at low speed with an electric mixer 2 to 3 minutes or until well blended, scraping down sides.

- Divide dough into 2 portions; press each portion onto a cookie sheet to ¹⁄₁₆-inch thickness.

- Beat egg white in a small bowl with a fork until foamy; brush over dough and sprinkle with almonds.

- Bake at 350° for 12 to 15 minutes or until very lightly browned. Immediately cut into 2-inch squares and remove from pan.

- Let cool. Store squares in an airtight container.

Makes 12 to 18 squares

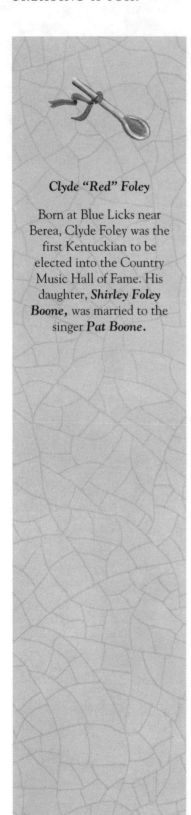

Clyde "Red" Foley

Born at Blue Licks near Berea, Clyde Foley was the first Kentuckian to be elected into the Country Music Hall of Fame. His daughter, **Shirley Foley Boone,** was married to the singer **Pat Boone.**

Mocha Cheesecake Squares

¼ cup all-purpose flour	1 tablespoon hot water
¼ teaspoon baking soda	1 (8-ounce) package cream cheese,
1 cup sifted powdered sugar	softened
½ cup cocoa	1 (14-ounce) can sweetened
¾ cup butter, cut into pieces	condensed milk
1 tablespoon instant coffee granules	2 large eggs

- Sift together flour, baking soda, powdered sugar, and cocoa in a large bowl; cut in butter with a fork or pastry blender until mixture is crumbly. Press into the bottom of a 9 x 13 x 2-inch pan.

- Bake at 350° for 15 minutes.

- Combine coffee granules and 1 tablespoon hot water, stirring to dissolve.

- Beat cream cheese at medium speed with an electric mixer until fluffy; gradually add sweetened condensed milk, beating well.

- Add coffee to cream cheese mixture, beating well. Add eggs, beating well. Pour over prepared crust.

- Bake 20 minutes or until set. Remove from oven and let cool on a wire rack.

- Cover and chill thoroughly. Cut into bars to serve.

Makes 18 to 24 bars

Cranberry Squares

The combination of cranberry and almond flavoring team up in this winning dessert square. Fresh cranberries give them a great texture!

1½ cups sugar	1 teaspoon almond extract
2 large eggs	1½ cups all-purpose flour
¾ cup unsalted butter, melted and	2 cups fresh cranberries
cooled slightly	½ cup chopped pecans

- Preheat oven to 350°.

- Beat sugar and eggs at medium speed with an electric mixer 2 minutes or until thickened; add butter and almond extract, beating well.

- Add flour to sugar mixture, beating well. Stir in cranberries and pecans. Pour batter in a buttered 9-inch square pan.

- Bake at 350° for 1 hour or until a wooden pick inserted in center comes out clean.

- Remove from oven and let cool on a wire rack. Cut into squares.

Makes 12 to 16 squares

Almond Brickle Bars

*Wow . . . are these good! Rich and buttery but slightly delicate,
they're a perfect addition for any dessert tray.*

2	large eggs	1	cup butter, melted
1	cup sugar		Almond Topping
1	cup all-purpose flour		

- Beat eggs and sugar at medium speed with an electric mixer until thick and pale; stir in flour and butter. Pour into a greased and floured 9 x 13 x 2-inch pan.

- Bake at 350° for 30 minutes.

- Spread Almond Topping over prepared cake. Broil 4 inches from heat (with electric oven door partially open) 3 to 5 minutes or until golden brown and bubbly.

- Let cool on a wire rack and cut into squares.

Almond Topping

½	cup butter	1	tablespoon all-purpose flour
½	cup sugar	1	tablespoon milk
½	cup sliced almonds		

- Cook all ingredients in a small saucepan over low heat, stirring constantly, until sugar is dissolved and mixture is thickened.

Makes 2 dozen bars

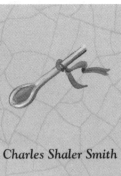

Charles Shaler Smith

Charles Smith designed High Bridge in 1877. The original bridge was dedicated by President Rutherford B. Hayes and was at the time the highest bridge in North America and the highest railroad bridge in the world. Its design introduced the beginning of more scientific bridge building.

Auntie's Brown Sugar-Walnut Squares

Preparation for this deliciously chewy square is a breeze!!

½	cup margarine, softened	1	teaspoon vanilla extract
1	(16-ounce) box brown sugar	2	cups self-rising flour
3	large eggs	2	cups chopped walnuts

- Beat margarine and brown sugar at medium speed with an electric mixer until creamy; add eggs and vanilla, beating well.

- Add flour to sugar mixture, beating well. Stir in walnuts. Spoon mixture into a lightly greased 9 x 13 x 2-inch pan.

- Bake at 325° for 40 minutes.

Makes 15 to 18 squares

Chocolate-Raspberry-Coconut Squares

These are divine! A pretty square that boasts a spectacular blending of flavors.

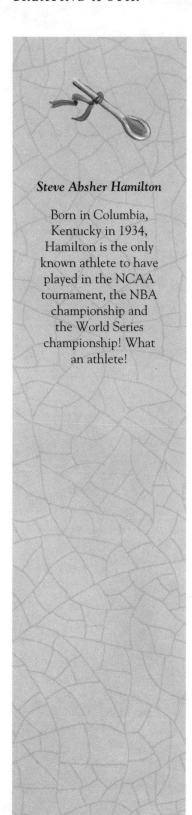

Steve Absher Hamilton

Born in Columbia, Kentucky in 1934, Hamilton is the only known athlete to have played in the NCAA tournament, the NBA championship and the World Series championship! What an athlete!

1	cup all-purpose flour	Chocolate-Raspberry-Coconut Topping
¼	cup firmly packed brown sugar	
½	cup butter, chilled and cut into pieces	½ cup raspberry preserves
		⅓ cup flaked coconut, toasted

- Preheat oven to 350°.
- Combine flour and brown sugar in a large bowl; cut in butter with a fork or pastry blender until mixture is crumbly. Press into a greased 9-inch square pan.
- Bake at 350° for 20 minutes.
- Pour Chocolate-Raspberry-Coconut Topping over prepared crust. Bake 25 minutes.
- Spread preserves over top of warm cake and sprinkle with coconut. Let cool completely on a wire rack.
- Cut into 1½-inch squares to serve.

Chocolate-Raspberry-Coconut Topping

1	cup sweetened condensed milk	1	cup (6 ounces) semisweet chocolate morsels
½	cup all-purpose flour		
½	teaspoon baking powder	1	cup flaked coconut
¼	teaspoon salt	½	cup chopped pecans
2	large eggs		

- Combine condensed milk, flour, baking powder, salt, and eggs in a large bowl, stirring well. Stir in chocolate morsels, coconut, and pecans.

Makes 16 squares

Cranberry Jewels

This has a ruby red layer that makes it wonderful for a holiday dessert bar!

2 cups all-purpose flour	2 large eggs
1½ cups uncooked regular oats	1½ teaspoons vanilla extract
¾ cup firmly packed brown sugar	1 teaspoon grated orange zest
1 cup butter, chilled and cut into pieces	1 tablespoon brown sugar
1 (14-ounce) can sweetened condensed milk	2 tablespoons cornstarch
1 cup ricotta cheese	1 (16-ounce) can whole berry cranberry sauce

- Preheat oven to 350°.

- Combine flour, oats, and brown sugar in a large bowl; cut in butter with a fork or pastry blender until mixture is crumbly. Set 2 cups mixture aside.

- Press remaining oat mixture into the bottom of a 9 x 13 x 2-inch pan.

- Bake at 350° for 15 minutes.

- Beat milk, ricotta cheese, eggs, vanilla, and grated orange zest at medium speed with an electric mixer until smooth; spread evenly over prepared crust.

- Combine 1 tablespoon brown sugar and cornstarch in a small bowl; stir in cranberry sauce. Spoon over cheese layer and top with reserved 2 cups oat mixture.

- Bake 40 minutes or until lightly browned. Remove from oven and let cool on a wire rack.

- Chill thoroughly. Garnish as desired and cut into bars. Store covered in the refrigerator.

Makes 20 to 24 squares

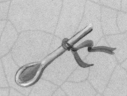

Harlan Boys Choir

From Harlan, Kentucky, the choir is made up of 100 boys in grades four through twelve. *David L. Davies* and *Marian Maxwell* organized the choir in 1965 and in 1969 Marilyn Schraeder joined Davies as an associate conductor and accompanist. The group performs throughout the U.S. and has traveled to Canada and Austria. They were awarded top rating in the Graz, Austria International Youth Music Festival. Their highest honor came when they sang "This Is My Country" at the 1989 presidential inauguration of George Bush.

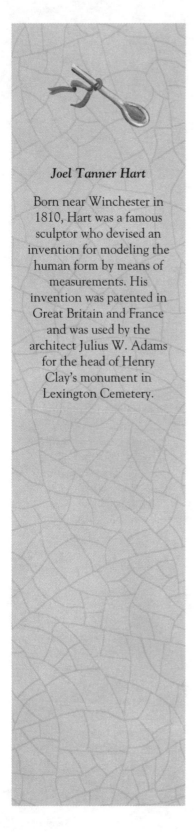

Joel Tanner Hart

Born near Winchester in 1810, Hart was a famous sculptor who devised an invention for modeling the human form by means of measurements. His invention was patented in Great Britain and France and was used by the architect Julius W. Adams for the head of Henry Clay's monument in Lexington Cemetery.

Layered Chocolate Chip–Cream Cheese Bars

1¼ cups firmly packed brown sugar
¾ cup butter-flavored shortening
3 large eggs, divided
2 tablespoons milk
1 tablespoon vanilla extract
2 cups all-purpose flour
1 teaspoon salt
¾ teaspoon baking soda

1 cup semisweet chocolate mini-morsels
1 cup finely chopped walnuts
2 (8-ounce) packages cream cheese, softened
¾ cup granulated sugar
1 teaspoon vanilla

- Beat brown sugar and shortening at medium speed with an electric mixer until creamy; add 1 egg, milk, and 1 tablespoon vanilla, beating well.

- Combine flour, salt, and baking soda; gradually add to sugar mixture, beating at low speed. Stir in chocolate morsels and walnuts with a wooden spoon.

- Divide dough into 2 portions; set 1 portion aside. Spread remaining portion in a greased 9 x 13 x 2-inch pan.

- Bake at 375° for 8 minutes.

- Beat cream cheese, remaining 2 eggs, granulated sugar, and 1 teaspoon vanilla in a separate bowl at medium speed until smooth; pour over prepared crust.

- Roll remaining dough portion into a 9 x 13-inch rectangle between 2 sheets of wax paper. Remove top sheet and flip dough over filling. Remove bottom sheet.

- Bake 40 minutes or until top is set and light golden brown. Remove from oven and let cool completely on a wire rack.

- Cut into bars and chill.

Makes 18 to 20 bars

Lemon Bars with Coconut Glaze

Coconut gives this traditional favorite flair!

½   cup butter, softened
1   cup all-purpose flour
¼   cup powdered sugar

Lemony Filling
Coconut Glaze

- Preheat oven to 350°.
- Beat butter and flour at medium speed with an electric mixer until combined; add sugar, beating well. Press into a 9-inch square baking dish.
- Bake at 350° for 15 minutes.
- Pour Lemony Filling over prepared crust. Bake 25 minutes.
- Spread Coconut Glaze over filling and cut into small squares.

Makes 16 squares

Lemony Filling

Grated zest of 1 lemon
2   tablespoons fresh lemon juice
2   large eggs

1   cup granulated sugar
2   tablespoons all-purpose flour
½   teaspoon baking powder

- Beat all ingredients at medium speed with an electric mixer until smooth.

Coconut Glaze

¾   cup powdered sugar
1   teaspoon vanilla extract
1   tablespoon butter

1   tablespoon milk
1   cup flaked coconut

- Beat all ingredients at medium speed with an electric mixer until blended.

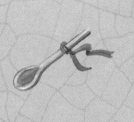

"Golden Boy"

Paul Hornung

Known as the "Golden Boy", Hornung was born in Louisville in 1935. While at Notre Dame Hornung was an All-American quarterback (1955-1956) and won the Heisman Trophy in 1957. He led the NFL in scoring in 1959-1961 and was elected to the Professional Football Hall of Fame in 1986.

Perfect Lemon Bars

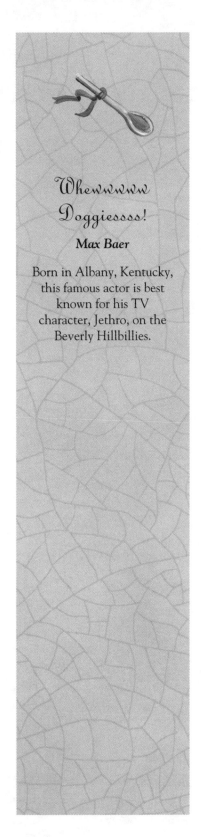

Whewwwww Doggiessss!

Max Baer

Born in Albany, Kentucky, this famous actor is best known for his TV character, Jethro, on the Beverly Hillbillies.

1¾ cups all-purpose flour
⅔ cup powdered sugar
¼ cup cornstarch
¾ teaspoon salt

¾ cup unsalted butter, cut into 1-inch slices and softened
Lemon Filling
Powdered sugar

- Preheat oven to 350°.

- Lightly butter a 9 x 13 x 2-inch pan and line with parchment paper; dot paper with butter and lay a second sheet of parchment paper crosswise over it.

- Pulse flour, sugar, cornstarch, and salt in a food processor to blend; add butter and process 8 to 10 seconds. Pulse 3 times or until mixture resembles coarse meal.

- Press mixture into a ¼-inch layer on bottom and 2 inches up sides of prepared pan. Chill 30 minutes.

- Bake at 350° for 20 minutes.

- Pour Lemon Filling over prepared crust. Bake 20 minutes or until filling feels firm when lightly touched.

- Remove from oven and let cool on a wire rack 30 minutes. Remove from pan and cut into 1½- to 2-inch square bars. Sprinkle with powdered sugar, if desired.

Lemon Filling

4 large eggs
1⅓ cups granulated sugar
3 tablespoons all-purpose flour
2 teaspoons grated lemon zest

⅔ cup fresh lemon juice, strained
⅓ cup milk
Dash of salt

- Whisk together eggs, sugar, and flour in a medium bowl; add lemon zest, lemon juice, milk, and salt, stirring well.

Makes 2 dozen squares

Southern Pecan Pie Squares

The perfect bar interpretation of a Southern favorite . . .
pecan pie lovers will ask for them again and again!

3 cups all-purpose flour	¾ teaspoon salt
¼ cup plus 2 tablespoons sugar	Pecan Pie Filling
¾ cup margarine, softened	

- Preheat oven to 350°.

- Beat flour, sugar, margarine, and salt at medium speed with an electric mixer until crumbly (mixture will be dry). Press firmly into a greased 10 x 15-inch jelly-roll pan.

- Bake at 350° for 20 minutes.

- Pour Pecan Pie Filling over prepared crust. Bake 25 minutes or until filling is thickened.

- Remove from oven and let cool on a wire rack. Cut into 1½-inch squares.

Pecan Pie Filling

4 large eggs	3 tablespoons margarine, melted
1½ cups sugar	½ teaspoon vanilla extract
1½ cups corn syrup	2½ cups chopped pecans

- Beat eggs, sugar, corn syrup, margarine, and vanilla at medium speed with an electric mixer until creamy; stir in pecans.

Makes 6 dozen squares

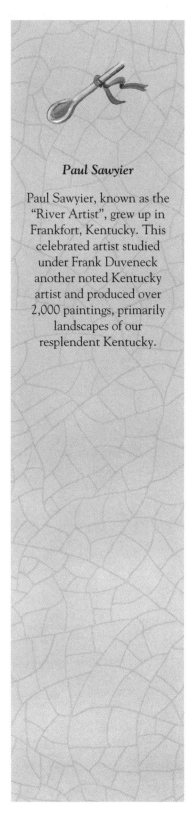

Paul Sawyier

Paul Sawyier, known as the "River Artist", grew up in Frankfort, Kentucky. This celebrated artist studied under Frank Duveneck another noted Kentucky artist and produced over 2,000 paintings, primarily landscapes of our resplendent Kentucky.

Toffee Squares

These are a snap to make and boy are they gooooood!

12 whole graham crackers	1 cup brown sugar
1 cup butter	1½ cups chopped pecans

- Line a 10 x 15-inch jelly-roll pan with graham crackers.

- Melt butter and brown sugar in a saucepan over medium heat; bring to a boil and cook exactly 2 minutes. Pour mixture over graham crackers. Sprinkle with nuts.

- Bake at 350° for 8 to 10 minutes. Remove from oven and let cool slightly on a wire rack.

- Cut into small squares to serve.

Makes 4 dozen squares

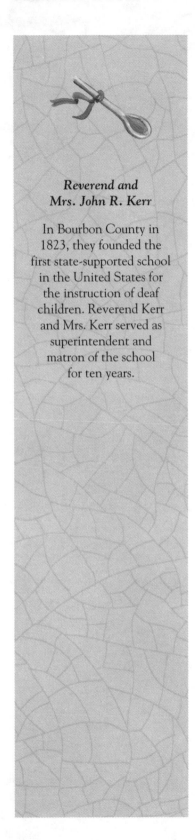

Peanut Butter Brownies

These chewy brownies go beyond basic with the addition of creamy peanut butter!

½	cup peanut butter	1	cup all-purpose flour
⅓	cup butter or margarine	1	teaspoon baking powder
1	cup granulated sugar	¼	teaspoon salt
¼	cup firmly packed brown sugar	1	cup (6 ounces) semisweet chocolate morsels
2	large eggs	½	teaspoon vanilla extract

- Beat peanut butter and butter at medium speed with an electric mixer until blended; gradually add sugars, beating until fluffy. Add eggs, 1 at a time, beating well after each addition.

- Combine flour, baking powder, and salt; add to peanut butter mixture, beating well. Stir in chocolate morsels and vanilla. Spread into a greased 9-inch square baking dish.

- Bake at 350° for 25 minutes or until done.

Makes 16 squares

Mimi's Tea Time Tassies

The pastry that cradles the filling for these bite-size delectables is outstanding!

½	cup butter	¾	cup firmly packed brown sugar
1	(3-ounce) package cream cheese, softened	1	large egg
1	cup all-purpose flour	1	teaspoon vanilla extract
1	teaspoon butter, melted	1	cup finely chopped pecans

- Process butter, cream cheese, and flour in a food processor until a dough forms. Chill dough at least 1 hour.

- Pinch off pieces of dough and press into bottom and up sides of miniature muffin pan cups.

- Combine melted butter, brown sugar, egg, vanilla, and pecans, stirring well; pour evenly into muffin pan cups.

- Bake at 350° for 15 minutes. Reduce oven temperature to 250° and bake 30 minutes. Remove from oven and let cool on wire racks.

Makes 2 dozen tassies

Caramel Brownies

This is Ann Wheeler's (one of our Auxiliary members) recipe for
"Yummy Bars." It was submitted to and published by Southern Living magazine!
They truly are yummy and have been enjoyed by folks all over the country!

1	(14-ounce) package caramels	¾	cup butter or margarine, melted
1	(5-ounce) can evaporated milk, divided	1	large egg
		1	cup (6 ounces) semisweet chocolate morsels
1	(18.25-ounce) package German chocolate cake mix with pudding	1	cup coarsely chopped pecans

- Cook caramels and ¼ cup evaporated milk in a small saucepan over low heat, stirring occasionally, until smooth.

- Combine cake mix, butter, egg, and remaining evaporated milk, stirring well; spoon half of mixture into a greased 9 x 13 x 2-inch pan.

- Bake at 350° for 6 minutes.

- Sprinkle prepared crust with chocolate morsels and pecans; spoon caramel mixture over top. Spoon remaining half of cake mixture over caramel.

- Bake 20 to 25 minutes.

- Remove from oven and let cool on a wire rack. Cut into bars to serve.

Makes 3 dozen

Beth's Best Sugar Cookies

You better double the recipe for this one!

1	cup powdered sugar	1	teaspoon vanilla extract
1	cup granulated sugar	1	teaspoon salt
1	cup butter	1	teaspoon baking soda
1	cup vegetable oil	1	teaspoon cream of tartar
2	large eggs	4	cups all-purpose flour

- Beat powdered sugar, granulated sugar, butter, and oil at medium speed with an electric mixer until creamy; add eggs, beating until fluffy.

- Add vanilla, salt, baking soda, and cream of tartar, beating well. Beat in flour.

- Drop dough by heaping teaspoonfuls onto ungreased cookie sheets or roll into balls and press with the bottom of a glass dipped in sugar.

- Bake at 350° for 8 to 10 minutes. (Do not brown edges.)

Makes 3 dozen cookies

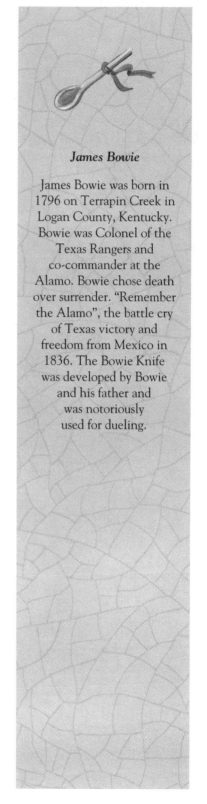

James Bowie

James Bowie was born in 1796 on Terrapin Creek in Logan County, Kentucky. Bowie was Colonel of the Texas Rangers and co-commander at the Alamo. Bowie chose death over surrender. "Remember the Alamo", the battle cry of Texas victory and freedom from Mexico in 1836. The Bowie Knife was developed by Bowie and his father and was notoriously used for dueling.

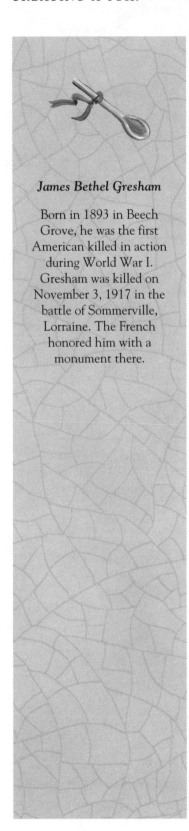

James Bethel Gresham

Born in 1893 in Beech Grove, he was the first American killed in action during World War I. Gresham was killed on November 3, 1917 in the battle of Sommerville, Lorraine. The French honored him with a monument there.

Coconut and Rolled Oat Cookies

These are like sweet macaroons!

1	cup butter	2	cups all-purpose flour, sifted
2	cups firmly packed light brown sugar	2	teaspoons baking soda
		1	teaspoon baking powder
2	large eggs	1	teaspoon salt
2	cups flaked coconut	1	teaspoon vanilla extract
2	cups uncooked quick-cooking oats		

- Beat butter and sugar at medium speed with an electric mixer until creamy; add eggs, beating well. Add coconut and oats, beating well.

- Combine flour, baking soda, baking powder, and salt. Add flour mixture and vanilla to butter mixture, beating well. Chill.

- Shape level tablespoonfuls of dough into balls and place on cookie sheets.

- Bake at 325° for 12 to 15 minutes or until lightly browned.

Makes 6 dozen cookies

Spiced Oaties

1½	cups butter	1	teaspoon salt
¾	cup firmly packed brown sugar	1	teaspoon ground cinnamon
½	cup granulated sugar	½	teaspoon ground nutmeg
1	large egg	3	cups uncooked regular oats
1	teaspoon vanilla extract	½-1	cup raisins
1½	cups all-purpose flour	1	cup chopped walnuts
1	teaspoon baking soda		

- Beat butter, brown sugar, and granulated sugar at medium speed with an electric mixer until creamy; add egg and vanilla, beating well.

- Combine flour, baking soda, salt, cinnamon, and nutmeg; add to butter mixture, beating well. Stir in oats, raisins, and walnuts.

- Drop dough by rounded tablespoonfuls onto cookie sheets.

- Bake at 350° for 10 to 12 minutes. (Do not overbake.)

Six ounces semisweet chocolate morsels can be substituted for raisins, if desired.

Makes 3 to 4 dozen cookies

Pumpkin Cookies with Chocolate Chips and Walnuts

Pumpkin adds a spicy twist to the traditional chocolate chip cookie.

2	cups all-purpose flour	1	large egg
1	teaspoon baking soda	1	teaspoon vanilla extract
1	teaspoon baking powder	1	cup canned pumpkin
½	teaspoon salt	½	cup chopped walnuts
1	teaspoon ground cinnamon	½	cup chocolate morsels
1	cup butter, softened		Brown Sugar Frosting
1	cup sugar		

- Sift together flour, baking soda, baking powder, salt, and cinnamon in a bowl.

- Beat butter and sugar at medium speed with an electric mixer until creamy; add egg, vanilla, and pumpkin, beating well.

- Stir walnuts and chocolate morsels into butter mixture; fold in flour mixture. Drop dough by teaspoonfuls onto ungreased baking sheets.

- Bake at 350° for 15 minutes. Remove from oven and let cool completely on wire racks.

- Ice cooled cookies with Brown Sugar Frosting.

Brown Sugar Frosting

3	tablespoons butter	3	tablespoons milk
½	cup firmly packed brown sugar	¾	teaspoon vanilla extract
1-1½ cups powdered sugar			

- Melt butter in a saucepan over medium heat; add brown sugar, powdered sugar, milk, and vanilla, beating with a hand held mixer until smooth and thickened.

Makes 3 to 4 dozen cookies

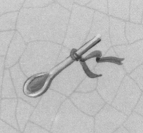

Austin Gollaher

Born in 1806 in Larue County, Austin Gollaher was Abraham Lincoln's favorite childhood friend. Lincoln was overheard saying, "I would rather see him than any man living." They were best buddies and Gollaher is credited with saving Lincoln from flooded waters of Knob Creek.

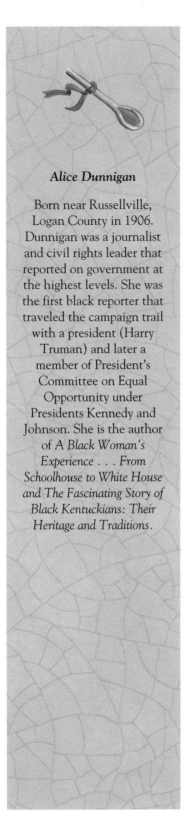

Alice Dunnigan

Born near Russellville, Logan County in 1906. Dunnigan was a journalist and civil rights leader that reported on government at the highest levels. She was the first black reporter that traveled the campaign trail with a president (Harry Truman) and later a member of President's Committee on Equal Opportunity under Presidents Kennedy and Johnson. She is the author of *A Black Woman's Experience . . . From Schoolhouse to White House* and *The Fascinating Story of Black Kentuckians: Their Heritage and Traditions*.

Snickerdoodles

A timeless cookie classic!

2¾ cups all-purpose flour	1 cup butter
1 teaspoon baking soda	1¾ cups sugar, divided
¼ teaspoon salt	2 large eggs
2 teaspoons cream of tartar	4 teaspoons ground cinnamon

- Combine flour, baking soda, salt, and cream of tartar in a bowl.

- Beat butter, 1½ cups sugar, and eggs at medium speed with an electric mixer until creamy; add flour mixture, beating well.

- Combine remaining ¼ cup sugar and cinnamon in a shallow dish.

- Shape dough into 1-inch balls; roll balls in cinnamon mixture and place on ungreased cookie sheets.

- Bake at 400° for 8 to 10 minutes. (Do not overbake.)

Cookies will rise up while baking, then flatten after being removed from the oven

Makes 6 dozen cookies

Molasses Cookies

A wonderful Autumn treat

¾ cup butter	½ teaspoon salt
1 cup sugar	½ teaspoon ground cloves
¼ cup molasses	½ teaspoon ground ginger
1 large egg	1 teaspoon ground cinnamon
2 cups sifted all-purpose flour	Sugar
2 teaspoons baking soda	

- Melt butter in a saucepan over low heat; remove from heat and let cool. Add 1 cup sugar, molasses, and egg and beat at medium speed with a hand held mixer until blended.

- Sift together flour, baking soda, salt, cloves, ginger, and cinnamon; add to butter mixture, beating well. Chill.

- Shape dough into 1-inch balls and roll in sugar; place on greased cookie sheets.

- Bake at 375° for 8 to 10 minutes.

Makes 4 dozen cookies

Cream Filled Sandwich Cookies

Outstanding!

1 cup butter, softened	Sugar
⅓ cup whipping cream	Cream Filling
2 cups all-purpose flour	

- Beat butter, whipping cream, and flour at medium speed with an electric mixer until blended; cover and chill 1 hour or up to 2 days.

- Roll one-third of dough to ⅛-inch thickness on a lightly floured surface with a rolling pin. Cut with a 1½-inch round cookie cutter and place rounds on wax paper.

- Dredge both sides of rounds in sugar and place on ungreased baking sheets. Prick rounds 3 to 4 times with a fork. Repeat procedure with remaining dough portions.

- Bake at 375° for 7 to 9 minutes or until lightly browned. (Watch carefully-do not overbake or underbake.)

- Remove from oven and let cool on wire rack. Spread half of cookies with Cream Filling and top with remaining half of cookies.

Cream Filling

¼ cup butter, softened	Liquid or paste food coloring (paste
¾ cup powdered sugar	will give a deeper color)
1 teaspoon vanilla extract	

- Beat butter, powdered sugar, and vanilla at medium speed with an electric mixer until creamy; add desired amount of food coloring

Makes 4 dozen cookies

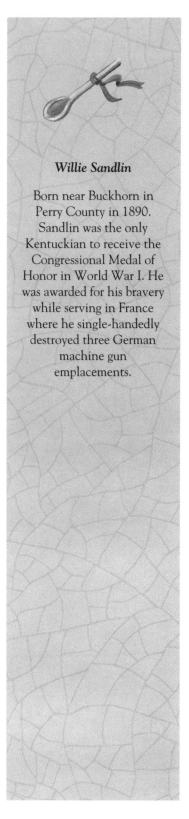

Willie Sandlin

Born near Buckhorn in Perry County in 1890. Sandlin was the only Kentuckian to receive the Congressional Medal of Honor in World War I. He was awarded for his bravery while serving in France where he single-handedly destroyed three German machine gun emplacements.

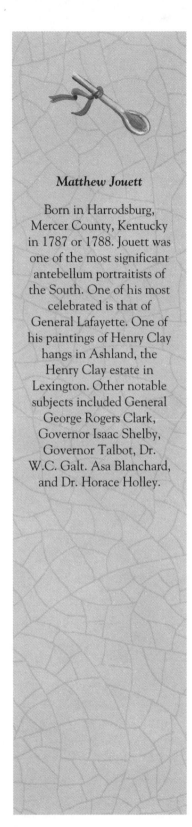

Matthew Jouett

Born in Harrodsburg, Mercer County, Kentucky in 1787 or 1788. Jouett was one of the most significant antebellum portraitists of the South. One of his most celebrated is that of General Lafayette. One of his paintings of Henry Clay hangs in Ashland, the Henry Clay estate in Lexington. Other notable subjects included General George Rogers Clark, Governor Isaac Shelby, Governor Talbot, Dr. W.C. Galt, Asa Blanchard, and Dr. Horace Holley.

Coconut and Oat Chocolate Chippers

1	cup flaked coconut	2	large eggs
1	cup uncooked regular oats	2	cups all-purpose flour
1	tablespoon cocoa	1	teaspoon baking soda
1	cup butter, softened	2	cups semisweet chocolate morsels
1½	cups firmly packed brown sugar	1½	cups chopped nuts
2	teaspoons vanilla extract		

- Process coconut, oats, and cocoa in a food processor until smooth.
- Beat butter, brown sugar, and vanilla at medium speed with an electric mixer until creamy; stir in eggs, 1 at a time, with a wooden spoon.
- Combine coconut mixture, flour, and soda; add to butter mixture, ½ cup at a time, beating well after each addition. Stir in chocolate morsels and nuts.
- Mold 2 tablespoonfuls of dough to ½-inch thickness and place on lightly greased cookie sheets.
- Bake at 350° for 10 to 12 minutes or until lightly browned. Remove from oven and let cool on wire racks.

Makes 2 dozen cookies

Dough can be formed into balls and frozen before baking. Bake frozen balls according to directions above.

White Chip-Oatmeal Cookies

1	cup butter, softened	2	cups self-rising flour
1	cup sugar	1	teaspoon vanilla extract
1	cup firmly packed brown sugar	1	teaspoon almond extract
2	large eggs	1	(8-ounce) package white chocolate morsels
2½	cups uncooked regular oats		

- Beat butter, sugars, and eggs at medium speed with an electric mixer until creamy.
- Sift together oats and flour; add to butter mixture, beating well. Add extracts, beating well. Stir in white chocolate morsels.
- Drop dough by spoonfuls onto greased cookie sheets.
- Bake at 375° for 10 minutes.

Makes 2 dozen cookies

Meringue Chocolate Chip Cookies

An interesting variation on America's favorite cookie!

2	egg whites, at room temperature	¾	cup sugar
⅛	teaspoon cream of tartar	1	cup milk or semisweet chocolate
1	teaspoon vanilla extract		morsels

- Preheat oven to 300°.

- Beat egg whites, cream of tartar, and vanilla at medium speed with an electric mixer until soft peaks form; gradually add sugar, beating until stiff peaks form.

- Fold chocolate morsels into egg white mixture and drop by spoonfuls onto brown paper-lined cookie sheets (grocery bags will do).

- Bake at 300° for 25 minutes.

Makes 2 dozen

Lee Collins

A native of Princeville, Kentucky, Collins is credited with over 100 inventions of electrical, radio, television and national defense equipment.

Chewy Noels

A Christmas bar with true holiday spirit!

2	tablespoons butter	1	(8-ounce) package chopped dates
⅔	cup lightly packed brown sugar	2	large eggs, lightly beaten
6	tablespoons all-purpose flour	1	teaspoon vanilla extract
	Pinch of baking soda	½	cup powdered sugar
1	cup chopped nuts		

- Preheat oven to 350°.

- Melt butter in hot oven in a 9-inch square pan.

- Toss together brown sugar, flour, baking soda, nuts, and dates; add eggs and vanilla, stirring well. Pour mixture over butter and DO NOT STIR.

- Bake at 350° for 30 minutes or until lightly browned. Remove from oven and let cool.

- Cut into bars and sprinkle lightly with powdered sugar.

Makes 2 dozen bars

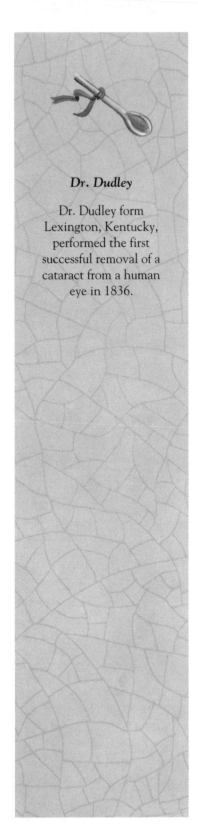

Dr. Dudley

Dr. Dudley form Lexington, Kentucky, performed the first successful removal of a cataract from a human eye in 1836.

Date-Nut Pinwheel Cookies

1	pound dates	1	cup butter
1	cup water	3	large eggs, lightly beaten
1	cup sugar	4	cups all-purpose flour
1	cup finely chopped nuts	1	teaspoon baking soda
2	cups firmly packed brown sugar		

- Cook dates, 1 cup water, and sugar in a saucepan over medium heat 10 minutes; let cool.

- Combine nuts, brown sugar, butter, eggs, flour, and soda in a bowl, stirring well; chill.

- Divide dough into 2 portions. Roll 1 portion to ¼-inch thickness on a lightly floured surface; spread with half of date mixture. Roll up, jelly roll fashion, starting at a long end; chill.

- Repeat procedure with remaining dough portion.

- Slice chilled rolls and place on a cookie sheet.

- Bake at 425° for 10 minutes.

Makes 4 dozen

Crispy Butter Pecan Sticks

A crispy shortbread type cookie that will generate a multitude of raves!
Eat them plain or with a scoop of your favorite ice cream!

½	cup butter, softened	3	teaspoons vanilla extract
1	cup all-purpose flour	1	cup chopped pecans
3	tablespoons sugar		Powdered sugar

- Beat butter, flour, sugar, vanilla, and pecans at medium speed with an electric mixer until blended.

- Roll dough out on a lightly floured surface and cut into sticks. Place sticks on cookie sheets.

- Bake at 300° for 30 minutes or until crisp and brown.

- Roll sticks in powdered sugar.

Makes 2 to 3 dozen

Truffles au Chocolate

An elegant candy dessert-great for finger food gatherings

1	cup heavy cream	¼	cup butter
10	(1-ounce) bittersweet chocolate squares, chopped	½	cup cocoa

- Bring cream to a boil in a saucepan over medium-high heat; stir in chocolate. Add butter and whisk until smooth. Chill overnight.
- Shape chocolate mixture into small balls; chill until set. Roll balls in cocoa to coat.

Makes 18 to 24 truffles

Dan Dan's Chocolate-Peanut Butter Fudge

This is the real thing! In our "jammies" watching the Miss America pageant with Dan Dan's fudge . . . it didn't get any better than that! The only addition to the original recipe . . . a pan! Daddy used to spread his on a plate!

2½	cups sugar	½	cup butter, divided
¼	cup cocoa	1	cup finely chopped pecans
1	cup milk	½	cup creamy peanut butter
1	tablespoon light corn syrup	2	teaspoons vanilla extract

- Cook sugar, cocoa, milk, and corn syrup in a heavy saucepan over medium heat, stirring constantly, until sugar is dissolved. Add 2 tablespoons butter, stirring until melted.
- Cover and boil 3 minutes. Uncover and cook without stirring until a candy thermometer registers 234° (soft ball stage). Remove from heat.
- Add remaining butter, pecans, peanut butter, and vanilla. Do not stir. Let cool 10 minutes.
- Beat mixture until well blended. Pour immediately into a buttered 9-inch square pan.
- Let cool and cut into ½-inch squares.

Makes 3 dozen squares

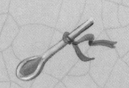

Now That's Taste!

Ruth Hanley Booe/Rebecca Gooch

The Creators of Rebecca Ruth Candies. The two ex-schoolchums got their idea for the famous mint candies from the chance comment of a friend who pointed out that the two best tastes in the world were a sip of bourbon whiskey and a piece of Ruth's mint candy! Their business and friendship persevered through fire, babies, the Great Depression, and sugar rations during WWII. Their comical antics proved a winning marketing strategy. Often times they could be found outside their store peering back into the front window extolling the virtues of their candy until a curious crowd would gather and buy every piece! Booe purchased the business from Gooch in 1929 and remained active until she retired. Rebecca-Ruth candies is still family-owned and operated by Booe's grandson in Frankfort out of the same clapboard house with the striped awning.

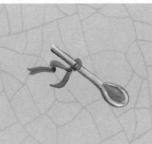

George Keats

Born in London, England in 1797, George Keats was the brother of **John Keats,** one of England's most noted poets. Keats moved to Henderson, Kentucky in 1818 and then to Louisville in 1819 and with his brother Thomas' inheritance, successfully invested in a lumber mill and a boat. He subsequently became one of Louisville's wealthiest citizens. Among his accomplishments were his revision of the Louisville school system, he ran several railroads, helped to print the first city directory, and promoted the construction of the first bridge from Louisville to cross the Ohio River.

Chocolate-Nougat Balls

½	cup butter, softened	1	teaspoon vanilla extract
1	(14-ounce) can sweetened condensed milk	3	cups chopped walnuts
2	(16-ounce) packages powdered sugar	2	(12-ounce) packages semisweet chocolate morsels
1	teaspoon salt	4	ounces Paramount Crystals or shredded baking wax

- Beat butter and sweetened condensed milk at medium speed with an electric mixer until smooth. Stir in powdered sugar, salt, vanilla, and walnuts.

- Roll nougat mixture into 1-inch balls and place on wax paper-lined cookie sheets. Chill until firm.

- Cook chocolate and crystals in a medium saucepan over low heat 4 to 5 minutes or until melted; dip nougat balls in chocolate, coating evenly. Place on wax paper.

- Store chocolate-covered balls in refrigerator.

Makes 6 dozen balls

Chocolate Covered Cherries

2	(16-ounce) packages powdered sugar	½	cup heavy cream Maraschino cherries
6	tablespoons butter, softened Dash of salt	1-2	(8-ounce) packages semisweet chocolate morsels
½	teaspoon vanilla extract	1	(2-inch) paraffin square Pecan halves

- Beat 1¾ packages powdered sugar, butter, salt, and vanilla at medium speed with an electric mixer until creamy; beat in just enough cream so mixture will hold its shape and be stiff. Beat in remaining ¼ package powdered sugar.

- Form mixture into small balls, placing a cherry or piece of cherry in the middle of each. Place balls on a buttered platter. Chill until firm.

- Place chocolate and paraffin in the top of a double boiler; bring water to a boil and cook, stirring often, until melted.

- Dip cherry balls in chocolate using a wooden pick, coating well. Place a pecan half on the top of each chocolate-covered ball. Place on wax paper and let dry.

- Store balls in a cookie tin in the refrigerator or a cool place.

Cinnamon Glazed Pecans

A nice treat for coffee or tea parties or as a side dish for a dessert buffet.

1	egg white	1	cup sugar
1	tablespoon water	1½	teaspoons salt
1	pound pecans	1-1½	teaspoons ground cinnamon

- Preheat oven to 300°.
- Beat egg white in a 1-quart bowl at medium speed with an electric mixer until stiff peaks form; fold in 1 tablespoon water and pecans.
- Combine sugar, salt, and cinnamon; sprinkle over pecans, mixing well.
- Spread pecans on aluminum foil-lined baking sheets.
- Bake at 300° for 30 minutes. Remove from oven and stir pecans to separate.
- Let cool and store tightly covered.

Makes 1 pound

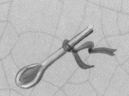

Laura Clay

Born at White Hall in Richmond, Kentucky in 1849, Laura Clay was one of the most controversial figures in the national women's rights movement. Clay was a graduate of Sayre School in Lexington and later attended the universities of Michigan and Kentucky. Known for her work in winning the coeducational, property and joint guardianship rights for Kentucky women. One of her associates was Susan B. Anthony. She was the daughter of Cassius M. Clay, founder of the Republican party.

Pretty Party Mints

These creamy mints are easy to make and they freeze beautifully!

4	ounces cream cheese, softened	1	(16-ounce) package powdered sugar
3	drops peppermint, wintergreen, lemon, or spearmint extract		Few drops liquid food coloring
			Granulated sugar

- Combine cream cheese and extract in a bowl, stirring until creamy; add powdered sugar, mixing well using your hands. Knead in desired amount of food coloring.
- Shake candy mold in granulated sugar; press a small amount of dough into mold, pressing to even off top. Flip out onto wax paper. Repeat procedure with remaining dough.
- Let mints stand at room temperature overnight or until firm. Freeze, if desired.

Remember that food coloring darkens when it dries.

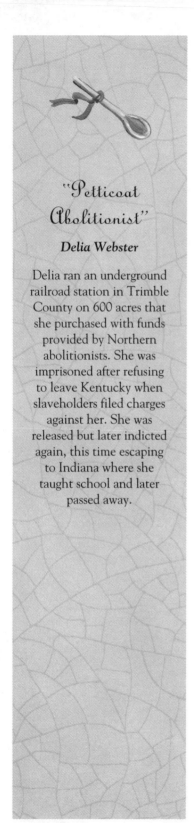

"Petticoat Abolitionist"

Delia Webster

Delia ran an underground railroad station in Trimble County on 600 acres that she purchased with funds provided by Northern abolitionists. She was imprisoned after refusing to leave Kentucky when slaveholders filed charges against her. She was released but later indicted again, this time escaping to Indiana where she taught school and later passed away.

Sugared Nuts

No baking required for these!

1½ cups sugar	1 teaspoon vanilla extract
¼ cup honey	Liquid food coloring (optional)
½ cup water	2 cups unsalted nuts

- Bring first 3 ingredients to a boil in a saucepan; boil until a candy thermometer registers 234° (soft ball stage). Add vanilla and beat slightly with a wooden spoon. Stir in food coloring, if desired.
- Add nuts and beat until stiff; turn out onto wax paper. Break into pieces.

Makes 2 cups

Nanny's Twisted Hard Candy

3 cups sugar	1 teaspoon liquid food coloring
1 cup corn syrup	1 teaspoon desired extract
1 cup water	Powdered sugar

- Boil sugar, corn syrup, and 1 cup water until a candy thermometer registers 300° (hard crack stage). Remove from heat.
- Stir food coloring and extract into candy. Spread mixture into a buttered 10 x 15-inch jelly-roll pan.
- Let candy cool slightly and cut quickly into ½- to ¾-inch strips using sharp kitchen shears. (It helps to have 2 people cutting.) Twist candy and roll in powdered sugar.

Orange Pecans

A nice change from the traditional sugar and cinnamon recipes

2 cups sugar	1 tablespoon grated orange zest
¾ cup fresh orange juice	3 cups pecan halves

- Cook sugar and juice in a saucepan over medium-high heat until a candy thermometer registers 234° (soft ball stage). Turn off heat.
- Add orange zest and pecans, stirring with a wooden spoon until cream colored. Turn out onto wax paper and let cool.

Makes 2 cups

Children's Favorites

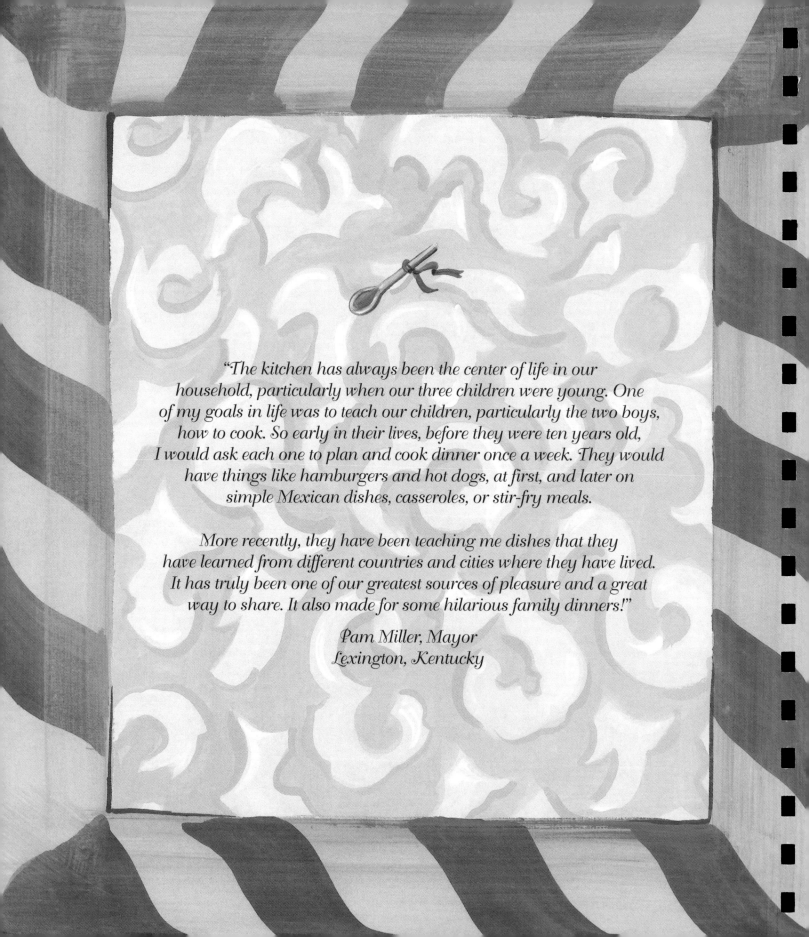

"The kitchen has always been the center of life in our household, particularly when our three children were young. One of my goals in life was to teach our children, particularly the two boys, how to cook. So early in their lives, before they were ten years old, I would ask each one to plan and cook dinner once a week. They would have things like hamburgers and hot dogs, at first, and later on simple Mexican dishes, casseroles, or stir-fry meals.

More recently, they have been teaching me dishes that they have learned from different countries and cities where they have lived. It has truly been one of our greatest sources of pleasure and a great way to share. It also made for some hilarious family dinners!"

Pam Miller, Mayor
Lexington, Kentucky

Claire's White Chocolate Crunch

That wonderful combination of sweet and salty . . .
everyone loves this mix and always requests the recipe!

1	package white almond bark	3	cups crispy corn cereal squares
3	cups pecan halves	3	cups crispy rice cereal squares
3	cups small pretzels ("trees" are best)		

- Microwave almond bark in a bowl at HIGH 3 minutes or until melted, stirring after every minute.

- Combine pecans and next 3 ingredients in a large bowl; pour melted bark over top, folding in gently to coat. Pour onto wax paper and let cool completely.

- Break mixture into chunks.

Package mixture in decorative bags or tins for a great holiday gift!

Chocolate Pizza

A pretty and fun dessert that kids love!

1	(12-ounce) package semisweet chocolate morsels	1	(6-ounce) jar red maraschino cherries, drained and cut in half
1	pound white almond bark, divided	½	(6-ounce) jar green maraschino cherries, drained and cut in half
2	cups miniature marshmallows		Flaked coconut
1	cup crispy rice cereal		
1	cup peanuts		

- Microwave chocolate morsels and three-fourths of almond bark in a bowl at HIGH 2 minutes; stir mixture well and continue to microwave until smooth.

- Add marshmallows, cereal, and nuts to chocolate mixture, stirring to coat. Pour onto a 12-inch pizza pan. Sprinkle evenly with cherries and coconut.

- Microwave remaining almond bark in a small bowl at HIGH 1 minute or until smooth. Drizzle over pizza. Chill until firm.

- Store pizza at room temperature. Cut into small pieces to serve.

Serves 10 to 12

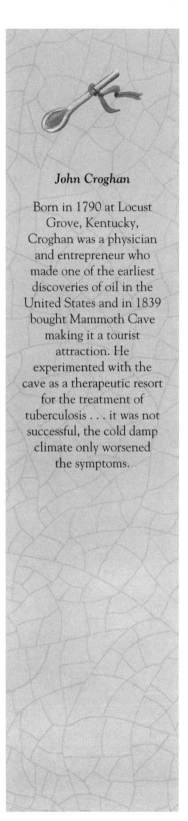

John Croghan

Born in 1790 at Locust Grove, Kentucky, Croghan was a physician and entrepreneur who made one of the earliest discoveries of oil in the United States and in 1839 bought Mammoth Cave making it a tourist attraction. He experimented with the cave as a therapeutic resort for the treatment of tuberculosis . . . it was not successful, the cold damp climate only worsened the symptoms.

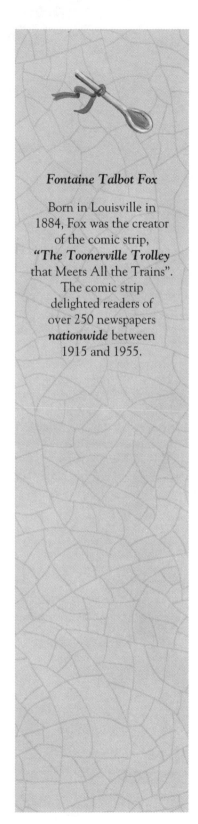

Dizzy Lizzies

These tasty little treasures are extremely easy to make . . . little ones will love helping!

1	pound vanilla candy coating, chopped	1	pound white chocolate morsels
		1	pound salted Spanish peanuts

- Microwave candy coating and chocolate morsels at HIGH 3 minutes or until melted, stopping at 1-minute intervals to stir.
- Add peanuts, stirring well. Drop by tablespoonfuls onto wax paper-lined baking sheets. Chill until firm.

Makes 36 to 48

Milk chocolate morsels can be substituted for white chocolate morsels.

Meredith's Fruit Dip for Apples and Berries

1	cup cream cheese, softened	¼	teaspoon vanilla extract
¾	cup firmly packed brown sugar	4	teaspoons milk
¼	cup powdered sugar		Apple slices and strawberries

- Beat all ingredients at medium speed with an electric mixer until smooth. Serve in mixing bowl.

Nutty Noodle Clusters

These disappear quickly!

1	(12-ounce) package semisweet chocolate morsels	2	(3-ounce) cans chow mein noodles
1	(12-ounce) package butterscotch morsels	½	cup favorite nuts

- Microwave chocolate and butterscotch morsels in a bowl at HIGH, stirring often, until melted. Add noodles and nuts, stirring to coat.
- Drop mixture by spoonfuls onto wax paper. Chill until firm.

Makes 2½ dozen clusters

Peanut Blossoms

Scrumptious peanut butter cookies with sparkly sugar and a kiss on top!

½	cup butter	1	teaspoon vanilla extract
½	cup peanut butter	¾	cup all-purpose flour
½	cup granulated sugar	1	teaspoon baking soda
½	cup firmly packed brown sugar	½	teaspoon salt
1	large egg		Granulated sugar
2	tablespoons milk		Milk chocolate kisses

- Beat butter, peanut butter, granulated and brown sugar at medium speed with an electric mixer until creamy; add egg, beating well. Add milk and vanilla, beating well.

- Stir flour, baking soda, and salt into butter mixture, blending well. Chill dough 1 hour.

- Form dough into 1-inch balls and roll in granulated sugar; press a chocolate kiss firmly in the center of each ball and place on a cookie sheet.

- Bake at 375° for 10 to 12 minutes or until golden (do not overbake).

Makes 3 to 4 dozen

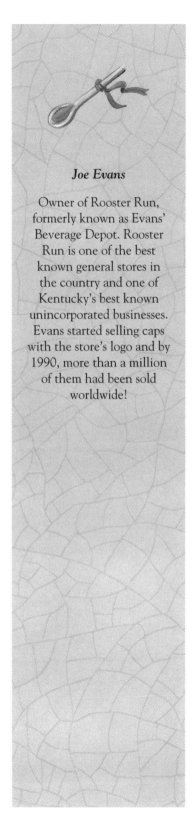

Joe Evans

Owner of Rooster Run, formerly known as Evans' Beverage Depot. Rooster Run is one of the best known general stores in the country and one of Kentucky's best known unincorporated businesses. Evans started selling caps with the store's logo and by 1990, more than a million of them had been sold worldwide!

Buster Bar Dessert

1	small package cream-filled chocolate sandwich cookies, crushed	1	(10-ounce) can salted Spanish peanuts
½	cup margarine, melted	1	(9-ounce) container frozen whipped topping, thawed
½	gallon vanilla ice cream, softened		
1	(12-ounce) jar hot fudge sauce		

- Combine crushed cookies and margarine, stirring well; set aside 1 cup mixture. Press remaining mixture into the bottom of a 9 x 13 x 2-inch pan.

- Spread ice cream over prepared crust and freeze until firm.

- Spread fudge sauce over ice cream and sprinkle with nuts. Spread whipped topping to cover and sprinkle with reserved 1 cup cookie mixture. Freeze until firm.

- Let stand at room temperature 10 minutes before serving.

Serves 15

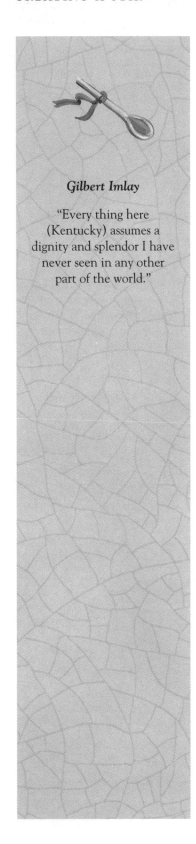

Gooey Buttercake Bars

These chess bars are rich and delicious!

1	(18.25-ounce) package yellow cake mix	1	(8-ounce) package cream cheese, softened
1	large egg	3	large eggs
½	cup butter, melted	1	(16-ounce) package powdered sugar
			Powdered sugar

- Combine cake mix, egg, and butter, stirring well; press into the bottom of a lightly greased 9 x 13 x 2-inch baking dish.

- Beat cream cheese and 3 eggs at medium speed with an electric mixer until creamy; add sugar, beating well. Pour over prepared crust and sprinkle lightly with powdered sugar.

- Bake at 350° for 35 to 40 minutes.

Makes 18 to 24 bars

Chunky Peanut Butter-Chocolate Bars

1	(18.25-ounce) package yellow cake mix	1	cup (6 ounces) semisweet chocolate morsels
2	large eggs	1	(14-ounce) can sweetened condensed milk
1	cup chunky peanut butter		
½	cup butter		

- Beat cake mix, eggs, peanut butter, and butter at medium speed with an electric mixer 2 to 3 minutes; press three-fourths of mixture into the bottom of a 9 x 13 x 2-inch pan.

- Bake at 350° for 10 minutes.

- Remove from oven and sprinkle with chocolate morsels; drizzle with condensed milk and sprinkle with remaining one-fourth of peanut butter mixture.

- Bake 30 more minutes.

- Cool and cut into bars.

Makes 16 to 20 bars

Easy Peanut Butter Fudge

3	cups sugar	1¼ cups peanut butter	
¼	teaspoon salt	1	teaspoon vanilla extract
2	tablespoons corn syrup	3	tablespoons butter
1½	cups milk		

- Cook sugar, salt, corn syrup and milk in a heavy 4-quart saucepan over medium heat, stirring constantly, until sugar is dissolved.

- Cook over medium heat until a candy thermometer registers 234° (soft ball stage). Remove from heat.

- Stir in peanut butter, vanilla, and butter. Let stand at room temperature 10 minutes or until slightly thickened. Pour into a buttered pan.

- Let fudge cool and cut into squares.

Nuts and Bolts

This quick and easy snack mix puts everyone in a festive mood!

2	cups crispy wheat cereal squares	½	cup butter or margarine
2	cups crispy rice cereal squares	1	teaspoon garlic salt
2	cups small cheese crackers	1	teaspoon onion salt
2	cups pretzel sticks	1	teaspoon celery salt
2	cups mixed nuts	1	tablespoon Worcestershire sauce

- Combine wheat and rice cereal squares, cheese crackers, pretzel sticks, and nuts in a large roasting pan.

- Melt butter in a saucepan over medium heat; add garlic salt, onion salt celery salt, and Worcestershire sauce stirring well. Pour over cereal mixture, stirring well to coat.

- Bake at 300° for 1 hour, stirring every 15 minutes.

Makes 12 cups

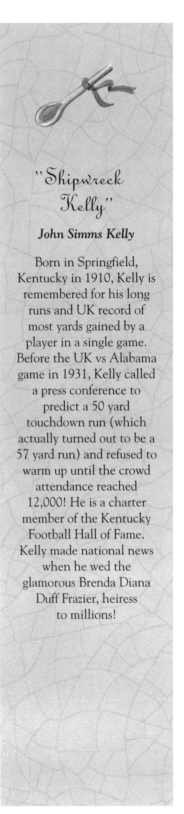

"Shipwreck Kelly"

John Simms Kelly

Born in Springfield, Kentucky in 1910, Kelly is remembered for his long runs and UK record of most yards gained by a player in a single game. Before the UK vs Alabama game in 1931, Kelly called a press conference to predict a 50 yard touchdown run (which actually turned out to be a 57 yard run) and refused to warm up until the crowd attendance reached 12,000! He is a charter member of the Kentucky Football Hall of Fame. Kelly made national news when he wed the glamorous Brenda Diana Duff Frazier, heiress to millions!

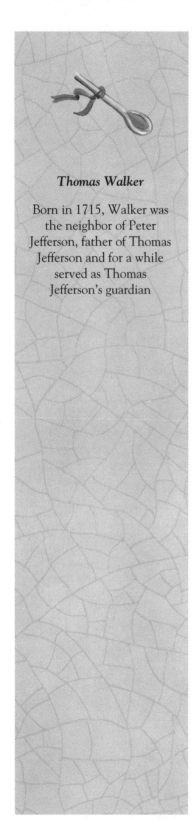

Thomas Walker

Born in 1715, Walker was the neighbor of Peter Jefferson, father of Thomas Jefferson and for a while served as Thomas Jefferson's guardian

Soft Pretzels

*These thick and chewy pretzels "tie the knot"
with creamy cheese dip and make for great nibbling at casual gatherings.*

1 teaspoon active dry yeast	1¾ cup all-purpose flour
¾ cup warm water	1 large egg, lightly beaten
1¼ teaspoons sugar	1 teaspoon kosher salt
½ teaspoon salt	

- Combine yeast and ¾ cup warm water in a large bowl, stirring to dissolve; let stand at room temperature 5 minutes.

- Combine sugar, salt, and flour; add to yeast mixture, stirring until smooth.

- Turn dough out onto a lightly floured surface; knead 3 minutes or until smooth and elastic. Cut dough into 18 pieces.

- Roll each piece into a 9-inch rope and shape as desired (twist or tie into a knot). Cook pretzels in boiling water 3 minutes.

- Place pretzels on a baking sheet. Brush with egg and sprinkle with salt.

- Bake at 425° for 10 to 12 minutes or until golden.

Makes 18 pretzels

Juicy Summer Fruit Salad

A refreshing fruit salad that's very juicy

3-4 oranges, sectioned and shredded	1 pint strawberries, sliced
3-4 apples, chopped	1 cup chopped pecans
1 bunch seedless red grapes, sliced	Sugar to taste
3-4 peaches, peeled and cut into small pieces	

- Combine all ingredients in a large bowl. Chill until ready to serve.

Serves 10 to 12

Cheesy Mixed Vegetable Bake

A great way to get children to eat their vegetables

1   (16-ounce) package frozen mixed
    vegetables
1   cup (4 ounces) shredded process
    cheese spread loaf
¾   cup chopped onion
¾   cup mayonnaise

Dash of salt and pepper
1   can sliced water chestnuts, drained
    (optional)
¼   cup butter, melted
1   cup crumbled buttery round
    crackers

- Cook vegetables according to package directions until tender; drain. Place in a greased baking dish.

- Combine cheese, onion, mayonnaise, salt, pepper, and, if desired, water chestnuts; spread over vegetables.

- Combine butter and cracker crumbs; sprinkle over cheese mixture.

- Bake at 350° until bubbly and golden brown.

Serves 8 to 10

Bite-size Sloppy Joes with Cheese

Easy to make, easy to eat . . . watch them disappear!

1   (10-ounce) can refrigerated
    buttermilk biscuits
1   pound ground chuck
1   (6-ounce) can tomato paste

1   cup water
1   package Sloppy Joe seasoning mix
2   cups (8 ounces) shredded cheddar
    cheese

- Flatten biscuits into greased muffin pan cups.

- Brown ground chuck in a skillet over medium heat, stirring until it crumbles and is no longer pink; drain and return to skillet.

- Add tomato paste, 1 cup water, and seasoning mix to meat, stirring well. Spoon mixture evenly into muffin pan cups and sprinkle with cheese.

- Bake at 375° for 15 to 20 minutes or until golden. Let cool before removing from pan.

Serves 6 to 8

Henry Watterson

Born in 1840, he was an editor for the Louisville Courier Journal and knew personally, every president, with only one exception, from John Quincy Adams to Franklin Delano Roosevelt!

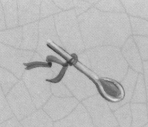

Chicken Pot Pie and I Don't Care

This savory chicken pie provides a fast and easy family-pleasing meal.

¼	cup butter	¼	cup chopped celery
½	cup all-purpose flour	¼	cup chopped onion
1	cup chicken broth	1	(10-ounce) package frozen peas and carrots, thawed
1	cup milk		
½	teaspoon salt	1	(15-ounce) package refrigerated pie crusts, divided
⅛	teaspoon pepper		
⅛	teaspoon celery salt	2	cups cubed cooked chicken or turkey
¼	teaspoon garlic powder		

- Preheat oven to 350°.

- Melt butter in a saucepan over medium heat; add flour, stirring until smooth. Add broth and cook, stirring often, until thickened.

- Add milk, salt, pepper, celery salt, and garlic powder to butter mixture and cook, stirring often, until smooth and bubbly. Stir in vegetables.

- Unfold 1 pie crust and fit into a 2-quart baking dish; place chicken in crust.

- Pour vegetable mixture over chicken and top with remaining pie crust, pressing edges to seal and fluting.

- Make an aluminum foil cuff and place over edge of pastry to keep from burning.

- Bake at 350° for 35 minutes. Remove foil and bake until golden.

Serves 6 to 8

Ranch Chicken Legs

A favorite among little cowpokes!

½	cup butter, melted	3	tablespoons Ranch dressing mix
3	tablespoons vinegar	½	teaspoon paprika
12-16 chicken legs, skinned			

- Combine butter and vinegar in a shallow dish. Dip chicken legs in butter mixture and place in a 7 x 11 x 2-inch baking dish coated with vegetable cooking spray.

- Pour remaining butter mixture over chicken and sprinkle with Ranch dressing mix.

- Bake at 350° for 1 hour. Sprinkle with paprika before serving.

Serves 4 to 6

Tamale Casserole

Ole! Really delicious . . . even big kids love this!

1	pound ground beef	1	(15-ounce) can corn kernels, drained
1	(16-ounce) jar mild salsa	3	teaspoons chili powder
1	(15-ounce) can kidney beans, rinsed and drained	½	teaspoon ground cumin
1	(15-ounce) can Mexican-flavored stewed tomatoes	1	(8.5-ounce) package cornbread mix
		⅓	cup shredded cheddar cheese
		1	tablespoon sliced green onions

- Brown beef in a large skillet over medium heat, stirring until it crumbles and is no longer pink; drain.

- Add salsa, beans, tomatoes, corn, chili powder, and cumin to beef; reduce heat and simmer, stirring occasionally, 10 minutes.

- Preheat oven to 400°.

- Prepare cornbread batter according to package directions; spoon around the edges of a 7 x 11 x 2-inch baking dish coated with vegetable cooking spray.

- Spoon beef mixture into center of batter, spreading to edge of batter but not over.

- Bake at 400° for 18 minutes. Sprinkle with cheese and bake 4 to 5 more minutes or until cheese is melted.

- Sprinkle with green onions just before serving.

Serves 6 to 8

Favorite Pork Chops

7-8 pork chops, trimmed
¼   cup apple cider vinegar
¼   cup water
7-8 onion slices

Ketchup
Salt and pepper to taste
Garlic powder to taste

- Place pork chops flat in a 9 x 13 x 2-inch baking dish; pour vinegar and ¼ cup water into dish.

- Top each pork chop with an onion slice and spread a large dollop of ketchup over the onion. Season to taste.

- Bake at 350° for 45 to 60 minutes or until tender and browned.

Serves 5 to 6

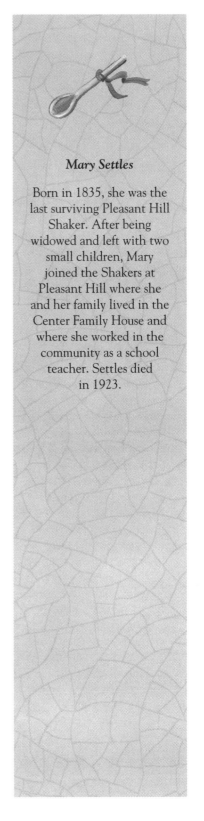

Mary Settles

Born in 1835, she was the last surviving Pleasant Hill Shaker. After being widowed and left with two small children, Mary joined the Shakers at Pleasant Hill where she and her family lived in the Center Family House and where she worked in the community as a school teacher. Settles died in 1923.

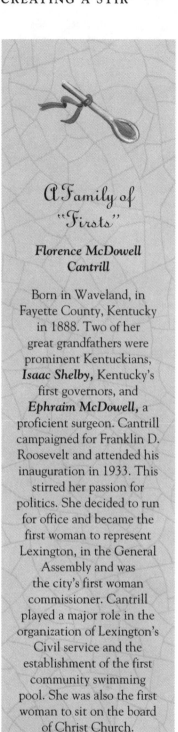

Spaghetti Pizza

A wonderfully delicious way of combining two of their favorites . . .
spaghetti and pizza . . . to our picky little pals, it doesn't get much better than this!

½	cup milk	1	teaspoon dried Italian seasoning
1	large egg	1	teaspoon lemon pepper
7	ounces spaghetti, cooked	¼	teaspoon pepper
1	pound ground chuck	1	(4-ounce) package pepperoni slices
1	medium onion, chopped		Pizza toppings of choice
1	medium-size green bell pepper, chopped	2	cups (8 ounces) shredded mozzarella cheese
2	garlic cloves, minced	2	cups (8 ounces) shredded cheddar cheese
1	(15-ounce) can tomato sauce		

- Whisk together milk and egg in a large bowl; add hot cooked spaghetti, tossing to coat well. Spread into a 10 x 15-inch jelly-roll pan.
- Cook ground chuck, onion, bell pepper, and garlic in a saucepan over medium heat, stirring often, until meat crumbles and is no longer pink; drain and return to pan.
- Add tomato sauce, Italian seasoning, lemon pepper, and black pepper to pan; reduce heat and simmer, stirring occasionally, 5 to 10 minutes. Spoon evenly over spaghetti.
- Top tomato sauce with pepperoni slices.
- Sprinkle with desired pizza toppings and cheese.
- Bake at 350° for 20 minutes.

Serves 10 to 12

Creamy Chicken Soup

4	chicken breasts, cooked and shredded	½	cup onion, chopped
6	cups chicken stock (fresh or bouillon)	2	tablespoons margarine, melted
3	tablespoons chicken flavored soup base or bouillon granules	5-6	tablespoons flour
3	bay leaves	4	cups milk, heated and divided
¾	teaspoon pepper	1½	tablespoons parsley (dried)

- Heat 6 cups of chicken stock, chicken flavored soup base or bouillon base, bay leaves, and pepper in a Dutch oven. Bring to a boil, reduce heat, and simmer 10 minutes.
- Sauté onion in margarine and add to stock.
- Add 2 cups of milk to stock. Add flour to the remaining 2 cups of heated milk, stir to prevent lumping. Add to stock mixture. Simmer 10 minutes.
- Remove the bay leaves, add parsley and chicken. Simmer 10 minutes and serve.

Serves 8

Baked Macaroni and Cheese

They'll never eat boxed again!

½	pound elbow macaroni		Pinch of ground white pepper
1	tablespoon salt	3	cups milk
¼	cup butter	4	cups (16 ounces) shredded cheddar
1	small onion, minced		cheese, divided
¼	cup all-purpose flour	¾	cup fine, dry breadcrumbs
½	teaspoon dry mustard	2	tablespoons butter, melted
1½	teaspoons salt		

- Boil macaroni and salt in water to cover in a large saucepan 8 to 10 minutes; drain.

- Melt butter in the top of a double boiler over boiling water; add onion and cook a few minutes. Add flour, mustard, salt, and white pepper, stirring well. Gradually add milk and cook, stirring constantly, until smooth and thoroughly heated.

- Add 3 cups cheese to flour mixture and cook, stirring constantly, until melted. Pour sauce over macaroni, tossing gently to coat well.

- Pour mixture into a buttered 2-quart baking dish. Sprinkle with remaining 1 cup cheese.

- Combine breadcrumbs and butter, stirring well; sprinkle over cheese.

- Bake at 400° for 20 minutes. Let stand at room temperature 10 to 15 minutes before serving.

Serves 8 to 12

Susan Bradley-Cox

Born in 1937, Susan Bradley-Cox was a five time World Triathlon Championship gold medal winner.

Sidewalk Chalk

Plaster of Paris	**Water**
Powdered tempera paint	

- Fill individual small plastic cups two-thirds full with plaster of Paris; add 1 teaspoon tempera paint to each cup.

- Gradually add water to each, stirring with a wooden craft stick until consistency of cake frosting. Add more plaster of Paris and proportionate water to fill cups, stirring well to evenly distribute tempera. Let harden.

- Cut cups off of chalk to use.

This is not edible. Do not use paper cups.

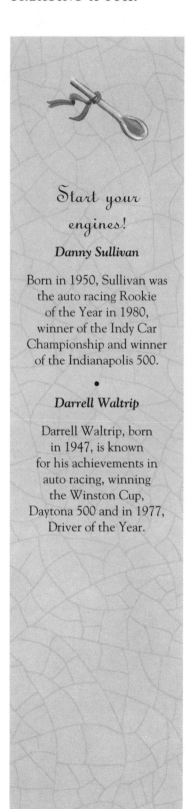

Cookie Jars

A darling gift that's as much fun to make as it is to eat.

64 ounce plastic jar
3 sandwich-size zip-top plastic bags
  Cute material cut into a 10-inch circle
  Rubber band
  Twine, string, or ribbon

  Wooden spoon
2 recipe cards (with hole punched in the far left corner)
  Chocolate Chip-Oatmeal Cookies Recipe

- Wash and thoroughly dry the jar and lid.

- Pour 2 cups oats into jar, making level. Pour 1 cup chocolate morsels over oats, making level.

- Pour 1½ cups sugar into zip-top bag; place bag on top of chocolate morsels to the side of the jar.

- Pour 1½ cups flour, 1 teaspoon salt, and 1 teaspoon baking soda into zip-top bag. Place this bag on the other side of jar on top of the chocolate morsels.

- Place 1 cup pecans into remaining zip-top bag; place bag between the bags with sugar and flour in them. Place the lid on the jar and seal tightly.

- Place the 10-inch circle of material evenly over jar lid; secure in place with the rubber band. Wrap the rubber band with twine, string, or ribbon.

- Slide recipe card with Chocolate Chip-Oatmeal Cookies Recipe on it onto the string. Place wooden spoon on top of recipe card and tie a knot. Tie into a bow.

Chocolate Chip-Oatmeal Cookies Recipe

1 cup shortening
1½ cups sugar
2 large eggs
1 teaspoon vanilla extract
1 tablespoon water
1½ cups all-purpose flour

1 teaspoon salt
1 teaspoon baking soda
2 cups uncooked regular oats
1 cup chocolate morsels
1 cup chopped pecans

- Beat shortening and sugar at medium speed with an electric mixer until light and fluffy; add eggs, 1 at a time, beating well after each addition.

- Add vanilla and 1 tablespoon water, beating well. Add flour, salt, and baking soda, mixing well. Stir in oats, chocolate morsels, and nuts.

- Drop batter by spoonfuls onto cookie sheets.

- Bake at 350° for 12 to 15 minutes. Remove to wire racks to cool.

Makes 4 dozen

Cheeseburger Soup

This recipe received a thumbs-up from our pint-size panel!

1	sandwich bread slice, processed into crumbs	1	cup cubed potato
1	large egg	1	cup sliced celery
1	pound ground beef	½	cup chopped onion
1	teaspoon salt	½	cup sliced carrot
1	(16-ounce) can beef consommé	1	(16-ounce) jar processed cheese spread (we used Cheez Whiz)
1	cup corn kernels		

- Combine breadcrumbs, egg, ground beef, and salt; shape mixture into small nickel-size balls.

- Bring meat balls and consommé to a simmer in a saucepan over medium heat; simmer 5 minutes. Add corn, potato, celery, onion, and carrot and simmer 2 to 3 hours or until vegetables are tender and meat balls are done.

- Add processed cheese spread, stirring until blended.

- Serve soup with breadsticks or French bread.

Magic Reindeer Dust

On Christmas Eve, sprinkle the Magic Reindeer Dust on your lawn where you want Santa to land his sleigh. The Reindeer will smell the oats and the glitter will catch Santa's eye. He'll be sure to visit your house on Christmas Day!

8	cups uncooked regular oats	12	tags with the directions for use (see above)
1½-2	cups green glitter	12	yards decorative ribbon (plaids, checks, stripes, polka dots, etc.)
1½	cups iridescent glitter or confetti		
18-20	decorative or cellophane bags (we used clear so that you can see)		

- Combine oats and green and iridescent glitter, mixing well. Pour 1 cup mixture into each bag.

- Tie a tag to each bag with ribbon.

Makes 12 gift bags

This is not edible.

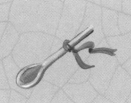

George Ella Lyon

George Ella Lyon grew up in a Kentucky mountain town and now lives in Lexington, KY with her husband and son. Her critically acclaimed books include the picture books *AB Cedar: An Alphabet of Trees, The Outside Inn, Come a Tide, Who Came Down That Road? Dreamplace, Mama Is a Miner* and *A Day at Damp Camp.* Her books for middle readers include *Borrowed Children*— winner of the Golden Kite Award—and *Here and Then.*

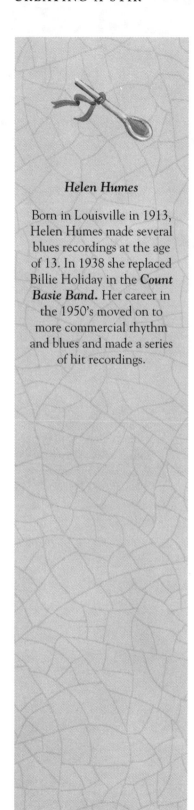

Helen Humes

Born in Louisville in 1913, Helen Humes made several blues recordings at the age of 13. In 1938 she replaced Billie Holiday in the **Count Basie Band.** Her career in the 1950's moved on to more commercial rhythm and blues and made a series of hit recordings.

Gingerbread House Dough with Royal Icing

½   cup butter, softened
½   cup shortening
1   cup sugar
2   teaspoons ground ginger
2   teaspoons ground allspice
1   teaspoon baking soda
½   teaspoon salt

1   large egg
½   cup molasses
2   tablespoons lemon juice
2   cups all-purpose flour
1   cup whole wheat flour
    Royal Icing

- Beat butter and shortening at high speed with an electric mixer 30 seconds; add sugar, ginger, allspice, soda, and salt, beating well. Add egg, molasses, and lemon juice, beating well.

- Combine flours; gradually add to butter mixture, beating in as much as possible. Stir in remaining flour with a wooden spoon.

- Divide dough into 2 portions; chill at least 3 hours.

- Roll dough out to ¼-inch thickness. Cut out according to desired pattern and place on baking sheets.

- Bake at 375° for 10 to 12 minutes.

- Pipe Royal Icing out of a cake decorating bag to assemble and decorate house.

Royal Icing

3   egg whites
1   (16-ounce) package powdered sugar

1   teaspoon vanilla extract
½   teaspoon cream of tartar

- Beat all ingredients at high speed with an electric mixer 10 minutes or until stiff peaks form.

- Use icing immediately, keeping bowl covered with a paper towel to keep icing from drying out.

Finger Paint

Powdered tempera paint

Weak liquid detergent or liquid starch

- Combine tempera and detergent, stirring well.

This is not edible.

No School... Snow Cream

Great winter day entertainment

All by Myself

2	quarts freshly fallen snow		Sugar
	Cream	1	camera
	Vanilla		

- Send children out to get the whitest snow they can find; you mix cream and vanilla to taste. (There are no proportions-flavor to taste!)

- Place a layer of snow in a large chilled bowl; sprinkle with sugar. Repeat layers until bowl is filled.

- Fold cream mixture into snow mixture, making so cream doesn't fall to the bottom of the bowl. Toss snow constantly to freeze the cream.

- Eat immediately and use the camera for pictures.

With Mom's Help

1	(14-ounce) can sweetened condensed milk	1	teaspoon vanilla
1	(5.33-ounce) can evaporated milk	2	quarts freshly fallen snow

- Combine condensed milk, evaporated milk, and vanilla, stirring well. Gradually add snow, beating at medium speed with an electric mixer until ice cream is desired consistency.

Serves 5 to 6

Silly Putty

¼	cup white glue (do not use school glue)	2	tablespoons starch

- Combine glue and starch, mixing well. Let dry until pliable. Store in an airtight container.

This is not edible.

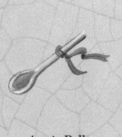

Annie Belle Goddard/Pauline Dedman

Annie Belle Goddard opened the Beaumont Inn in 1918 to accommodate former students of Beaumont College, formerly Daughters College, who returned to visit their alma mater. The Inn is located in Harrodsburg, Kentucky and is known for its traditional Kentucky cooking and its graceful furnishings and accommodations. Pauline Dedman, Goddard's daughter later took over ownership of the popular Inn, followed by her son, **T.C. Dedman** and grandson Charles.

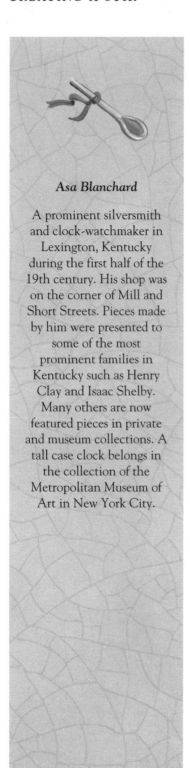

Gak

Always a hit . . . especially at Halloween parties!
They'll love making this creepy, slimy, gooey "stuff"!

2 cups white school glue (do not use "no-run")	Borax Solution
3 cups distilled water	Liquid food coloring

- Combine glue and 3 cups water, stirring well.
- Place 2½ tablespoons glue mixture each into small containers with plastic lids. Pass out to children.
- Let them pick their food color and add 1 to 2 drops to each cup.
- Add 2 teaspoons "magic" (Borax Solution) to each cup and let them stir with wooden craft sticks. Watch the laughter as it turns to Gak.

Borax Solution

1 quart distilled water	¼ cup borax

- Combine water and borax, stirring well.

For individual amounts combine 1 tablespoon glue and 1½ tablespoons water. Add 2 teaspoons Borax Solution and 1 to 2 drops of food coloring; let the child stir with a wooden craft stick.

This is not edible.

Perfect Playdough

Doesn't crumble!

2 cups all-purpose flour	2 tablespoons vegetable oil
1 cup salt	2 cups water
4 teaspoons cream of tartar	Desired liquid food coloring

- Cook all ingredients in a saucepan over medium heat, stirring constantly, until dough leaves sides of pan.
- Turn out onto a lightly floured surface and knead with a little flour. Let cool.
- Store playdough in airtight bags.

This is not edible.

Bibliography

Crowe-Carraco, Carol, *Women Who Made a Difference*, ed. Judy Cheatham
(Lexington, Kentucky: The University Press of Kentucky 1989).

Fradin, Dennis B. et al., eds., *From Sea To Shining Sea; Kentucky* (Chicago:
Children's Press, 1993).

Harrison, Lowell H., James C. Klotter, *A New History of Kentucky*
(Lexington, Kentucky: The University Press of Kentucky 1997).

Kerr, Bettie L., John D. Wright, Jr., *Lexington: A Century in Photographs*
(Lexington, Kentucky: Lexington-Fayette County Historic Commission 1984).

Kleber, John E. et al., eds., *The Kentucky Encyclopedia*
(Lexington, Kentucky: The University Press of Kentucky 1992).

McConnell, John Ed, *A Compendium of Kentucky Humor*, ed. Ken Hart
(Lexington, Kentucky: Host Communications Printing 1987).

Smith, Adam, Katherine Snow Smith, *A Historical Album of Kentucky*
(Brookfield, Connecticut: The Millbrook Press 1995).

Thompson, Kathleen, *Portrait of America: Kentucky*
(Austin, Texas: Raintree Steck-Vaughn Publishers 1996).

INDEX

D

N

O

P

Creating A Stir

FCMA Publications
2628 Wilhite Court, Suite 201
Lexington, Kentucky 40503-3304

Telephone: (859) 293-9100   FAX: (859) 277-3919
E-mail: creatingastir@mindspring.com
Visit our web page at www.creatingastir.com

Name _____

Address _____

City _____ State _____ Zip _____

Please send _____ copies   @ $22.95 each _____
Kentucky residents add sales tax   @ $ 1.38 each _____
Postage and handling   @ $ 4.00 each _____

                                         Total Enclosed _____

Make checks payable to Creating A Stir

Please charge to: ❏ Visa   ❏ Mastercard

Card Number: _____ Expiration Date: _____

Signature: _____

To open a wholesale account, call (859) 293-9100

Creating A Stir

FCMA Publications
2628 Wilhite Court, Suite 201
Lexington, Kentucky 40503-3304

Telephone: (859) 293-9100   FAX: (859) 277-3919
E-mail: creatingastir@mindspring.com
Visit our web page at www.creatingastir.com

Name _____

Address _____

City _____ State _____ Zip _____

Please send _____ copies   @ $22.95 each _____
Kentucky residents add sales tax   @ $ 1.38 each _____
Postage and handling   @ $ 4.00 each _____

                                         Total Enclosed _____

Make checks payable to Creating A Stir

Please charge to: ❏ Visa   ❏ Mastercard

Card Number: _____ Expiration Date: _____

Signature: _____

To open a wholesale account, call (859) 293-9100